Health and Human Behaviour

Health and Human Behaviour

FOURTH EDITION

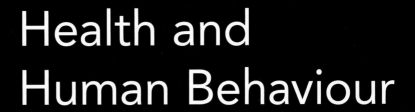

KEN JONES

DEBRA CREEDY

KATRINA LANE-KREBS

FLORIN OPRESCU

OXFORD

UNIVERSITY PRESS

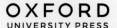

OXFORD
UNIVERSITY PRESS

Oxford University Press is a department of the University of Oxford.
It furthers the University's objective of excellence in research,
scholarship, and education by publishing worldwide. Oxford is a registered
trademark of Oxford University Press in the UK and in certain other countries.

Published in Australia by
Oxford University Press
Level 8, 737 Bourke Street, Docklands, Victoria 3008, Australia.

First published 2003
Second edition published 2008
Third edition published 2012
Reprinted 2013
Fourth edition published 2023

A catalogue record for this
book is available from the
National Library of Australia

ISBN 9780190309893

Reproduction and communication for educational purposes
The Australian *Copyright Act 1968* (the Act) allows educational institutions that
are covered by remuneration arrangements with Copyright Agency to reproduce
and communicate certain material for educational purposes. For more information,
see copyright.com.au.

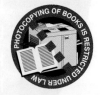

Edited by Adrienne de Kretser, Righting Writing
Typeset by Integra Software Services Pvt. Ltd
Proofread by Allison Lamb
Indexed by Puddingburn Publishing Services Pty Ltd
Printed in China by Golden Cup Printing Co Ltd

Disclaimer
Aboriginal and Torres Strait Islander peoples are advised that this publication may
include images or names of people now deceased.

Links to third-party websites are provided by Oxford in good faith and for information only.
Oxford disclaims any responsibility for the materials contained in any third-party website
referenced in this work.

Brief Contents

List of Figures and Tables	xi
Preface	xii
Guided Tour	xiv
About the Authors	xvi
Acknowledgments	xviii

PART I » FOUNDATIONS OF HEALTH AND BEHAVIOUR — 2

1	Who is Sick? Defining and Applying Concepts of Illness, Disease and Health	4
2	Infant, Child and Adolescent Development	17
3	Adult Development and Ageing	35
4	Reactions to Illness	50
5	Understanding Reactions to Chronic Conditions	72

PART II » HEALTHY AND RISKY BEHAVIOUR — 88

6	Understanding Health Behaviour	90
7	Thinking about Health Behaviour: Cognition and Health	113
8	How to Change Health Behaviour	137
9	A Complex Example: Activity, Eating and Body	160

PART III » PSYCHOPHYSIOLOGICAL ASPECTS OF HEALTH — 176

10	Understanding Mind and Body Interactions	178
11	A Complex Example: Understanding Pain	194
12	Stress and Trauma	206
13	Coping: How to Deal with Stress	222

OXFORD UNIVERSITY PRESS

PART IV » FACTORS AFFECTING HEALTH AND BEHAVIOUR   240

14   Socio-cultural Influences and Inequalities   242

15   Health Literacy   258

16   Promoting Health and Preventing Illness   275

Glossary   291

References   298

Index   312

OXFORD UNIVERSITY PRESS

Contents

List of Figures and Tables   xi
Preface   xii
Guided Tour   xiv
About the Authors   xvi
Acknowledgments   xviii

PART I » FOUNDATIONS OF HEALTH AND BEHAVIOUR   2

**1   Who is Sick? Defining and Applying Concepts
of Illness, Disease and Health**   4
    Health and illness   5
    Who is sick?   5
    How do illness and disease compare?   10
    Health   12
    Well-being   12

2   Infant, Child and Adolescent Development   17
    Introduction   18
    Determinants of health and illness   18
    Measurement of age   20
    Stages of development   21

3   Adult Development and Ageing   35
    Adulthood   36
    Death and grieving   45
    The five stages of dying   46

4   Reactions to Illness   50
    Introduction   51
    Illness behaviour   53
    The sick role   56
    Abnormal illness behaviour   57
    Factors affecting reactions to illness   59
    Vulnerability and capability   60
    Behavioural strategies   64
    Illness perceptions   66

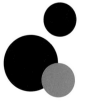

5   Understanding Reactions to Chronic Conditions   72

Chronic conditions   73

Prevalence of chronic conditions   74

Impact on daily life   75

Variations in individual coping   78

Models of self-care   79

Practical care and interventions   81

PART II » HEALTHY AND RISKY BEHAVIOUR   88

6   Understanding Health Behaviour   90

The relationship between behaviour and health   91

Risky behaviours   91

Health behaviours and risk-reduction behaviours   95

The basis of learning and memory: The changing brain   97

Interconnectedness of the nervous system   97

Learning   99

Memory   105

7   Thinking about Health Behaviour: Cognition and Health   113

Introduction   114

Rational decision-making   115

Heuristics   116

Clinical decision-making   119

Health beliefs   120

Too many theories?   123

Social cognitive theory   124

The steps to health behaviour change   125

Compliance   127

Expectations and healing   127

8   How to Change Health Behaviour   137

Introduction   138

Motivation for change   138

Genetic factors   140

Biological factors   140

Cognitive factors   142

Strategies for behaviour change   144

Changing behaviour by changing stimuli | 147
Increasing and decreasing behaviours | 149
Changing behaviour by changing reinforcements | 151
Positive reinforcement approaches | 152
Managing lapses | 156

9   A Complex Example: Activity, Eating and Body | 160
Activity and eating as behavioural health issues | 161
Body image as a health issue | 171
Intervention | 172

PART III » PSYCHOPHYSIOLOGICAL ASPECTS OF HEALTH | 176

10   Understanding Mind and Body Interactions | 178
Introduction | 179
Emotion | 180
Psychophysiology | 188

11   A Complex Example: Understanding Pain | 194
A broader understanding of pain | 195
Reporting pain | 196
Factors affecting the experience and reporting of pain | 197
Physiology of acute pain | 198
Neurochemical basis of acute pain | 199
Psychological responses | 200
Pain control techniques | 201
Behavioural activation | 203

12   Stress and Trauma | 206
What is stress? | 207
Stress as a stimulus | 207
Trauma | 217

13   Coping: How to Deal with Stress | 222
Introduction | 223
Types of coping | 223
Stress management techniques | 225
Managing COVID-19 stress | 237

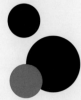

PART IV » FACTORS AFFECTING HEALTH AND BEHAVIOUR   240

14   Socio-cultural Influences and Inequalities   242

Introduction   243
Culture   243
Race and ethnicity   244
Culture and health beliefs   245
Three-tier system of socialisation   247
Health care as a culture   249
Inequalities and inequities   250
Social determinants of health   251
Implications of inequalities for health care: Challenges
   for the individual   255

15   Health Literacy   258

What is health literacy?   259
Prevalence of poor health literacy in the community   260
Socio-cultural factors associated with low health literacy   263
Implications of low health literacy   264
Theoretical considerations to enhance health literacy   266
Getting the most from existing health services   271

16   Promoting Health and Preventing Illness   275

Introduction   276
Strategies to prevent serious illness and death due to smoking   276
Strategies to prevent and address injury   276
Illness prevention   279
Types of prevention   279
Levels of prevention   282
Health promotion   283
Health and human behaviour   288

Glossary   291
References   298
Index   312

OXFORD UNIVERSITY PRESS

List of Figures and Tables

List of Figures

2.1	Reaction range	18
3.1	The grieving cycle	47
6.1	Types of memory	105
7.1	Health belief model	121
7.2	The Theory of Reasoned Action	122
7.3	The Theory of Planned Behaviour	122
8.1	Maslow's hierarchy of needs	139
8.2	Drive cycle	141
8.3	The pleasantness of an unfamiliar temperature	143
9.1	An ecological model for understanding obesity	164
12.1	The arousal–performance curve	209
12.2	A biopsychosocial model of stress	210
12.3	Demands and resources	212
12.4	Effects of stress on health	215
14.1	Equality vs equity	250
15.1	Five steps necessary for learning to take place	266
15.2	Mastery learning	268
15.3	Teach-back learning cycle	270
16.1	Health as the focus of three complementary areas of action for health professionals: health promotion, illness prevention and clinical treatment	285

List of Tables

2.1	Erikson's stages of child and adolescent psychosocial development	24
2.2	Piaget's stages of child cognitive development	25
3.1	Erikson's stages of adult development	37
8.1	Summary of stimulus control	149
16.1	Examples of health promotion interventions	284

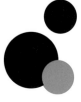

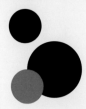

Preface

Each of us experiences health and illness as essential conditions of life. Our experience of health and illness affects our physical status as well as our feelings, thoughts and actions. We see constant evidence of the impact of health and illness on individuals, their families, institutions of health care and the wider community through the media and personal and fictional accounts. As the biomedical sciences have increased our knowledge about what regulates health at a biological level, individuals have become more interested in maximising their own health as well as reducing illness. We are also learning that health and illness involve much more than just our physical well-being. Psychological, cognitive, cultural and family issues are also intimately involved, and are frequently more important than the biological components of illness and health. The treatment of illness and maintenance of health consume an ever-increasing proportion of personal and public expenditure. As a result, health and illness have become central social and political concerns. This intersection is clearly demonstrated by the impact of the COVID-19 pandemic on health and behaviour, which is discussed in several chapters. Future health professionals and scientists need to understand and address all the personal and social issues involved in health, illness and human behaviour.

THE AIM OF THIS BOOK

Health and Human Behaviour has been written with entry-level students in the health professions, biomedical sciences and other health-related disciplines in mind. For this fourth edition, two new authors have been brought in to expand the range of expertise, and ensure that the material suits the needs of students. Topics have been carefully selected to cover the range of relevant psychological, physiological and sociological concepts, without trying to be comprehensive or detailed in the coverage of those concepts.

The book introduces concepts in ways that are usable for students. It is intended to attract students without a background in health, psychology and sociology to that material, and provide enough information, without overwhelming them with details of those disciplines. If you already have a background in these disciplines, you may be able to skip over sections of the material to focus on areas that are new to you.

THE CASE STUDIES

Each chapter includes case studies that illustrate issues arising in that chapter. The case studies are not intended to cover every kind of health problem, but to illustrate the experiences of those who are ill or who want to protect their current wellness. As in real life, the case studies are about individuals, each of whom experiences health and illness differently. Some may vary from standard presentations for a condition in order to make points more clearly. Again, this parallels real life.

We encourage you to go beyond these simple cases and look at the real experience of individuals of your own acquaintance in the light of material in this book. There is no better way to understand the interaction of health and human behaviour. Nearly all students in health-related programs are required to carry out a case study of an individual with a chronic condition or medical illness as part of their course work. Many students are initially concerned that they will not be able to find such a person, but they soon come to realise that chronic conditions and medical illness are extremely common. The search for a suitable case rapidly becomes a problem of selection rather than identification. Common conditions, such as asthma, arthritis and depression, have a high incidence among otherwise healthy individuals. However, it is also true that rare conditions—due to the very large number of them—are also common in spite of the small number of individuals experiencing each one.

The difficulty with much of the traditional study of the individual in health and illness is that it has usually been compartmentalised into biological, psychological and sociological specialities. These compartments are usually taught by discipline specialists with little interest in a whole-person perspective. Books tend to be specialised, each presenting more detail within the speciality than most readers will need at the introductory level. Basing the study of health and illness on the experience of the individual by the use of case studies overcomes this compartmentalisation and aims to increase the interest and accessibility of the material. The cases raise issues that we can all relate to, without including biomedical detail that most first-year students would find difficult to understand.

CONCLUSION

Miller (1990), a prominent educator in the health professions, identified levels of performance with regard to the content of education: *knows, knows how, shows how* and *does*. Our aim in presenting material in this book to students in the health professions and biomedical sciences is to have an impact on what you actually do in your professional activities. The self-test material addressed in the Guided Tour can provide only an indication of what you *know*, and what you *know how* to do. Looking in depth at an individual can provide an indication of whether you can demonstrate an ability to use the material; that you can *show how* to use it. We will never know whether you have learnt how to put your knowledge from this book into practice—how to do something in a better way—but it is our hope that this book will prompt some positive changes in your eventual professional practice.

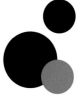

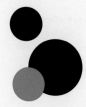

Guided Tour

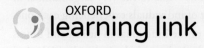

YOUR FREE DIGITAL STUDENT RESOURCES

Keep an eye out for this icon throughout the text. Integrated into this book are carefully designed learning features, presented both within the text and online, to help you gain a deeper understanding of the topics being discussed, and develop the essential knowledge and skills you'll need for your future career. This icon indicates that additional digital resources, relevant to the chapter you are reading, are available.

Go to **www.oup.com/he/jones4e** to access these resources.

Each chapter begins with a list of **Chapter Objectives** indicating the core knowledge, attitudes and/or skills you will learn in the chapter.

CHAPTER OBJECTIVES

By the end of this chapter, you should be able to:

» understand how the behaviour and lifestyle of the individual can influence health and illness

» recognise differences between behaviours that improve health and those that minimise harm

» apply basic principles of learning and memory to explain the development and maintenance of behaviour

---

Key words appear throughout the text to assist your understanding as you read. These terms are presented in a helpful list at the beginning of each chapter, defined in the margin where they first appear, and then collated in the **glossary** at the back of the book.

KEYWORDS

» aversive conditioning
» avoidance learning
» classical conditioning
» confabulation
» habit
» health behaviours
» learning
» learned helplessness

» lifestyle diseases
» memory
» neuroplasticity
» phobia
» punishment
» reinforcement
» risk-reduction behaviours
» risky behaviours

» secondary gain
» shaping
» stimulus
» stimulus generalisation
» synaptic cleft
» unsafe sex

Biofeedback
The control of internal processes through conditioning, using mechanical devices to make those internal processes perceptible.

Pause and Reflect activity boxes are presented throughout the book to encourage the extension of knowledge and deeper thought about the concepts being addressed.

PAUSE & REFLECT

What is it that motivates you to do well at university?
Where do think your motivation comes from?

8.1 CASE STUDY

DANIELLE AND SLEEP

Danielle is a 19-year-old university student enrolled in a Bachelor of Nursing degree, and she hopes to eventually work in intensive care. She has read in textbooks and on social media that older teenagers—like her—and young adults need seven to nine hours of sleep each night in order to perform at their best. She has been getting only about five hours or less on weekdays, because of classes, a busy social life, part-time work, and studying. Until recently she had thought she was coping, as long as she slept in for a few hours on Sunday mornings to catch up. Lately, she has noticed that she is finding it hard to stay awake during lectures, and frequently loses concentration while studying. However, a lot of her fellow students follow the same sort of low-sleep lifestyle and seem to be coping. She also knows an ICU nurse who claims that she can cope perfectly well on four hours sleep a night. At this point, Danielle's behaviour is unlikely to change unless there is a change in her motivation.

1 What might stimulate such a change for her?

2 Who should be responsible for making sure that students training for high-pressure health professions get enough sleep?

> **Case Studies** are presented throughout each chapter and used to illustrate the issues being discussed. Recurring case studies give you the opportunity to test your grasp of concepts before moving on, while longer cases at the end of the chapters give you a deeper understanding of the chapter material. Each case study is accompanied by **Questions**, inviting you to reflect on the content and encouraging independent thinking and reasoning.

> **Cross references** noted in the margin, direct you to related content in other chapters of the text to help connect ideas.

> *The influences of culture, social class and family are discussed in Chapter 14.*

CHAPTER SUMMARY

- Understanding motivation—the factors that arouse, sustain and direct behaviour—is important in changing behaviour. Motivation has genetic, biological and cognitive components, but is also strongly influenced by learning.

- Primary drives are based on the biological needs of the organism. Acquired drives arise out of experience with the environment.

- Opponent–process theory and optimal level theories suggest that the organism is motivated to maintain balance as well as to satisfy needs.

- Successful strategies for behaviour change involve picking appropriate behaviours and methods, not expecting too much, giving methods a chance to work, and recognising that methods may be failures but people are not.

> Each chapter ends with a clear **Chapter Summary** which draws together important ideas into a list, and links back to the Chapter Objectives to reinforce what has been covered.

FURTHER READING

Hughes S, Lewis S, Willis K, Rogers A, Wyke S & Smith L (2020) How do facilitators of group programmes for long-term conditions conceptualise self-management support? *Chronic Illness* 16(2), 104–18.

Lynch S, Shuster G & Lobo M (2018) The family caregiver experience: Examining the positive and negative aspects of compassion satisfaction and compassion fatigue as caregiving outcomes. *Aging & Mental Health* 22(11), 1424–31.

Marrie R (2017) Comorbidity in multiple sclerosis: Implications for patient care. *Nature Reviews Neurology* 13(6), 375–82.

Shulman R, Arora R, Geist R, Ali A, Ma J, Mansfield E, Martel S, Sandercock J & Versloot J (2021) Integrated community collaborative care for seniors with depression/anxiety and any physical illness. *Canadian Geriatrics Journal* 24(3), 251–7.

> A list of **Further Reading** concludes each chapter, providing you with the opportunity to expand your knowledge by exploring related concepts or reading about the findings of current research in the area.

Learn more
Access additional resources to broaden your understanding of this chapter. See the Guided Tour for access details.

> Further resources are available online through **Oxford Learning Link** and arranged by chapter. **Self-Test Multiple Choice Questions** enable you to determine whether you have understood some of the essential points of each chapter. Annotated **Weblinks** encourage you to gain further insights into particular health conditions and illness responses, or access the latest facts and figures presented on government and health websites.

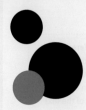

About the Authors

KEN JONES

Retired after 40 years of teaching behavioural sciences to students in health and biomedical sciences, Kenneth V. Jones, PhD, is now Adjunct Associate Professor in the Department of Psychiatry, Faculty of Medicine, Nursing and Health Sciences, Monash University. One of the first psychologists employed by a medical school to develop behavioural sciences content, he filled a variety of roles including Director of Behavioural Sciences, First Year MBBS Coordinator, Head of the Clinical Teaching Administrative Unit, Foundation Co-chair of the Personal and Professional Development Theme for the MBBS degree, and Director of the university-wide Transition Program for Monash University. The first edition of this book arose out of courses he developed for Medicine, Radiography, Nutrition and Dietetics, and Biomedical Sciences. His contributions to the education of health professionals through the Australian and New Zealand Association for Health Professional Education (formerly ANZAME) include serving as President, Vice-President and Membership Secretary, and Editor of ANZAHPE's journal— *Focus on Health Professional Education*. He is an Honorary Life Member of ANZAHPE and recipient of the ANZAME Award for Achievement in Education, the ANZAME Award for Service and the Silver Jubilee Prize for Education (FMNHS, Monash). He was a signatory of the 1988 Edinburgh Declaration on Medical Education. He has published many refereed journal articles and chapters on education, on his research area of psychophysiology, and supervised postgraduate students in psychology, medicine and nursing.

DEBRA CREEDY

Professor Emeritus Debra Creedy is a nurse and psychologist with expertise in Perinatal Mental Health at Griffith University. Professor Creedy has conducted clinical and education research for 35 years. Her clinical research involves successful mixed methods studies and randomised controlled trials on the effectiveness of counselling interventions to assist distressed women, support programs for couples becoming parents, and reducing childbirth fear in pregnant women. Her recent educational research involves the development of tools to measure the clinical learning environment, critical thinking, awareness of cultural safety and development of cultural capability. To promote evidence-based practice, Professor Creedy has conducted systematic reviews through the Cochrane Collaboration, Joanna Briggs Institute and independently with research higher-degree students. Professor Creedy was named 'Best in Field' for the discipline of Midwifery in *The Australian* newspaper in 2022. She has authored four books and nearly 300 peer-reviewed articles.

KATRINA LANE-KREBS

Katrina Lane-Krebs is a lecturer at CQ University and a cluster lead for psychosocial well-being related research. She specialises in family and lifespan studies specifically, disability, rehabilitation and inclusion. Her PhD explored the biopsychosocial impact of trauma and disability. Dr Lane-Krebs is an established author and reviewer for prominent journals. As a registered health practitioner, she has extensive experience delivering acute and community-based care within a variety of environments. She also has qualifications in Early Childhood

Education, Health Science, Tertiary Education and Correctional Management. She holds a Masters degree, for which her dissertation related to welfare and mental health and well-being.

FLORIN OPRESCU

Florin Oprescu is Associate Professor in Public Health: Health Promotion at the University of the Sunshine Coast. He specialises in mixed methods research (both qualitative and quantitative) in the areas of health promotion and education. He is passionate about educational development, teaching and learning; health education; health communication and capacity building. He is a strong advocate for the translation of scientific evidence into practice, and of good practice into evidence.

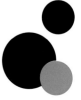

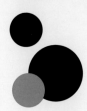

Acknowledgments

This fourth edition of *Health and Human Behaviour* has taken several months to prepare and would not have been completed without the support of a few special people. We give heartfelt thanks to our employers, the School of Nursing & Midwifery at Griffith University; the School of Nursing, Midwifery & Social Sciences at Central Queensland University; and the School of Health and Behavioural Sciences at the University of the Sunshine Coast, which supported us with time and resources to write.

Our sincere thanks to the editorial staff at OUP, Helen Carter, and our editor Adrienne de Kretser for turning our writing into a book.

The author and the publisher wish to thank the following copyright holders for reproduction of their material.

Figure 7.1, Rosenstock IM. Historical Origins of the Health Belief Model. Health Education Monographs. 1974;2(4):328–335. doi:10.1177/109019817400200403; Figure 7.2 based on Fishbein, M. & Ajzen, I. (1975) Belief, Attitude, Intention and Behavior: An Introduction to Theory and Research. Used with permission; Figure 7.3, Reprinted from Ajzen, I. & Madden, T. (1986) Prediction of Goal-directed Behavior: Attitudes, Intentions, and Perceived Behavioral Control. Journal of Experimental Social Psychology, 22, 453–74, with permission from Elsevier; Figure 9.1, Reprinted from Swinburn, B., Egger, G. & Raza, F. (1999) Dissecting Obesogenic Environments: The Development and Application of a Framework for Identifying and Prioritising Environmental Interventions for Obesity. Preventive Medicine, 29, 563–70, with permission from Elsevier; Figure 12.1, based on Yerkes, R.M. & Dodson, J.D. (1908) The Relation of Strength of Stimulus to Rapidity of Habit-formation. Journal of Comparative Neurology and Psychology, 18, 459–82; Figure 12.2, from Frankenhaeuser, M. (1991) The Psychophysiology of Workload, Stress and Health: Comparison between the Sexes. Annals of Behavioral Medicine, 13, 197–201, by permission of Oxford University; Figure 12.3, based on Fisher, S. (1986) Stress and Strategy. Reproduced by permission of Taylor and Francis Group, LLC, a division of Informa plc.; Figure 12.4, Cohen, S., Kessler, R. & Gordon, L. (1995) Conceptualising stress and its relation to disease. In Cohen, S., Kessler, R. & Gordon, L. (Eds.) Measuring Stress: A Guide for Health and Social Scientists (pp. 3–26) New York: OUP, by permission of Oxford University; Page 230, Principles of mindfulness, adapted from The Foundations of Mindfulness Practice: Attitudes and Commitment, in Full Catastrophe Living: Using the Wisdom of Your Body and Mind to Face Stress, Pain, and Illness, by Jon Kabat-Zinn, Penguin RandomHouse, New York, 2013, pp. 19–38. For guided mindfulness meditation practices with Jon Kabat-Zinn, see www.mindfulnessapps.com; Figure 14.1, Interaction Institute for Social Change | Artist: Angus Maguire, released under a creative commons CC BY-SA 4.0 license https://creativecommons.org/licenses/by-sa/4.0/

Cover image: Shutterstock

PART I

FOUNDATIONS OF HEALTH AND BEHAVIOUR

» Chapter 1: Who is Sick? Defining and Applying Concepts of Illness, Disease and Health...4
» Chapter 2: Infant, Child and Adolescent Development...........................17
» Chapter 3: Adult Development and Ageing 35
» Chapter 4: Reactions to Illness...50
» Chapter 5: Understanding Reactions to Chronic Conditions.................72

WHAT IS HEALTH AND ILLNESS?

While behaviour has a central role in health, many of the things required to maintain health and avoid illness are beyond our ability to control. This could be due to our individual physical and/or psychological characteristics, social factors and barriers. As biomedical sciences advance our understanding of biological processes (e.g. the human system), it becomes evident that psychological and social processes need to be understood in order to make sense of what it means to be sick, to be healthy or to be well. Part I of this book begins with an exploration of these concepts.

The connections between health and behaviour are complex and it is widely acknowledged that our individual habits affect health. Healthy media campaigns present the links between obesity and disease, provide warnings about misuse of alcohol, tobacco and other drugs and try to promote healthy behaviours such as screenings and good parenting. It is equally important to recognise that health and illness affect our behaviour. The most fundamental place to begin the examination of the connections between health and behaviour is with an understanding of the concepts of health, illness and disease (i.e. what it means to be well, healthy or sick). These concepts are not absolute values but rather social constructs, ideas or mental schemas that we share with the people around us.

OXFORD UNIVERSITY PRESS

Chapter 1 defines some key terms and describes ways in which well-being, health and illness can be measured and understood. Additionally, the importance of identifying appropriate health status measurements for an individual, community or population is discussed. The chapter introduces readers to two models (medical and biopsychosocial) that provide different ways of thinking about managing illness and promoting health.

Chapter 2 draws on major developmental theorists such as Piaget, Erikson and Vygotsky who offered important observations and concepts relating to healthy child, adolescent and young adult development. In addition to physical growth, childhood and adolescence are times of tremendous cognitive, social and emotional development. It is also interesting to consider how children of different ages conceptualise illness. Understanding of each individual's cognition, evaluation and behaviours towards health and illness, needs to be presented in age-appropriate and culturally sensitive ways that are supported by the community in which the child lives, so as to foster optimisation of health outcomes. The chapter also introduces readers to adverse childhood experiences and to basic principles of trauma-informed care as these factors can influence behaviours in later stages of the lifespan.

Adulthood and ageing are discussed in Chapter 3. As individuals progress from childhood to adulthood, they develop habitual ways of behaving, responding to stimuli and thinking. During adulthood, these habitual patterns of response begin to influence individuals' health, their families and significant others. During adulthood, age can affect an individual's behaviour in different ways. Decline of capabilities in seniors is often thought of as a consequence of age itself; however, it frequently links to a disease process that happens coincidentally with ageing. The chapter also discusses issues related to death, dying and grieving. These are important considerations for high-quality end-of-life care for clients as well as for the family members and health professionals.

Chapter 4 explores how people react to being sick and looks at the influence that a change in health status can have on people's feeling, thinking and behaviours. Reactions vary between people, and this can be explained by the vulnerabilities and capabilities that a person brings to the experience. Vulnerabilities and capabilities can include cognitive, emotional and behavioural strategies adopted for dealing with life situations. The chapter explores processes (cognitive, emotional, behavioural) that a person goes through to think of themselves as being ill. It also discusses the roles of illness perceptions that allow a person to 'learn' what it means to be sick.

Chapter 5 discusses in more detail people's reactions to chronic conditions. While episodes of illness are often short and acute, there are more and more people who live a long time with chronic health challenges. Chronic events often elicit a different response in comparison to those arising from acute experiences.

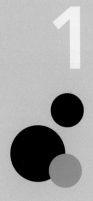

1 Who is Sick? Defining and Applying Concepts of Illness, Disease and Health

Health and illness

Health and **illness** are dynamic concepts that have a significant impact on how an individual perceives (thinks), experiences (feels) and behaves (acts). Being either 'sick' or 'well' is influenced by perceptions of the person as well as by perceptions of others towards them. There is a common expectation of a state of wellness. Consider, for example, an everyday greeting to someone we believe is well. Although we ask 'How are you?' we presume a response of 'Fine'. We rarely expect to receive a negative or detailed response. In greeting someone who we know to be experiencing reduced health, our social greeting remains the same. 'How are you?' In this situation, we may expect to get specific information but also have an expectation that over time the person will eventually become 'well'.

As people tend to be reasonably well most of the time, the concept of health does not normally occupy a large place in our thoughts. During times of reduced health, the desire to return to a state of wellness becomes a priority. The importance of health and quality of life (QoL) only becomes obvious to individuals when they experience a deficit in their usual state of health. Health is a valued asset and in the presence of dramatic life-changing events (e.g. divorce, flood and loss of possessions, loss of employment) it is not uncommon to find the prioritisation and value of health expressed as 'At least I've got my health'.

For many people, there is not a clear distinction between being well or having a disease or illness. Most people do not consider themselves to be unwell (sick) even when there may be signs and symptoms of underlying disease or illness. The state of wellness rests with the individual's perspective and is termed a subjective experience. The meaning of health varies over the course of a person's life, and can differ between social groups, cultures, countries, families and individuals. People living with major disabilities may consider themselves well, despite living with pain or disability that would make most of us feel very unwell indeed. Similarly, many older individuals consider themselves to be well, despite diminished vision and hearing, limitations of mobility, or loss of significant others leading to altered emotional health because of grief. The experience of health is therefore a dynamic process.

Health
A dynamic concept that varies over time and is influenced by social situations, cultures, ethnicities, families and individuals.

Illness
A subjective experience on the part of an individual that something is not quite right with their health.

Differences about the meaning of health are discussed in Chapter 7.

PAUSE & REFLECT

Defining health and illness is an important first step in determining its importance for a person. Your individual definition will also influence how you view and react to others' concepts of health.

Do you consider yourself to be well or sick right at this moment? Why?

Who is sick?

Being sick is not a fact: it is a social definition. The problem of defining who is sick has significance not just for the individual but also for others who are important in their daily lives. It even has a moral dimension. Many people believe, for example, that smokers deserve less medical care than, say, innocent accident victims because smokers contribute to their own illness. Others see this attitude as an example of blaming the victim for their illness.

There are two definitions commonly used to decide whether someone is sick; namely, the illness definition and the disease definition.

ILLNESS DEFINITION: THE SICK ARE THOSE WHO HAVE SYMPTOMS

We are all familiar with the experience of feeling unwell or ill. Being unwell or ill is essentially a change in a person's sense of normal, balance or equilibrium. These changes are identified by symptoms. Symptoms are felt by the individual. This personal, or subjective, feeling that something is not quite right is the most important indicator of illness. It relates to having symptoms that are not usually present, or a worsening of symptoms that the person experiences but is usually able to adequately manage.

Being unwell may be based on our personal beliefs of normality for various stages of the lifespan. If we have a symptom that others around us do not have, or that they consider abnormal, we feel unwell or sick. Consider, for example, that in older adults a deterioration of vision is commonly experienced and prescription glasses, laser surgery or cataract procedures are regularly undertaken. Therefore, a deficit of vision is not necessarily considered abnormal in this cohort. An elderly person requiring corrective lenses probably does not consider themselves unwell as their situation does not deviate from that of many others at the same stage of life. In comparison, an adolescent who has experienced an event leading to lowered mood, feeling negative about the future, and reduced self-esteem may be perceived as different from most adolescents and therefore see themselves as unwell. These contrasting examples also highlight that reduced health (illness or a state of unwellness) is not always visible. Even if others may not recognise our feelings or we display no outward signs of illness, we may still feel ill and find it difficult to deal with the demands of the world around us.

Generally, whenever we are feeling 'not quite right', it is reasonable that we will want to understand why and then try to return to our usual state of wellness. We commence this process by seeking a cause or an explanation for our changed situation. The kinds of causes that we accept as reasonable will depend on our own personal view of how the world works. Imagine, for example, trying to explain the symptoms of a cold to one of your ancestors from several centuries in the past. They would never have heard of terms such as germs or virus, and subsequently would not understand that a cold was caused by a virus. Depending on where your ancestors came from, when they feel ill they could draw very different conclusions about why they feel that way and (equally importantly) what to do about it. We are likely to discuss our symptoms with those living around us (e.g. our family and friends) to understand a cause because we tend to be exposed to similar information and shared experiences. These concepts also relate to culture, which is defined as shared characteristics within a group.

Some individuals experience illness in the absence of a clear physical cause. Remember, illness is subjective. As an example, there is no definitive test for a headache—this event is experienced within the individual and the symptoms are only identifiable by the person experiencing the headache. The headache would produce an altered state of what that person normally experiences. As there are no measurable signs of headache, people around that person may feel that the person is not really sick, or even believe that the person is faking illness. None of this makes the illness any less real to the person experiencing it. This links to the rights and obligations of the sick role.

Symptoms contrast with signs. Signs are externally validated elements of illness (Berman et al., 2020). For example, an elevated temperature of 39°C is a validated sign whereas feeling hot and feverish are subjective symptoms. The notion of illness as the presence of

Culture is explored in Chapter 14.

The sick role is explored in Chapter 4.

disease (Manderscheid et al., 2010) or the concept of identifiable pathology (e.g. blood test results outside of a recommended range) is a dominant view in Western health systems.

There has been ongoing debate regarding a definition of illness based on the presence of symptoms. Armstrong (1980) suggests that broader consideration about what it means to be ill is necessary for the following reasons.

- *Symptoms are very common.* It is quite likely that you will have had a potentially treatable or self-rectifying symptom in the past few days (e.g. a headache, cough or runny nose, anxiety, a cut or scrape). Would you consider yourself to be a sick person? Most will not. Children and older people are even more likely to have symptoms but not think of themselves as sick (Armstrong, 1980; Bueter, 2019).

- *Most symptoms are trivial and easily forgotten.* If you woke up with a cough this morning but it got better in a couple of hours, you would probably not even remember it tomorrow. Many people live with regular symptoms (e.g. chronic pain); however, they have adapted and normalised the presence of these symptoms. The symptoms have been shifted into a background level of awareness, so a person does not consider themselves to be sick unless the symptoms are greater than, or different from, their normal experience. Even in the presence of a variety of recurrent or constant symptoms, individuals may trivialise, minimise the significance of, or discount the symptoms and therefore exploration of an underlying illness or causal factors is not undertaken by the individual or a health care professional (Bontempo, 2021).

- *It is usually not the symptom (or even its severity or persistence) that matters to the individual.* What matters is the meaning of the symptom (Armstrong, 1980; Bueter, 2019). A person who experiences a perceptual distortion such as blurred vision, or a lump or pain that is unexpected or new, may be far more worried by it than the person with diabetes who experiences the symptoms of low blood glucose levels on a regular basis, or the person living with arthritis who has swelling and severe persistent pain in their joints. These experiences may be normalised and absorbed into their concept of stable health. Again, these symptoms can be negated or explained away even during interactions with health professionals (Bontempo, 2021).

- *Even for a given individual and symptom, perception of meaning will vary according to the mood of the individual, context of the symptom, the individual's level of knowledge and experience, their usual coping strategies and many other factors* (Armstrong, 1980; Bueter, 2019). A symptom that looks serious to an individual may suddenly lose all significance when the individual is given a satisfactory explanation for it. Imagine waking to find a large warm lump behind your ear. You might have panicky thoughts of cancer, and because you cannot examine the lump might become preoccupied with thoughts that severely disrupt your daily activities and sleep. A great sense of relief may be experienced if you are told by a knowledgeable person that the lump is a fatty cyst produced by a blocked sebaceous gland, which is very common and often self-rectifying.

Strategies for dealing with illness are discussed in Chapter 7.

Sometimes an individual may not perceive that they have a symptom. People who live with bipolar or unipolar disorder may experience a condition known as mania. During a manic episode the individual may feel exceptionally well, full of energy, require less sleep and/or have grand plans that they believe can only be completed by themselves (Berman et al., 2020). In the eyes of others, these behaviours are outside what is socially considered to be 'normal' and the individual's plans may seem unrealistic or reckless. The individual may not be aware that their behaviour is unusual even though they may actually require urgent psychiatric treatment.

Strategies for coping with stress are in Chapter 13.

DISEASE DEFINITION: THOSE WHO ARE DEEMED SICK, AND HAVE BEEN GIVEN A DIAGNOSIS BY A HEALTH PROFESSIONAL

In contemporary Western society, it is generally assumed that illness arises from pathophysiological changes in the body. In most cases, these changes can at least be observed and substantiated by health professionals. Altered pathology is identifiable through measuring and charting trends in a person's vital signs such as blood pressure, respiration rates, heart rate, temperature and so forth. Medical science can detect viruses, bacteria and other pathogens in samples of various body tissues, including blood, urine and sputum. Radiologists interpret X-rays, MRIs, CTs, ultrasounds or other imaging to identify abnormalities or injuries deep inside the body organs, bones and tissues. The test findings are used to determine the presence or absence of disease. This is an objective determination of pathology by an independent and qualified observer. Altered pathology, therefore, underlies the concept of **disease**—that there is something biomedically wrong.

Disease
An abnormal state of a person's body or mind, as identified by a qualified observer.

The nature of pathological findings has evolved over time in keeping with emerging scientific processes. New technologies assist in detection; for example, testing of the amniotic fluid (amniocentesis) can detect a wide range of abnormalities in a developing foetus (Queensland Health, 2018). Similarly, genome sequencing of the COVID-19 virus has revealed detailed variations such as a Delta strain (CDGN, 2020) and later an Omicron strain. Other strains are likely to be identified using these techniques.

Epidemiological studies have revealed that abnormal pathology, such as cholesterol level, may vary according to ethnicity and geographical location. European countries like Iceland and Germany have the highest cholesterol levels in the world, with mean serum total cholesterols of around 5.5 mmol/L.

1.1 CASE STUDY

MELISSA

The aim of this case study is to examine how health, illness and disease concepts may apply to one person's experience.

Melissa is 32 years old. She carries out a routine breast self-examination each month. Recently she felt a lump in her breast. Melissa may experience a range of responses when she discovers this lump. If she has felt a lump previously or believes that the cause is trivial, she may ignore the lump and experience no change in her concept of herself as a well person. If the lump is new, has changed in size or shape or represents to her the possibility of serious disease, she may start thinking about whether she is ill; that is, she may experience a feeling that something is not quite right.

Melissa had previously found lumps in her breasts when she was breastfeeding. Occasionally, a lump would also appear around the time of her menstrual period. Melissa weaned her child 12 months ago. She is becoming increasingly concerned about the lump because her mother was diagnosed with breast cancer at the age of 45.

Melissa decides that something is not right and sees her doctor to get a medical opinion. A mammogram is undertaken. The radiology report indicates that most presentations of this nature are benign (non-cancerous); however, based on Melissa's family history, a biopsy is recommended (BreastScreen Victoria, 2021).

Before Melissa's mother was diagnosed with breast cancer, she had been in good health. Melissa recalls that her mother had the lump detected at an annual breast screening. Within a matter of weeks, her mother had a biopsy then surgery and was having chemotherapy for the affected breast and lymph tissue. This was a very worrying time for everyone, and her mother broke down and cried several times with Melissa. Her mother felt sick from the treatment, and for years afterwards needed to protect her arm on the affected side. Melissa found herself thinking often about her mother's experience and wondered how she would cope if she had breast cancer.

1   Does Melissa have an illness or disease? Explain your answer based on the illness definition or the disease definition.

2   Melissa witnessed her mother's experience of breast cancer. How might that experience influence Melissa's response to her current situation?

However, the disease definition has some problems. Unknown pathologies continue to be found. HIV/AIDS, for example, was not originally identified by pathology. A number of people, with similar signs and symptoms, went to see their doctors feeling ill, and only then did medical scientists start looking for a common cause. Furthermore, there are other factors.

- *Health professionals tend to accept a patient's definition that they are sick.* Upon consulting a health care professional, people may be issued certificates for absence from work or study even when the cited symptoms were minor, difficult to classify as disease or easily faked. Doctors and other health professionals tend to respond to the patient's feelings as true expressions of subjective illness, such as feeling unwell, tired and stressed, or even feeling burnt out from overwork. These experiences, while subjective, are no less significant than identifiable signs such as elevated temperature. It would be far more concerning if health professionals dismissed subjective information and regarded the person as wasting their time, or malingering (lying). Help-seeking is seen by health professionals in most cases as justifying the giving of help, and it would be hard to argue that this is unreasonable.

- *The diagnosis and treatment of medical conditions varies from time to time and place to place.* Not long ago, a child with tonsillitis living in one state in Australia was twice as likely to have surgery as a child with tonsillitis in another state. Caesarean deliveries are more common in women with private health insurance than in women attending a public maternity service. It could be argued that, in either case, high rates of intervention do not reflect real medical need. Behaviours and diagnosis may also be influenced by political, religious or cultural beliefs such as grief processes and mental health conditions (Dorrian et al., 2017).

- *Diagnosis and treatment depend on concepts of normality.* These concepts may be cultural, subcultural or even family-based. For example, in some cultures women cope with labour pains in silence, while other cultures encourage the vocalisation of pain. DiTomasso (2019) highlights changes in social influences relating to pain management and childbirth, indicating that giving birth with minimal medical intervention is considered essential in some cultures, and that obstetricians advocate the use of pharmacological pain relief (e.g. pethidine or epidural anaesthesia) while the Natural Childbirth movement advocates for a woman's right to choose how and where birth takes place. There will always be differences in beliefs between religious groups, locations and genders across a wide variety of health situations.

1.2 CASE STUDY

MELISSA (CONT.)

Deciding whether someone has a disease sometimes means deciding what to do next. In Melissa's case, the consequences of doing nothing to further investigate her symptom could be severe. If her breast lump is cancerous, the probability of her dying could be greatly increased by inaction. Conversely, doing something about the symptom could save her life. It is likely in this case that the doctor would do everything possible to persuade Melissa that if her lump is cancerous, it would be worth treating, and that treatment should begin as soon as possible. This reflects evidence-based practice in breast cancer.

Melissa talked over the initial results with her husband, Peter, and her sister, who were supportive for Melissa to undergo the biopsy and be treated if necessary. Melissa faced a dilemma. She wanted to have further testing to be reassured that everything was okay, but she was also worried about the possibility of having cancer. She kept thinking about her mother's experience and the long-term consequences of treatment. She was worried about losing part or all of her breast. She and Peter still had an active sex life and Melissa was worried that Peter may not find her attractive if she required breast surgery. She was concerned about whether she would still feel feminine if she had surgery.

After several nights of talking things through, Melissa and her husband made an appointment with her doctor. They agreed that her lump should be removed and examined to determine whether it was cancerous. During the appointment, the doctor informed her that, with appropriate treatment, even if the lump was cancerous her chance of long-term survival was good and that she could lead a full life.

1   Will treatment make Melissa healthy again?
2   How might this experience affect Melissa's view of her health in the short and long term?

How do illness and disease compare?

Usually, disease and illness go together, and we feel unwell because we have a disease. This is not always the case, and problems may arise for the individual when disease and illness do not go together. High blood pressure (hypertension), for instance, is dangerous as people with high blood pressure are at increased risk of stroke and heart attack. Yet many people who have undiagnosed high blood pressure probably do not feel any symptoms at all. Most people diagnosed with high blood pressure usually find out because a health professional tested for it during a routine examination. An individual who experiences no symptoms is less likely to accept treatment. This is an example of a person with a disease who is not experiencing an illness. In contrast, another person may experience repeated headaches, which is a sign of hypertension. In this case, the person is experiencing an illness but does not yet know they have an underlying disease.

PAUSE & REFLECT

The definitions presented in this chapter suggest that high blood pressure would be considered a disease, not an illness.

How might this affect whether or not a person diagnosed with high blood pressure would treat it as a serious health problem?

A third consideration is the possibility of having an illness without having a disease. Think about a young man who notices that his hair is falling out. He feels that something is not right and fears the consequences—he does not want to be bald. When he goes to his doctor, however, he is told that there is nothing wrong with him and that he is simply displaying normal male pattern baldness, which is largely determined by his genes. Some men are satisfied with this definition of themselves as being well, and adapt to the change in their appearance. They consider themselves normal and bald. Others are dissatisfied and may pursue treatment with drugs or even with surgery, to avoid being bald.

If the individual's need to define baldness as a disease is strong enough, they will find professionals who will agree that they need treatment or seek to discover a causal factor other than genetics; for example, a thyroid disorder could be the underlying cause. Because baldness is not generally considered to be a disease, the person wanting to address their baldness will probably have to pay for treatment out of their own pocket.

There are other conditions that most societies do not consider to be diseases. Take the woman who considers her breasts to be too small and wants implants, or the person with discoloured but otherwise healthy teeth. The boundaries become very unclear in some instances. Is male circumcision a procedure that doctors should conduct? If the foreskin is too tight or chronic infections occur then there is a clear medical reason; however, male circumcision is infrequently performed in Australia (Qin et al., 2021). In most societies, female genital circumcision would be considered mutilation. It is prohibited in many countries and considered a crime if performed in Australia (Ogunsiji et al., 2018). Yet, there remain some cultures and societies where female circumcision is considered not only acceptable but desirable.

Confusion about whether illness equals disease is common in the early stages of symptoms before a cause has been established. Someone with anaemia may experience headaches, lethargy, weakness, dizziness and pallor but require a blood test to determine the cause. Conversely, there are some conditions where the disease classification is identified prior to the individual experiencing any symptoms of illness (e.g. ovarian cancers). These are often termed 'silent diseases' (Tan et al., 2021). In this case, pathology tests can identify a disease in the absence of symptoms. Some disease to illness or illness to disease processes

Cultural impacts on health behaviours are discussed in Chapter 14.

have short intervals; for example, a consequence of COVID-19 (disease) is chronic fatigue syndrome (illness) (Araja et al., 2021). This highlights the importance of routine screening for individuals with risk factors.

As medical science progresses, the classification of disease becomes clearer. More causes are identified and links between causes and symptoms are better understood. Sometimes, because of new evidence, we find that we must go back to ideas that have previously been rejected by medical science.

Health

Negative definition of health
The absence of disease equates with being healthy.

Commonly, we think of health as the normal state, experienced whenever we are not actually ill. This pertains to the **negative definition of health**—a person is considered healthy in the absence of disease. The negative definition of health has some criticisms. Consider the usefulness of a definition that potentially classifies whole groups or even populations as sick (unhealthy). Do members of those groups consider themselves to be sick? One of the main reasons why they do not is that we all tend to measure our health against the health of those around us. Older people are likely to experience a variety of health conditions, sensory problems (hearing or vision), reduced mobility, hypertension (high blood pressure), arthritis or diabetes, yet often express a sense of sound well-being as they go about their daily lives (AIHW, 2018b). These measures relate to pathophysiological health. In addition to physical health, psychological and social domains of life significantly contribute to the sense of well-being. Subjective well-being is the appraisal of the individual; it is their perspective of health and considers the biological (physical), psychological, social and often spiritual domains of their environment (Weinberg et al., 2018). Similarly, people in low-income countries where parasites are common may see themselves as well, despite having a condition that would be considered a serious health problem for people in high-income countries.

The World Health Organization (WHO, 2021a) defines health as "a state of complete physical, mental and social well-being and not merely the absence of disease or infirmity". This definition is positive, dynamic and intended to be applicable globally. Challenges to this definition arise, however, due to different economies and the available scope of health care. The concept of health also needs to be responsive to new and acute events such as pandemics, natural disasters and war, where urgent action is needed to protect the populations experiencing the event.

Another way of thinking about health is in terms of what it enables the individual to do. The *Ottawa Charter for Health Promotion* (WHO, 1986) talks about health as a "resource for everyday life, not the objective of living". Health and well-being allow individuals to live to the best of their abilities, while disease and illness produce barriers to those activities. Individuals have 'enough' health when it no longer is of particular concern or focus for them, as they go about daily life.

Well-being

Well-being
A state of complete physical, social and mental health that is consistent with living a full and satisfying life.

The concept of **well-being**—included in the WHO definition of health given above—entered the discussion of what health means in the 1960s. It could be said that if health is the opposite of disease, well-being represents the opposite of illness; that is, well-being comprises a subjective sense that there is basically nothing wrong. Like illness, well-being can be completely independent of our objectively measured health or disease status.

Individuals who have capabilities and coping strategies that allow them to manage their lives without much difficulty, tend to feel that their disease status is irrelevant to their sense of being as a person and control of their life. Similarly, individuals may have a sense of personal well-being in very deprived circumstances, while dealing with chronic or acute disease, and even in the face of very stressful events. It is useful to keep in mind that an individual's **appraisal** of their situation is critically important. It will affect how they think and feel about health, and what behaviours they carry out.

Appraisal
The cognitions that an individual holds about the situation they are in at a given time.

MEASUREMENT OF HEALTH AND ILLNESS

Decisions about the existence, significance and priority of areas for action are usually made by the community, based on information about the occurrence of disease within that community. Contemporary decision-making is based on more objective measurements of health and illness within the community. The science of **epidemiology** has taken over the measurement task. The aim is to inform the decision-makers within a community about the health status of the specified population and various groups within that community.

Epidemiology
The science of measuring the health status of a community.

The health of a population is usually measured by looking at two characteristics: **morbidity** (amount of sickness) and **mortality** (number of deaths). It is possible to imagine a case where these two do not go together, but it is far more common for them to be closely associated. Where people experience high rates of disease, they tend not to live as long.

Morbidity
The amount of disease observed within a group.

There are two aspects of morbidity we will consider. First, how many people are experiencing a particular disease over a period of time? An example would be the number of cases of arthritis in a community in a year (the **prevalence** of that disease). Second, how many new cases are observed over a period of time? An example would be how many people are first diagnosed as having arthritis in a community during a year (the **incidence** of that disease). The fact that these can differ is quite significant.

Mortality
The number of deaths observed within a group.

Prevalence
The number of existing and new cases of a specific disease present in a particular population at a certain time.

PAUSE & REFLECT

Following a change in the kinds of pesticides used on farms in a particular area, it is observed that a large number of babies are born with birth defects.

How would the concepts of prevalence and incidence help you to understand this observation?

Incidence
The rate at which new cases of a specific disease occur in a particular population during a specified period.

One very good reason for keeping a watch on the incidence and prevalence of disease in the community is that changes can help us to identify new problems or changed health conditions. An outbreak of polio in Papua New Guinea in 2018 had implications for Australia and alerted experts to review immunisation and environmental factors. A public health warning was issued and recommendations regarding travel to this area were updated (Hall et al., 2019).

Monitoring of a population also enables other trends to be predicted. The ageing of the population in Australia has led to an increase in the prevalence of problems of older adults that will affect health care funding and decisions about the number of doctors, hospitals and nursing homes that will be needed in future.

Knowledge about health and illness within a society is obtained by looking at the causes of death. One problem with mortality measurement is that eventually everyone dies. This means that if fewer people die from, say, infections during the first year of life, more people must eventually die of other causes later in life. If we look back at statistics taken from death certificates over hundreds of years, it appears that we are in the midst of cardiovascular, diabetes and cancer epidemics (AIHW, 2018c). As larger proportions of people are dying of these conditions, investigating the age at which people die of these causes informs policy-makers about what types of interventions are needed and the age group at which to target the interventions. Interventions are not only focused on improving lifespan, they also consider quality of life (QoL).

Interventions for health-related behaviours such as obesity and drug intervention among young people may increase the lifespan of the people concerned, and at the same time greatly improve the QoL of those people over many years. Interventions with older people may not increase length of life but may increase QoL. Considering what can be done to improve QoL is equally as important as increasing longevity.

MODELS OF HEALTH AND ILLNESS

Medical model
A model of health that considers the individual as a case or patient, primarily the host for some sort of disease or malfunctioning organ.

The model of care that has dominated the thinking of health professionals is the **medical model** (or biomedical model) (Engel, 1977). This model considers the individual as a case or a patient, primarily the host for some sort of disease or malfunctioning organ. The solution to the individual's disease is to return the biological function to its healthy state by chemical or surgical means, or both. It is a powerful model, because it has led to substantial improvements in the development of diagnostic, management and treatment procedures.

If health professionals rely too heavily on the medical model, however, it can lead to serious consequences. These include:

* failure to consider the whole person, including feelings, needs and socio-economic factors that can affect health;
* overlooking the well person that exists between illnesses;
* failure to consider the past history of a particular episode of illness.

As the major threats to our health are linked to lifestyle and emotions, adopting a disease-centred view of people can have grave consequences for their treatment.

Biopsychosocial model
A model of health that considers the individual as a whole person in a social setting, who may or may not be ill at any given moment.

The **biopsychosocial model** considers the individual as a whole person within a social setting, who may or may not be ill at any given moment (Engel, 1977). This involves adding a variety of psychological and social factors to the biological ones. The biopsychosocial model emerged as an extension of the medical model to form a more comprehensive model of health.

Attitudes
An individual's thoughts, feelings and readiness to act in relation to any object, person or event.

The psychological domain relates to cognition, thoughts and perceptions. The beliefs we learn through our socialisation processes that are positive, tend to increase our self-esteem. In contrast, being the target of prejudice and discriminatory **attitudes** have the potential to reduce our sense of self-worth. Psychological responses to health and illness include how we perceive pain, how we communicate our experience (e.g. maintaining or avoiding eye contact) and our own attitudes to illness, disease, rights and obligations of the sick role, and opinions on conditions such as mental health, chronic illness and disability.

The social domain involves our networks and connections with others. Social domains can be in person or virtual (online). Social connections include relatives, friendships and interactions with providers of goods (e.g. in the supermarket) and services (e.g. hairdressers, taxi drivers and medical providers). On some level, everyone—even the most reclusive individual—maintains a level of social interaction with others and their environment.

Recently, the inclusion of spirituality has created the emergence of the **biopsychosocial-spiritual model**. Unlike the medical model, this model reflects a humanistic and holistic approach to the person and their environment as the focus of care. For example, application of the biopsychosocial-spiritual model for end-of-life care may involve facilitating the reconciliation of the person with their family and friends as a form of genuine healing.

Spirituality is a person's practice of creating meaning of their life, existence and purpose (Hoffnung et al., 2019). It can produce an awakening, new awareness, or renewal of perceptions (Salazar, 2018). Spirituality is not confined to religious beliefs and practices. While **religion** may contribute to spirituality, being a spiritual person is not restricted to religion. Religion is defined as an organised system of beliefs and practices associated with a divine or sacred entity and is often displayed by ceremony (e.g. attending a church and praying) (Berman et al., 2020). Spirituality does not necessarily have an origin in religion (and could be deemed non-religious). Spirituality does reflect a connection to something bigger than ourselves in a search for meaning, and is practised through reflection, meditation and connection to nature and other elements (Dorrian et al., 2017).

Some advantages of a biopsychosocial-spiritual approach are that it:

- recognises that the values of the person and the health professional must be considered;
- places the focus of thinking about health and illness on interactions between the physical, psychological, social and spiritual domains;
- facilitates consideration of the broader context of the individual and health, including familial, cultural, environmental and financial factors.

The biopsychosocial-spiritual model is not without deficits. By emphasising the role of lifestyle, this model may lead health professionals to overestimate the individual's control over and responsibility for their own health (Farre & Rapley, 2017). Further, it may reduce tolerance for those who do not behave in a healthy way (e.g. are obese or smoke), therefore leading to victim-blaming. The emphasis on the person as an active participant in their own care may create an unacceptable burden on someone whose resources are already limited.

Biopsychosocial-spiritual model
A humanistic and holistic view of a person and their environment.

Spirituality
A person's practice of creating meaning in their life, existence and purpose.

Religion
An organised system of beliefs and practices associated with a divine or sacred entity, often displayed by ceremony.

The impact of illness on the individual is discussed in Chapter 4.

PAUSE & REFLECT

How would the medical and biopsychosocial-spiritual models differ in thinking about the causes and management of childhood obesity?

1.3 CASE STUDY

ANH

Anh is 24 years old and works as a carpenter. He has been paying off his first home and his car loan. He has no other debts and no dependants. Anh fractured his leg while playing sport and required surgery to pin and repair the fracture. It will be eight weeks before he can begin physiotherapy and an estimated further six weeks to return to optimal function. Anh will not be able to work during this 14-week recovery period. He has only minimal savings.

1   Consider which model of health would fit this acute event.

2   Apply the domains of the biopsychosocial-spiritual model to the scenario.

3   Identify major potential issues for Anh.

Learn more
Access additional resources to broaden your understanding of this chapter. See the Guided Tour for access details.

CHAPTER SUMMARY

- Being sick is a social definition.
- The illness definition suggests that symptoms are the key to defining who is sick.
- The disease definition emphasises diagnosis by a health professional as the key element in deciding who is sick.
- Health cannot simply be defined as the absence of disease, but must take into account the social environment and sense of well-being of the individual.
- Health is measured using the amount of sickness (morbidity) and the number of deaths (mortality). The total number of cases (prevalence) and new cases (incidence) are important in ascertaining the health of a community.
- The medical and biopsychosocial-spiritual models provide different ways of thinking about the causes and management of illness, and how health can be maintained.

FURTHER READING

WHO (1986) *Ottawa Charter for Health Promotion.*

https://www.who.int/publications/i/item/ottawa-charter-for-health-promotion

2 Infant, Child and Adolescent Development

Introduction

Biopsychosocial model
A model of health that considers the individual as a whole person in a social setting, who may or may not be ill at any given moment.

A developmental approach of the individual fits well with the **biopsychosocial model** of health (as discussed in Chapter 1). Adopting a medical model often leads to overlooking important influences of age on health and illness. Our concept of 'acceptable health' differs according to the life stage. Older people may report that their symptoms of pain are dismissed by health professionals as aches and pains may be considered an expected part of ageing. Conversely, children may have their pain ignored because they have inadequate ways to express the nature of pain and may be fearful of their environment. An understanding of some of the differences occurring across the lifespan is useful to understanding the individual's experience of illness and health. An individual's perceptions of health can also assist health professionals in understanding their coping strategies in the presence of illness.

Determinants of health and illness

During a person's lifetime, the basic genetic building blocks of the individual (nature) are exposed to the influence of psychological and social experiences (nurture). We can see here that each domain of the biopsychosocial model is evident in guiding a child's development and behaviours. While there has been a great deal of debate over whether nature or nurture is more important, the answer depends on what aspect of the person you are considering, the uniqueness of the individual, and the complex and social environment in which they live. Nature and nurture both contribute to development and must be considered by health professionals dealing with children and adults.

Essentially, our genetic makeup and biology composes our nature—our biological living system. Numerous characteristics of the individual are relatively fixed by genes and little can be done to alter this pre-programming. Our height, weight, body shape, facial features, skin and eye colour are the result of DNA combinations during our creation. These physical characteristics tend to be well accepted. Less recognised is the fact that psychological features such as temperament, intelligence and predisposition to develop certain psychiatric and pathophysiological illnesses also have a substantial genetic component.

FIGURE 2.1 Reaction range

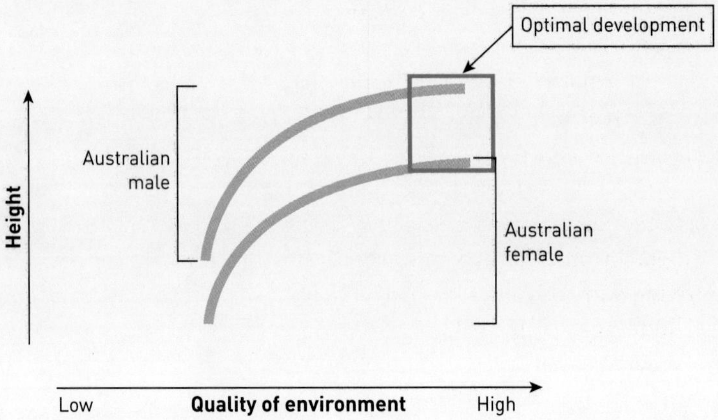

The quality of the environment can help individuals to reach their biologically possible potential or prevent them from doing so. Our **reaction range** (Fig. 2.1) dictates that while our genes pre-program a maximum height, the impact of our environment can either increase or decrease the potential to achieve our optimal height. In a severely deficient environment, including starvation (physical), war or abuse (psychological), development will tend to be at the lower end of the reaction range. As can be seen from Figure 2.1, a moderate to highly supportive environment tends to produce optimal development.

Speculative theories abound regarding turning children into geniuses by playing music to them while they are in the womb or teaching them maths by early intervention technology-based exposure before they can talk. Debate will undoubtedly continue in this area; however, the gains achieved by an overly enriched or stimulating environment compared to a satisfactorily stimulating one will likely be marginal. The major factors that distinguish academic superiority are hard work and obsessive fascination with the area of study. These relate to factors of motivation that can be nurtured. While our social environment shapes us to a large extent, it can only shape us as much as genetic potential permits (Barlow, 2019).

Genetics can also be responsible for illness. Prevention of some types of genetically transmitted conditions is possible, such as avoiding haemophilia through assisted reproduction with pre-implantation genetic screening (Lalezari et al., 2021). It is also possible to prevent some types of disease and **disability** by modifying diet or supplying missing hormones or minerals. An example is folic acid (B9) supplementation prior to conception and continuing into the early months of gestation; to reach recommended daily intake levels, reducing the risk of neural tube defects in the developing foetus (Argyridis, 2019).

It is further suggested that folic acid may also reduce the risk of congenital heart disease and reduce pregnancy complications for the mother. Trisomy 21 (Down Syndrome) can be genetically transmitted; however, this is rare. More commonly, the condition occurs as an anomalous event—an error in the division of reproductive cells results in an abnormal number of chromosomes (MedlinePlus, 2020).

In Chapter 1 we introduced the concepts of illness and disease. A further concept is disability. Disability is defined as "a limitation, restriction or impairment which restricts everyday activities and has lasted, or is likely to last, for at least six months" (ABS, 2019b, p. 1). It is important to note that disability is not only physical, but also includes cognitive and psychological impairments. Another defining aspect is the timeframe: a condition that has a duration of greater than six months (but that does not have a foreseeable conclusion) is classified as chronic.

Disability refers to a chronic health condition which cannot be rectified by medical or surgical interventions, but surgical procedures and pharmacological management are often utilised to reduce the severity of symptoms. Cerebral palsy is a lifelong neurological disorder with no cure, and affects 1 in 700 newborns in Australia (CPA, 2018). People with cerebral palsy have challenges with movement, posture and activities such as speech, communication and vision. They may also experience intellectual impairment. These challenges range from mild to severe.

Cerebral palsy meets the definition of a disability as it impacts on daily activities and is a chronic condition. In order to maximise the reaction range to active optimal health for the person living with this disease, interventions such as injections of botox (IncobotulinumtoxinA) into targeted muscle groups to reduce muscle spasticity, increase range of movement and reduce pain may be utilised (León-Valenzuela et al., 2020).

Reaction range
The total range of outcomes that are possible for a particular individual as a result of their genetic potential.

Disability
A chronic condition of the body, mind or senses that results in a limitation, restriction or impairment in performing activities of daily living.

The biopsychosocial model discussed above links the biological (neurological damage), psychological (emotions and cognition—pain) and social (reduced capacity to interact in their environment) domains. Østergaard et al. (2021) revealed that, for children living with cerebral palsy, the impact of pain influences their ability to interact and participate in physical leisure-based activities. There was a linkage across all domains considered by the biopsychosocial model of health.

Regardless of the presence or absence of illness, disease or living with a disability, understanding the concept of reaction range allows health professionals to consider the interactions between various determinants of development.

Measurement of age

A common error in dealing with children is to assume that they are just like adults, only smaller. Dramatic differences exist between children and adults, between children at different developmental ages and stages and between able-bodied children and children living with disability. Many of these differences are linked to biological changes, particularly neurological development.

Milestones is a term used for the sequence of observable skills achieved during various developmental stages. Milestones occur in scaffolded sequence, and at fairly similar times for each child. Age, therefore, is a fairly good measure of child development. Children are often assessed for attaining various tasks that indicate a milestone and therefore having reached a stage of development. Age as a general rule is a reasonable indicator of when a child will achieve the cognitive and physical ability to master certain tasks. Several different concepts of age have been developed that cater for variances in the mastery of milestones.

Chronological age
The number of years that have passed sequentially since a person was born.

Chronological age is a measure of how many years have passed since the person was born. Certain characteristics of individuals change more rapidly or slowly than others, and some developmental skills depends more on these rates of change than on the passage of time.

Physical age
The state of a person's biological machine.

Physical age (sometimes called biological age) refers to the state of the person's biological machine. We often hear terms like 'small for their age' or 'looking much older' that describe differences between chronological and physical age. For many teenagers, their physical age, as measured by appearance, is quite different from their chronological and social ages. Some females may still look like awkward adolescents but others may experience early development of secondary sex characteristics, the onset of menstruation and changes in body shape and thus look different from their more slowly developing peers. Some males at 13 years of age may grow to 180 cm, and have a full beard and the body development of an adult. In these examples, physical age does not correlate with chronological age.

Some events tend to happen at certain life points and have a powerful effect on our development, but they are not specifically linked to chronological or physical age. Examples include obtaining a driver's licence, finishing school, obtaining employment or commencing tertiary study. A person may experience such events at varied points in life, from earlier to much later, and so a range of chronological ages is relevant to reaching these achievements.

Social age
The points at which an individual has reached socially anticipated milestones in their life.

Social age refers to the points at which a person achieves a rite of passage or a milestone. Consider a high-school student who may be working in a casual job to increase household income, a teenager who may become a parent or take on family obligations of caring for a family member living with a disability, an adolescent who escapes a family violence situation and is considered independent, or perhaps enters into a partnered relationship and takes on family responsibilities. These examples represent elements of adulthood, and could be contrasted to adolescents who participate in schooling without any additional obligations.

PAUSE & REFLECT

Think back to your school days.

Can you identify someone who stood out as having a physical age that was far different from their chronological one?

Regarding social age, consider the situation of a talented 15-year-old boy whose sporting prowess enabled him to travel internationally and represent his country, with teammates who were aged up to 30 and possibly had children of their own.

Compare your perceptions of this athlete's confidence and social competence with those of a 15-year-old who lives at home, does not work or participate in any extracurricular activities, or who has not yet begun to shave.

Perhaps you know someone who became a parent at 16. How might their situation impact on the concept of age?

Stages of development

Some popular theories of development have looked at the human being in terms of the apparent stages that we all seem to move through as we age. These theories are popular because they are simple and reflect the ways in which Western countries think about typical activities of living. The main criticism is that they imply that the stages of development are fixed, and that they occur to the same extent and at the same time in everybody.

These theories also suggest that the shift from one stage to another happens rapidly—as if a switch was being turned on—whereas change is often gradual, partial, incomplete and even reversible. Theories of development suggest that what is typical is 'normal'; that is, it is the only healthy or desirable state for someone to be in at a given age. Theories, however, are useful as a foundation to explain human development and behaviours and to explore the variations that exist. The following discussion about age groups is based on a few stage theories; we encourage you to critically evaluate the conclusions that are drawn from them.

2.1 CASE STUDY

SEBASTIAN'S ENCOUNTER WITH BULLYING BEHAVIOURS

This case study aims to look at differences in an individual's experience of an ongoing disability at different ages.

Sebastian is a seven-year-old boy who lives with moderate cerebral palsy that impacts on his mobility and the development of his arms. On Sunday night, he complains of abdominal pain. There were no previous indications of illness. His mother takes him to a 24-hour clinic. She is aware that he is being bullied at school by some older boys. She believes that his recent onset of bed wetting is a result of this stress and mentions this to the GP. The GP agrees that these responses are a likely reaction to stress and manifest a desire to avoid the triggers in the school environment. They discuss the situation with Sebastian.

1   How would you expect Sebastian to react to the bullying behaviours at his current age?

2   How much would you expect Sebastian to understand about his health condition at his current age?

3   Would his current understanding of altered health status be greater than the understanding of those displaying the bullying behaviours? Why?

CHILDHOOD

Physical development

The most obvious component of development over the first 15 or so years of life is physical. A baby usually doubles its birth weight in five months and triples it in the first year of life. Over that same year, height increases by 50%. During middle childhood, the child adds about 5–7 cm and 2–3 kg per year until the **prepubertal growth spurt** when height and weight increase rapidly and dramatically.

Some of the early physical changes are not just steady increases in size; they also create dramatic change in the baby's behaviour. For example, **myelination** (the development of a fatty insulation on nerve cells that helps them work faster) is incomplete in a newborn. Although it does not reach its maximum levels until around age 15 or even later, most of the growth in myelination takes place in the first few years. One result of this is that the nervous system of the newborn is very primitive compared with that of the child it will become. The newborn is not capable of much control over movement, lacks the ability to perceive or interpret the world in any complex way, and is highly vulnerable to environmental change.

Newborns come equipped with some automatic behaviour patterns, called **reflexes**, that are essential to survival. These reflexes are unlearnt responses by the body to specific stimuli and do not require the intervention of higher brain functioning. Some, such as the breathing reflex, stay with us throughout our lives. Others are only useful in the earliest stages of life and, were we to retain them, could actually interfere with accepted ways of doing things.

Such reflexes include the **rooting reflex**, where stimulation of the lips and tongue leads the newborn to turn towards the stimulus and initiate sucking activity. Another well-known involuntary reflex is the laryngeal reflex (gag reflex) which exists at birth, causing the infant's larynx to close and block the airway when water is sensed on the face. These reflexes are gradually replaced by learnt behaviour that usually results in voluntary control becoming dominant over the reflexes. Without voluntary control over reflex actions, we could never learn to swim (gag reflex), be toilet trained (control over sphincter) or let go of objects we have grasped (motor control).

Development occurs simultaneously in physical, cognitive and social domains for each individual across the lifespan, and central themes for each stage can be identified. During the early years of life, developments are readily observable and most dramatic. In general,

Prepubertal growth spurt
A period of rapid and dramatic physical growth that occurs just before puberty.

Myelination
The development of a fatty insulation on nerve cells that accelerates their development and efficiency in electrical transmission.

Reflex
An unlearnt response to stimulus.

Rooting reflex
An automatic reaction where stimulation of the lips and tongue leads the newborn to turn towards the stimulus and initiate sucking activity.

the neonatal stage and early infancy involve growing larger and stronger, and bringing perception (cognition) under control. The second year of life involves gaining mastery over the motor functions of the body—walking and jumping (mobility), holding, dropping, throwing and catching (perception and object manipulation)—and the early stages of toilet training (learnt behaviour of voluntary control). The third year of life brings language (communication).

Though physical development continues steadily until just before puberty, the most significant areas of change occur in cognitive and social capacities. Reflecting on the biopsychosocial model of health, we see that development occurs in all domains (biological, psychological and social). There remains debate as to what characteristics are present at birth and the development and rate of occurrence that result from interaction with the physical environment and from social interactions.

Physical development tends to follow three basic principles: cephalocaudal, proximodistal and orthogenetic (Hoffnung et al., 2019). Initially, babies are very top-heavy, as the head of a newborn represents about 25% of total weight. Cephalocaudal is the first principle of development: growth proceeds from the head towards the extremities, so it is said that physical development follows a cephalocaudal (from head to tail) pattern. It is also noticeable that the arms and legs tend to lag behind the body in growth. The second principle, proximodistal growth (from near to far), is so named as the central parts approach their adult size and function faster than the extremities. The third principle, the orthogenetic principle, refers to the observation that the organism begins as undifferentiated but gradually changes in the direction of more differentiation and better integration of function. Most people are aware that stem cells can develop into a large variety of other cells: this adaptability has led to new treatments for many conditions including heart disease (undifferentiated cells are trained to become heart muscle) and Parkinson's disease (the cells are trained to become brain cells). This is a demonstration of the orthogenetic principle.

Social development

The most visible part of social development in the early years of life is the attachment that quickly develops between baby and parents (and regular caregivers). Attachment impacts the shaping of an infant's beliefs and understandings of people and the world around them. These foundational understandings of how things work take place in the primary agent of socialisation; that is, the home and family environment. These foundational beliefs and expectations continue as the child develops and, if left unchallenged, extend into adulthood, influencing future interactions with their own offspring and other individuals within their complex environments (Dorrian et al., 2017). Attachment helps to ensure the baby's survival through having its physical needs such as hydration, nutrition and elimination met. Attentive attachment by a caregiver also facilitates the development of a sense of safety, reliance and responsiveness of others. Attachment has two components for the baby. At first, the child attempts on several levels to maintain contact with or nearness to the caregiver; second, the child expresses anxiety when separated from the caregiver. Even in the very early days of life, babies maintain eye contact with their caregivers, recognise their individual smells and cling to them when distressed.

As the first year progresses, babies begin to smile, to tug and to make varying attempts to communicate through different-sounding cries or other sounds to attract attention. Some patterns of attachment are clearly desirable for the baby, such as dependability, consistency and responsive caregiving (creating positive attachment). Other patterns are clearly bad, such as neglect, unreliability and abusive caregiving (negative attachment). Variations in the care received can produce variations in attachment, with some babies being securely attached (the caregiver serves as a secure basis for exploring the world) and some being insecurely attached (fearful of loss of contact and of strangers, and anxious about the world). Some children even become avoidantly attached, preferring to disengage with caregivers and reject contact with others. They may even resort to conservation withdrawal from dysfunctional or abusive interactions. Children living with disability are at increased risk of negative attachment. They have increased vulnerability due to their higher care needs which they may not be able to communicate, and this may frustrate caregivers. Alternately the super normative caring that is required might cause caregivers to burn out (Howie et al., 2021).

Erikson (1950) proposed a theory of psychosocial development that helps us to consider together some of the strands of physical and social development (see Table 2.1). Erikson saw each stage as presenting the individual with a social task that needed to be achieved if development was to continue in an orderly fashion. For example, the task that the baby needs to achieve in the first year is to develop basic trust; if this is not accomplished, the child tends to distrust the world and may find it a frightening and incomprehensible place. If trust is developed, at least to some extent, the child is able to move into the second year and attempt to gain mastery over bodily functions and the self, producing a feeling of autonomy. Conversely, failure at this stage may produce self-doubt. A sense of autonomy allows the child to move on to developing initiative through the lifespan. The achievement of tasks is a scaffolding activity in which each sequential phase adds to the development of the whole self to become an autonomous individual.

TABLE 2.1 Erikson's stages of child and adolescent psychosocial development

Birth–1 year Trust vs mistrust	Babies learn to trust that others will care for their basic needs (e.g. nourishment, warmth, physical contact) vs learning to lack confidence in the capacity of others to care.
1–3 years Autonomy vs shame and doubt	Children learn to be self-sufficient in many activities (e.g. toileting, feeding, walking, exploring, talking) vs doubting their own abilities.
3–6 years Initiative vs guilt	Children try to undertake many adult-like activities (sometimes overstepping the limits set by parents) vs experiencing feelings of guilt.
7–11 years Industry vs inferiority	Children become competent and productive in mastering new skills vs feeling inferior and unable to do anything well.
Adolescence Identity vs role confusion	Adolescents try to figure out who they are by establishing sexual, political and career identities vs becoming confused about identity and role.

Hoffnung et al. (2019)

Cognitive development

Most people are less aware that the thinking of children gradually changes over a number of years, to become more like that of adults. Language, and the way in which children use language (and other forms of communication) to understand the world they live in, is critical to these changes in thinking. Psychologist Jean Piaget (1985) provided a stage theory of cognitive development (see Table 2.2) that can help to understand changes in thinking that take place during childhood. By comparing the ages in Table 2.1 and

Table 2.2 you should be able to see how these stages align with Erikson's, which will help you to understand how development in one area parallels development in others.

TABLE 2.2 Piaget's stages of child cognitive development

Birth–2 years Sensorimotor development	The infant uses senses and motor abilities to explore the world. No conceptual or reflective thought is evident (e.g. an object is understood in terms of what the child can do with it).
2–6 years Preoperational development	The child begins to use symbolic thinking, including language, to understand the world. Their thinking is predominantly egocentric, understanding the world only from one perspective—their own.
7–11 years Concrete operations	The child understands and applies logical operations, or principles, to help to interpret experiences from an objective and rational perspective, rather than intuitively.
12+ years Formal operations	The adolescent or adult thinks in abstract and hypothetical concepts, enabling speculation in thought about the possible as well as about the real.

Hoffnung et al. (2019)

Underlying Piaget's theory of development is the idea that children organise the world by the use of two strategies. When encountering an object or experience, they first try to deal with it by **assimilation**, which involves using a reflex or an existing habit (something learnt from previous experience) to deal with it (Dorrian et al., 2017). Babies, for instance, usually place newly encountered objects into their mouth. This is assimilation of new things into the existing behaviour. The other strategy, **accommodation**, generally arises if assimilation fails. The existing behaviours are modified to deal with the new experience or entirely new behaviours are developed that allow the baby to accommodate the new experience (Dorrian et al., 2017).

Piaget believed that play was accommodation, with the baby trying out a variety of new behaviours with objects or experiences and finding pleasure in this experimental activity. An example is a toddler mastering the skill of posting a square block into a toy with a single square block hole. If the toddler is presented with an oval and triangular block, they will try to use the same behaviours to insert the block. Eventually, there is a realisation that each shape has a corresponding hole.

Assimilation
The use of existing knowledge or habits to enable the individual to deal with a new experience.

Accommodation
The modification of existing behaviours or the development of entirely new behaviours to enable an individual to deal with a new experience.

Other viewpoints on cognitive development

Theories, as we emphasised earlier, are general explanations to help our understanding of situations. No one theory can be considered absolute. As increased understanding of behaviours is developed through research, critiques and criticisms of existing theories emerge. Piaget's theory and other theorists draw their conclusions from studying specific populations then apply those findings universally to all children. One emerging criticism of Piaget is that his theory does not adequately consider the influence of social and cultural influences or environments.

Alternative viewpoints have been offered for understanding the way children's cognitions develop. One focuses on the observation that learning takes place within a social and cultural context. The child learns rules ('coughs and sneezes spread diseases') and behaviours ('cover your cough and sneeze into the inner elbow') when engaged in interactions with adults and other children, through direct instruction (including social media) and/or through observation.

In the 1980s, Russian psychologist Lev Vygotsky's work emphasising a socio-cultural theory of cognitive development attracted the attention of Western psychologists and educators (Dorrian et al., 2017). According to Vygotsky, differences occurred when children were able to learn by independent exploration compared to what they could learn through guided participation in an activity with an adult or more capable peer. Development of cognitions was dependent on the interaction, and the guided participation that the child received during interactions. Speech between child and adult about the world, for example, eventually provides the basis for the child's language about the world, or the content of their thought processes. A child who grows up in an environment where there is engaging and instructive conversation (or other forms of communication) is more likely to have better-developed verbal (or alternate communication) and thinking skills than a child who is neglected.

Environments that are stimulating—that allow for opportunities to explore and provide role models to observe, imitate and interact—produce different developmental achievement from environments that lack these features. Interaction and engagement are influenced by inequalities, inequities, social advantage, culture and disability. These factors either enhance or restrain development.

The concepts of inequalities, inequities, culture and disability are explored further in Chapter 14.

2.2 CASE STUDY

SEBASTIAN (CONT.)

According to Erikson's theory, at the age of seven Sebastian is probably in the stage of developing initiative. According to Piaget's theory, he is using preoperational thinking. Sebastian will almost certainly understand that his life is different from that of other children of his age, but he is unlikely to understand the extent of that difference. Sebastian will need to have some assistance provided by an adult (e.g. teacher, parent, support worker) to be able to mobilise within and interact optimally within his school environment, for example. If Sebastian knows an adult (e.g. a teacher, sports hero) who has cerebral palsy, he might think that is cool. His classmates may react (either positively or negatively) to his mobility challenges, but not be able to understand the reason for his difference. Sometimes he is likely to find the constraints on his activities frustrating and he may become a target for bullying. Sebastian might even wonder what he has done wrong to be different (reasoning that bad consequences arise from bad actions).

1   How might Sebastian's understanding and behaviour change as he gets older?
2   How might Sebastian demonstrate his developing sense of initiative in managing the challenges of his mobility and dealing with the negative associations of others?

Many other processes, such as the development of moral reasoning and the development of concepts of health and healthy behaviour, follow cognitive development. In dealing with children, the environments of physical, social and cognitive development must all be considered. There are many tasks that young children (as a guideline, those under the age of about seven) simply cannot do, and other actions that they cannot understand in the same way that adults do. Trying to use adult modes of explanation simply will not work; behaviours that seem straightforward and sensible to you may seem threatening, illogical, unreasonable or unacceptable to a child. Even older children, who might understand the concepts, may not be able to understand the reasoning behind them. Although children might use adult concepts, they are likely to have a very limited understanding of the abstract meaning of those concepts and may be very literal and concrete in their thinking.

PAUSE & REFLECT

Consider the antics of children often displayed in popular media. You will have seen depictions or observed children undertaking activities as they learn about their world. Often these activities represent the 'failure' of a child in performing a task (e.g. stumbling when first attempting to walk, feed themselves or ride a bike), in developing understanding (e.g. exploring a new toy, explaining feelings and emotions of love, sadness or frustration, or correlating actions and consequences) or in acquiring communication (e.g. pronouncing words incorrectly or with incorrect meaning). Frequently, these situations are considered cute and comical.

Pause and reflect on your appraisal of these situations. You will be considering this from a logical, abstract and hypothetical perspective that is achieved in adulthood, therefore you have greater insight than if you had made this reflection during your adolescent stage of the lifespan.

Health in childhood

Generally, children in Australia are healthy and their burden of disease and injury remain low. Illness prevention strategies such as the Australian immunisation schedule enable children to access immunisation programs designed to eradicate many serious diseases. National indicators reveal that Australian children are faring well across the majority of domains considered by the Australian Institute of Health and Welfare [AIHW] people-centred data model. These domains are "health, education, social support, household income and finance, parental employment, housing, and justice and safety" (AIHW, 2020a). Australia remains roughly in the middle third of developed countries globally with regard to child health (AIHW, 2020a). We might think that Australia should be among the highest-performing developed countries; however, a significant reason for this middle ranking is the extremely poor health of the nation's First Peoples.

Inequalities, inequities and social influence greatly impact on First Peoples. Geographical diversity and difficulty in recruiting health care professionals to rural and remote areas of Australia produce added challenges for this already vulnerable population in accessing health care as well as culturally appropriate care. Infant mortality has decreased, but the comparative rates remain higher than those relating to non-Indigenous Australians. Birth rates in First Peoples communities remain high, with reduced birth weights and younger mothers (AIHIN, 2018). The health disadvantage for First Peoples children continues throughout childhood and adolescence, and contributes to the much higher rates of reduced health for First Nations people throughout Australia. Many health conditions are overrepresented in Indigenous populations. Examples include dental health (with associated deficits in speech, increased pain and reduced nutrition: Poirier et al., 2021), hearing (which links to education) and obesity (increased risk for diabetes and cardiovascular issues)

(AIHIN, 2021). The disadvantage in terms of survival is obvious from the beginning of life, with Indigenous infant mortality nearly twice that of non-Indigenous populations in Australia. Social and cultural determinants of health include education, employment, income, housing, access to health care and food security. Many issues in these areas compound the challenges in closing the gap in health disparity between Indigenous and non-Indigenous Australians.

Closing the Gap is an Australian government initiative designed to improve partnerships and autonomy for First Peoples. It "is underpinned by the belief that when Aboriginal and Torres Strait Islander people have a genuine say in the design and delivery of policies, programs and services that affect them, better life outcomes are achieved" (Australian Government, 2020). There have been improvements in health outcomes in target areas using illness prevention and health promotion programs; for example, Queensland's Deadly Ears program and oral health outreach for Northern Territory children. Much work is planned to further reduce the inequality in health status.

The main causes of altered health in Australian children are infectious diseases (e.g. commonly occurring respiratory system conditions) which are usually mild. As previously highlighted, immunisation programs in Australia have eradicated or significantly reduced the incidence and prevalence, and certainly the mortality rates, of diseases such as rubella, measles, mumps and polio. Chronic conditions in children are rare. Conditions such as asthma have relatively early diagnosis and therefore management plans can be developed that greatly improve the quality of life (QoL) and health outcomes for those living with those conditions. Childhood diabetes and cancer are relatively rare but contribute substantially to the burden of disease because of their impact on the normal physical and social development in the early years. Hereditary (genetic) conditions are transmitted through DNA from parent to developing child.

Examples of genetic conditions are haemophilia, cystic fibrosis and muscular dystrophy. Birth defects such as cleft palate and those with no known cause, such as Down Syndrome, do not have high incidence rates but certainly contribute to health challenges for the person living with the condition, and their family. Cerebral palsy is the most commonly presenting health challenge in Australia. Child injuries are predominantly sustained from recreation (e.g. fractures from skateboard falls), domestic (scalds, burns, falls in bathrooms) and farming (encounters with animals, injury from equipment) environments. Injuries from these sources were formerly the focus but this has been overshadowed by the increase in substance injuries including domestic violence. Trauma-informed approaches to improving health outcomes for vulnerable groups (particularly children) are gaining focus to address this escalating situation (Benjamin et al., 2019).

Inequality, inequity, culture and social impacts are discussed in Chapter 14.

2.3 CASE STUDY

SEBASTIAN (CONT.)

Now aged 12, Sebastian has received a lot of information about his condition, including what external supports will assist in improving his QoL (e.g. physio and occupational therapists). He has also received education about how his condition impacts on his body, and a self-management plan that increases his autonomy and ability to make decisions for himself. He may already have a better understanding of his condition than a typical adult would. The constraints placed on his behaviour due to the challenge of his condition are almost certainly a continued source of frustration.

Sebastian wants to do the same things as his friends (and this becomes increasingly important as he progresses into adolescence), but it is not easy. Sport and recreational activities are an important part of childhood that most children take for granted. Exercise contributes to physical fitness, weight management and a sense of accomplishment, and offers opportunities for Sebastian to mix with his friends. However, for Sebastian, exercise and recreation present added challenges. He is physically unable to keep up with his peers on the sporting field. Although he is keen to participate in school sports, his unique style of running serves to highlight his difference and he is prone to falls. This increases the risk of health complications and may cause him to be ridiculed by people who are unempathetic or less knowledgeable. Sebastian may develop a sense of isolation and difference, and as a result reduce his participation in physical activities. Withdrawal may occur. This will adversely impact on his psychological and social well-being.

As he moves towards adolescence, Sebastian may try harder to cover up his condition, except from those who are close and caring enough to understand he is a person first and that he just happens to have the added challenge of cerebral palsy.

1   What would you expect Sebastian to be able to do to manage his cerebral palsy as a 12-year-old?

2   As he moves into adolescence, how would you expect his behaviour and thinking to change?

3   What adaptations could be suggested for Sebastian's situation?

Behaviour and thinking, while established early as the primary agents of socialisation, change over time as the individual encounters new situations and environments that may challenge their earlier belief and value systems. If an individual remains in a fairly sheltered environment, they will retain many core values and beliefs. Different situations cause children to struggle with understanding the application of the 'rules' they have learnt.

Children are likely to have difficulty understanding, for example, that a behaviour such as undressing and letting another person touch your body may be considered wrong in most settings but it is acceptable in others, such as a medical appointment. This difficulty with abstract thinking generally continues into adolescence, until the development of formal operational thinking. Some adolescents and adults may never fully master abstract thinking and thus be unable to understand the distinctions that seem highly logical and obvious to most people.

ADOLESCENCE AND YOUNG ADULTHOOD

Physical development

The next major physical changes that do not involve a simple increase in size are those associated with **puberty**. Puberty is defined by the appearance of secondary sexual

Puberty
A developmental stage defined by the appearance of secondary sexual characteristics, such as body hair and deepening of the voice in males, and menstruation and breast development in females.

characteristics, such as body hair and deepening of the voice in males, and menstruation and breast development in females. Physical puberty is seen as ending when the long bones of the body, especially arm and leg bones, have reached their maximum length and the individual reaches their full adult height. It is hard to use physical changes to define the developmental stage called adolescence, however, because some people (especially girls) may have reached adult size and development by age 11 while others (especially boys) may not stop growing until they are aged 20 or more. This links with the earlier concept of using physical age to determine a stage of development.

Despite the obvious physical changes associated with puberty, it is important to recognise that adolescence is a psychosocial stage as well as a physical one. The biopsychosocial model of health considers the individual holistically, across the biological (physical), psychological and social domains. Each domain contributes to the development of the individual.

Social development

Adolescence represents the transitional time between childhood and adulthood. This has varied connotations that differ among societies and cultures. In adolescence, milestones can include finding a casual job or gaining a learner or provisional driver licence. Balancing these adult-like behaviours with the compulsory educational requirements is undertaken by many adolescents in urban areas. In rural communities, adolescents may also be expected to take on greater responsibilities on the family farm or cattle station.

Importantly, for those in regional and remote areas, this stage of adolescence may involve a move to boarding school or student accommodation for the senior years of high school or further education. These experiences and changes significantly affect the adolescent's lifestyle. In Western society, adolescence is often characterised by stress and rebellion as teenagers seek to establish a sense of individuality outside their family unit. Although adolescence tends to be a time of developing personal values and independence, it does not always involve rejection of parental values or large-scale conflict. Rather, it involves questioning and challenging to see if those established values and beliefs fit into the adolescent's new encounters. There is a duality in the role obligations of adolescence: establishing a unique sense of identity and self, while at the same time seeking to belong to groups and develop friendships.

Cognitive development

The theories held by Erikson and Piaget regarding the adolescent stage of the lifespan all involve the teenager navigating new ways of dealing with their increasing environment. During this time, development of formal operations can lead to conflicts between the adolescent's abstract understanding of what matters in life, their purpose and other people's understandings.

Adolescents adapt a flexible thought pattern and can consider complex and abstract subjects such as beauty, fairness, justice and empathy. The flexibility in their thinking enables them to take the learnt behaviours and concepts, and question whether they apply to new dimensions of their discovery of the lives of those outside their previously confined environments. Five general areas of advancement can be identified:

- the *speed* at which information is processed;
- *attention* span and intensiveness to focus on tasks;

- increased *memory* retention and recall;
- *organisation* (logic and sequencing);
- *metacognition* (awareness and understanding of their own thought processes) (Hoffnung et al., 2019).

Major influences on adolescent cognitive development are earlier parental–child relationships (this links to the concept of secure attachment), nutrition and environment. Dysfunctional environments and children who experienced domestic violence may exhibit a trauma response and withdrawal behaviours. It is important for health professionals to understand the important role that adverse childhood experience can have in the health and well-being of children, adolescents and adults alike (Felitti et al., 1998). It is also important for health professionals to be able to identify and address early any potential negative experiences that the child or a carer might face (Krinner et al., 2021).

Trauma response and withdrawal are explored further in Chapter 12.

Continuing through adolescence, cognitive development also involves the management of feelings and formation of relationships (socialisation) with others. **Emotional intelligence** is defined as an individual's ability to perceive, use, understand and regulate emotion (Dorrian et al., 2017). It demonstrates a person's overall emotional capacity and contributes to emotional health and social functioning. Individuals who are able to accurately detect, understand and appropriately respond to their feelings (insight) and the emotions of others (empathy) are more likely to be able to establish friendships and deep connections with others as well as adapt better in demanding social and emotional situations (Dorrian et al., 2017).

Emotional intelligence
The ability to perceive, use, understand and regulate emotion.

In addition, effective management of their own emotions (emotional regulation) enables the child to express feelings and act in ways that are socially appropriate. The extent to which a person develops emotional intelligence varies. Some disabilities, such as autism, are associated with lower emotional intelligence, and individuals living with this condition are likely to experience loneliness and depression. They may have reduced socio-emotional outcomes when compared to their peers who do not live with that health condition (Huggins et al., 2021). A high level of emotional intelligence is extremely important for becoming an effective health professional (Soto-Rubio et al., 2020).

Social development

For most people, adolescence involves a need to be independent and to move into different social relationships with other people. Friendships and emotional relationships become particularly important, and often can present challenges to the home environment. Adolescents seek to find a place where they 'fit in' and as such are susceptible to the pro-social (positive) or anti-social (negative) influences of peers.

Such peer influences, also labelled as social norms in some health behaviour theories (see Chapter 7), can lead to experimental and risk-taking activities such as using alcohol or illicit drugs, smoking and sexual exploration. In order to fit in, adolescents may adopt behaviours and opinions of the groups to which they seek to belong. This can include changing attitudes towards authority, the value of education and employment, and may be exhibited via a dress code (clothing, choice of colours) and body decoration (piercings, false nails, hair styles, tattoos). In learning how to deal with increasingly complex activities, adolescents may behave in ways that adults view as illogical or lacking in consideration of the consequences. While some risk is inherent in new adventures and trying unfamiliar things, adolescents generally have a highly developed sense of self-preservation. Mostly, they keep their experimentation to a minimum and learn very quickly from a lapse of good judgment.

There are many positives in the adolescent stage of the lifespan. Teenagers tend to have a good understanding of their health needs and are able to independently seek answers to their questions. They are savvy with technology and reasonably knowledgeable of the world. In physical strength and balance, they are often more confident and capable than younger or older people. In the early teen years, they may have been shy and uncertain in public situations or embarrassed by the physical development of their bodies. Generally, once the physical changes of puberty have been accepted, adolescents develop a strong sense of self. Their self-concept of correctness, newly developed confidence and sense of importance may make them prone to see everything through their **personal fable**—the belief that the world revolves around them. Any criticism, constructive or otherwise, is often taken very personally.

Throughout adolescence and into young adulthood, experimentations and ventures into new situations contribute to development of formal operational thinking in most people. However, it is important to keep in mind that not everyone develops formal operational thinking, and some individuals continue to function on the basis of concrete operational thinking throughout their lives.

Personal fable
A person's belief that the world revolves around them.

PAUSE & REFLECT

Why do some adolescents find it difficult to resist negative peer pressure, particularly with regard to unhealthy behaviours such as smoking and alcohol consumption?

2.4 CASE STUDY

SEBASTIAN (CONT.)

Sebastian is now 16 years old. He has been living with the reality of the restrictions of cerebral palsy all his life. Sebastian probably knows a great deal about his neurological condition by this stage (adolescence). He needs to incorporate his disability into his developing identity. He has a formal operational understanding of cerebral palsy— its causes, prognosis and management options. He may resent the fact that he has additional challenges when others do not.

As his condition is not always known to others, he is embarrassed when he trips or falls or has to decline to participate in physical contact sports. He tries to minimise these instances and socialises within a smaller group of friends who are mostly female and understand his situation. He attends a party held by some boys in his year at school. During the party, he joins in a drinking game. Later, he also decides to join an impromptu game of touch football. The combination of alcohol and his falls risk results in him taking a fall. He sustains a significant injury and an ambulance is called.

1   Elements of prosocial and antisocial activities are evident in this scenario. Select examples of each and explain why.

2   Why might Sebastian have decided to participate in these activities?

3   How might Sebastian's attitude towards his cerebral palsy change as he enters adulthood?

Health in adolescence

Data indicates that young people in Australia rate their health as good to excellent (AIHW, 2021a). The principal burden of disease in this age range is mental health conditions, primarily anxiety and depression. Substance abuse, schizophrenia and personality disorders are also represented in mental health conditions. Approximately 14% of youths aged 12 to 17 reported mental health concerns in the past 12 months (AIHW, 2021a). Mortality due to disease in this age group is rare; however, injuries (accidental or self-inflicted, such as alcohol or drug poisoning) accounted for 80 000 hospitalisations of those aged 15–24 (AIHW, 2021a). Overall, adolescence is the healthiest time of the lifespan, with the immune system working effectively and lifestyle disorders not yet playing a significant role in health and well-being. Interestingly, 93% of Australian children are fully immunised before commencing school and there are demonstrated benefits from this illness prevention program (AIHW, 2021a).

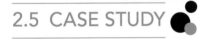

2.5 CASE STUDY

VANDHANA

This case study focuses on psychosocial stressors experienced during adolescence.

Vandhana is a 17-year-old student who has just completed Year 12. She is an only child and lives with her mother, who works as a cleaner. Vandhana was a high-achieving student throughout her senior schooling, and a school leader. She is eagerly awaiting the offer of a university place that requires an ATAR of 98, and will be the first in her family to begin tertiary study.

Vandhana has been on a three-week post-school celebration with many of her peers. Since her return she has been moody and uncommunicative with her mother, to whom she has always been very close. Vandhana has a number of new piercings including a belly-bar, dyed her hair and changed her style of clothing. A number of new friends with similar appearances, who Vandhana met during her Schoolies holiday, have been calling over to her house. Vandhana's mother has tried to embrace Vandhana's new look and has even purchased some jewellery as a surprise.

Vandhana is displaying signs of nervousness and is frequently heard crying in her room, but refuses to confide in her mother and physically pushes her mother from her bedroom when she comes to talk to her daughter. Yesterday, Vandhana was wearing an unusually short skirt and her mother noticed horizontal cuts on her thighs, that appear to be self-inflicted. In a state of tears, Vandhana disclosed to her mother, 'I don't know what to do anymore. Everything has changed'.

1   Can you identify possible psychosocial risk factors for Vandhana? Try to link these challenges to Piaget's stages of development.

2   As a teenager, Vandhana has reached the developmental stage of identity formation (Erikson, 1950). What might be some of the challenges Vandhana is now facing?

3   Why might she be displaying signs of increased anxiety and despair?

Learn more
Access additional resources to broaden your understanding of this chapter. See the Guided Tour for access details.

CHAPTER SUMMARY

- Behaviour, cognitions and emotions differ at different stages in the lifespan.

- Determinants of development include the individual's genetics and the biological, psychological and social experiences that they are exposed to.

- Reaction range describes the total range of outcomes that are possible for a particular individual as a result of their genetic potential.

- Age can be measured in terms of time from birth (chronological age), characteristics of the body (physical age) or events in the life of the individual (social age).

- During childhood, physical development (both growth in size and maturation of systems in the body) is rapid.

- Social development is influenced by the attachment of the child to caregivers.

- Erikson proposed that psychosocial development consisted of a series of tasks that must be resolved if the child is to develop in a healthy manner.

- Piaget considered the gradual development of thinking.

- During adolescence, identity is formed and the individual begins to develop strong relationships with others.

FURTHER READING

AIHW [Australian Institute of Health and Welfare] (2020) *Australia's Children: Population Groups.*
https://www.aihw.gov.au/reports-data/population-groups

AIHW [Australian Institute of Health and Welfare] (2020) *Queensland's Deadly Ears Program.*
https://www.aihw.gov.au/reports/indigenous-australians/queenslands-deadly-ears-program/contents/summary

AIHW [Australian Institute of Health and Welfare] (2020) *Oral Health Outreach Services for Aboriginal and Torres Strait Islander Children in the Northern Territory.*
https://www.aihw.gov.au/reports/indigenous-australians/oral-health-for-aboriginal-and-torres-strait-child/summary

Australian Indigenous Health InfoNet (2021) *Social and Cultural Determinants.*
https://healthinfonet.ecu.edu.au/learn/determinants-of-health/social-cultural-determinants/

3 Adult Development and Ageing

Adulthood

The concept of dynamic transition between stages of the lifespan was introduced in Chapter 2. Progression from adolescent to adult is more commonly based on behavioural achievements than an age range. The concept of rites of passage (activity milestones) is a **socio-cultural indicator** signifying transition from adolescence into adulthood. Examples of activity-based milestones into early adulthood include completing high school or commencing university, learning to drive, buying a car, commencing employment or taking on greater religious responsibilities (e.g. confirmation, bar mitzvah).

Some societies consider that biological development milestones signify the transition from childhood to adulthood. An example of a biological milestone includes onset of menstruation for females, growing a beard or the deepening of voice (males) and changes in body shape and height (males and females). Some biological developments (e.g. menstruation, nocturnal emissions) are not directly visible to a wider audience but many societies celebrate such activities openly by a direct announcement or by changes in behaviours and appearances.

A few examples of traditional socio-cultural signifiers of entry into adulthood are exclusion from the opposite gender at social events, wearing a hijab, the requirement to fast during Ramadan, Ritusuddhi (a Hindu ceremony for girls upon the first occurrence of menstruation, i.e. menarche) where they wear a sari for the first time, Rumspringa (a tradition in some Amish sects whereby adolescents are permitted to travel to other communities and explore the wider world for a period of time) and land diving (a South Pacific tradition where boys are tethered by a vine and jump off a cliff into the ocean to prove their courage and adult status).

Becoming an adult is a significant event which "provides self-confidence, identity, accountability, strength, a sense of belonging and purpose, emotional support, resilience, and agency" (Murrup-Stewart et al., 2021, p. 1833). The First Peoples use rich and deeply held traditions as part of the ceremonies to acknowledge rites of passage from child to adult. Generally, men's business and women's business are conducted separately. The rituals of First Peoples are often thought to exist only in rural and remote communities, but this is not entirely correct (Murrup-Stewart et al., 2021). The rituals are designed to emphasise the importance of ancestors and Elders, connection to Country and connection to Dreaming and Spirits. They are unique to each group and area, and often involve youths spending time on Country and being guided and instructed by Elders. This can be particularly significant for First Peoples who reside in metropolitan areas as it enables them to fully immerse themselves in their historical cultural context (Murrup-Stewart et al., 2021).

As a multicultural society, Australia mixes many old traditions with its own contemporary cultural identity. How well traditions of those from different backgrounds are accepted continues to be a source of debate. Most commonly, in Western society, attaining a legally significant age (in Australia, the age of 18) classifies a person as an adult. Legal adult status links to adulthood responsibilities such as voting, consuming alcohol, marrying and entering into legally binding agreements.

While these events may occur any time from puberty into the early 20s and later, in reality the change is most likely to be gradual and piecemeal. The usual experience reported by most people is that they were not specifically aware of becoming an adult, but simply started thinking of themselves as one somewhere along the line. The concept of independence

Socio-cultural indicators
Factors that shape or guide an individual's characteristics due to exposure to social and cultural norms within various environments.

Socio-cultural domains are explored in detail in Chapter 14.

varies among individuals. They may regard themselves as an adult in terms of responsibility and independence (e.g. earning an income, holding a highly regarded professional title such as Doctor) but not in regard to significant financial responsibilities such as a mortgage. An increasingly common trend in Australia is for **young adults** to pursue longer tertiary commitments (e.g. studying medicine or dentistry) while still residing at home with parents and without a spouse or children of their own. Another trend is for 'adult children' to return to their parents' house following a divorce.

Erikson's theory of psychosocial development (1968) describes milestones throughout the adult lifespan. As in childhood and adolescence, adulthood and old age present social and psychological tasks that need to be achieved if development is to continue in an orderly fashion. The tasks at these times of life involve forming intimate relationships, contributing to the next generation and being able to look back (reflect) on life and consider its meaningful satisfaction.

Young adulthood
Arbitrary classification of the transition time from adolescent to an independent adult; the earliest phase of adulthood.

Erikson's theory of psychosocial development was discussed in Chapter 2 in relation to child and adolescent development.

TABLE 3.1 Erikson's stages of adult development

Intimacy vs isolation	Young adults seek companionship and develop intimate connections with a significant person vs becoming isolated from others and fearful of rejection or disappointment.
Generativity vs stagnation	Middle-aged adults contribute to the next generation by performing meaningful work (security) or creative activities and/or raising a family vs becoming stagnant and inactive.

Hoffnung et al. (2019); Erikson (1968)

It is sometimes useful to divide the adult stage of the lifespan into young, middle and older adulthood. Behaviours of the young adult include tertiary or vocational study, commencing a career, generating an income and forming meaningful and often exclusive relationships. **Middle adulthood** can bring increased responsibility such as establishing and maintaining a family and gaining security through a house and savings. Transitioning to **older adulthood** (also known as the senior or ageing years) relates to ceasing work (retiring), enjoying leisure and recreational activities, and reflecting on life's journey.

There have also been changes to socio-cultural and biological indicators for transition into the various stages of adulthood. The start of adulthood as an independent person can be delayed by experiences such as university education, which is one of the most common factors in developed countries. The increased tendency for people to undertake tertiary study results in a longer period of dependence on others for training and support and produces a delayed sense of development in some areas. People undertaking tertiary education often postpone other adult experiences, such as marriage and relocation for work, until they have gained their qualification and developed a sense of a stable career path.

Middle adulthood
A general classification of adulthood where social and personal role expectations and goals are achieved, re-evaluated, challenged or forfeited, the major timespan of the adult lifespan.

Older adulthood
Subjective classification of adulthood generally coinciding with retirement from the workforce and more focus on leisure activities; the latter stage of the lifespan.

Those who do move into more adult experiences while still in full-time education often report difficulties in achieving a satisfactory work–life balance or feeling dissociated from other students. Progression to independent adult status may also be delayed due to economic issues (global financial crisis, high unemployment, increase in housing costs), political issues (employment and inflation control policies resulting in job insecurity) and health crises (COVID-19 pandemic or having to care for an ageing parent).

Many Australian university students remain in their parents' home instead of living independently.

What areas of adult life may be impacted by continuing to live at home?

Would there be some aspects of life where a person in this situation may not feel like an adult?

In most instances, responses to these questions would be negative.

Challenge your thinking and consider at least three positive outcomes of an adult-age student remaining in the family home.

3.1 CASE STUDY

SEBASTIAN'S UNIVERSITY YEARS

This case study discusses Sebastian, who was introduced in Chapter 2. It looks at the differences in a person's experience of a chronic health condition at different ages.

Sebastian is now 25. Having graduated from high school, he entered university and completed the seven-year program to become a general practitioner. During university he took up rowing as a sport. It helped him to manage stress and promoted his well-being, maintained his physical fitness and contributed to the management of his cerebral palsy by keeping his muscles, joints and bones stimulated. Sebastian found it difficult to maintain a social life. "Most of the time I was either studying or undertaking residency. I mixed mainly with other medical students and nursing students whose lives mirrored mine—except I also had to manage the CP complications." Sebastian continued to live at his parents' home except for when he was in residence at hospitals where on-site accommodation was provided. There has been no significant change in his cerebral palsy, and Sebastian continues to walk is a visibly different way. Associated care interventions such as regular specialists' appointments, physio and occupational sessions, and the occasional operation to maintain range of movement continue to be necessary but are also a source of frustration, taking up his limited free time. Although the bullying behaviours from school are a distant memory, Sebastian sometimes feels he is treated differently from others and has experienced discrimination in the workplace due to his health condition.

1   How has Sebastian's transition into adulthood differed from that of someone who perhaps commenced full-time work at the age of 15?

2   How can a supportive environment of family and friends help Sebastian to cope with his condition now and in the future?

3   What socio-cultural adult behaviours is Sebastian likely to adopt now that he has completed his medical degree?

4   What advantages and restrictions might Sebastian continue to experience in his adult life?

PHYSICAL DEVELOPMENT

Few of the physical changes of adulthood are obvious, and hardly any of them are apparent in early adulthood. There are exceptions, such as premature baldness or grey hair, that have a large genetic component and occur earlier for some people than for others. Most of the overt physical changes are gradual, such as loss of skin elasticity leading to wrinkles, the tendency to increase body weight or become malnourished and the loss of pigment in the hair. Most of the physical changes are internal, and not even the individual is aware of their occurrence until they begin to significantly affect the ability to do things. They include processes that may eventually result in significant health problems, such as atherosclerosis (the build-up of fatty deposits in the arteries) and a progressive decline in bone density (osteoporosis). The most common complaint about getting older is that people do not like their changed physical appearance.

Conversely, older adulthood has seen significant changes to our previously held ideas. The physical depiction of older adults has been challenged by advances in medicine (pharmacology and surgery), aesthetics (cosmetology) and lifestyle awareness. The stereotype (linked to physical age) of older adults as wrinkled, requiring glasses, obese or severely malnourished, confused, lacking mobility, with reduced cognitive ability and unable to live independently has changed somewhat.

Overall, life expectancy has increased from 79.4 years in 2000 to 83.5 years in 2021 for adult Australians (First Peoples average a shorter lifespan estimated at 76 years in 2021) (AIHW, 2021b). Advances in cosmetology and aesthetic surgery slow down the appearance of ageing, in that the increase in accessibility and affordability has increased the popularity of treatments such as lasering, injectables, fillers and cosmetic surgery. Advances in medicine have improved the pharmacological management of many conditions, such as arthritis, therefore delaying some decline in mobility and self-care. Other medical advances include surgical interventions for optical conditions, and replacement of worn or arthritic joints.

Health literacy is discussed in Chapter 15.

Health promotion and illness prevention programs have increased health literacy, so individuals can implement lifestyle changes early in order to maintain their health. Changes to delivery of health and well-being services with a community focus enable older adults to retain more independence by accessing services in their community rather than requiring nursing home facilities. Overall, older adults are on average looking 'less aged', living longer and remaining more independent in their own homes.

Illness prevention and health promotion are discussed in Chapter 16.

SOCIAL DEVELOPMENT

The key themes of adulthood tend to focus on responsibility: the adult gradually becomes enmeshed in a network of obligations to other people that can be summarised under the general headings of family, work, and society. **Self-care** is a new item on the agenda and can contribute to a person's well-being.

Self-care
Taking time out from the usual business of life to care and nurture yourself through relaxing and restorative pleasurable activities.

Family

Many adults form exclusive relationships at some time in their lives. However, the number of people who marry has slowly declined, there is an increase in divorce rates, a rise in single-parent households and a higher incidence of re-partnering after a relationship breakdown. In 2019, marriage rates in Australia were reported at 4.5 marriages per 1000 people (ABS, 2020c). There is a continuing decline in birth rates in Australia, approximating a 3% decrease each year from 2017 (ABS, 2020a). One in seven Australian households is composed of a single-parent family (ABS, 2020b). Family dynamics fluctuate in response to economic, political, financial and health environments.

Work

During adulthood, work serves a variety of functions. It occupies most of our waking hours, provides the income that determines lifestyle and status, and provides identity. These can be considered positive workforce participation outcomes (Werth & Brownlow, 2018). In general, society expects that adults will work to sustain themselves and those to whom they have obligations. Employment contributes to our sense of self-achievement, self-esteem and financial capacity (Werth & Brownlow, 2018). However, barriers may influence the type of work participation (casual, seasonal, part-time) and stages of the lifespan also impact on working capacity (pregnancy, access to childcare). People may desire work but be unable to obtain suitable employment due to disability or lack of the required skills or educational qualification.

Changes in the needs of a community also influence the types of jobs that are available; for example, during the COVID-19 pandemic there were shortages of nurses and doctors. The geographical disparity between different regions of Australia is also a consideration.

Society

There are various responsibilities in society, some of which are legal requirements. Australian adults must, for example, register with the electoral office and are legally required to vote. Many other responsibilities are inherent in chosen activities. Driving a car requires a licence, car registration and insurance. There are legal, moral and social obligations to provide adequate care for children including education, housing, food and clothing, immunisation and health care. A person who buys a property must pay council rates and meet financial obligations such as mortgage repayments and insurance. Those who are employed must pay taxes.

The more involved an individual is with other people, the more they become linked to social obligations. As with physical ageing, development of social involvement is often so gradual that a person only realises how involved they were when they look back on their lives, or find they are no longer able to carry out their obligations. In contrast to the early adult years when participation in group activities is common (e.g. sporting clubs, recreational pursuits), by middle adulthood most adults have formed an intimate partnership and their social cohort decreases as they focus more on the family environment. Friendships are often tied to their children's activities in sport, recreation and school, or to social responsibility and welfare-related activities such as Rotary, Lions and other community service clubs.

In older adulthood, the decline in social activities is often due to the death of friends and relatives, or having reduced capacity to socialise (access, mobility and the impact of illness, disease, disability). Group activities increase in popularity. Examples include sporting and recreational pastimes such as bowling, swimming, walking groups, birdwatching, art and craft groups and education for self-interest via institutions such as U3A (University of the Third Age) and CAE (Council for Adult Education).

Visit a U3A website.

What would be some benefits of belonging to a group such as U3A?

COGNITIVE DEVELOPMENT

Thinking (cognition) tends have gradual changes during mid to older adulthood. Rapid change in cognitive functioning may signify an underlying disease process and health professionals use symptoms of cognitive change as an early indicator. Cognitive decline can be subjective or mild. It is often associated with risk factors for further decline and the emergence of dementia and other neurodegenerative conditions (Lautenschlager et al., 2019).

There is a strong indicator that maintaining a degree of physical activity in older adulthood may improve cognitive function and prevent or reduce the rate of decline in older adulthood. The mind–body connection is quite evident here. Outside of maintaining physical activity, there is no treatment for dementia. On a positive side, the changes that occur in cognitive function in the absence of illness, disease or disability during adulthood are minor.

One gradual change in cognitive functioning throughout the lifespan relates to intelligence type. Researchers noted changes related to genetics and identified shifts from fluid intelligence towards more crystallised intelligence (Ding et al., 2019). **Fluid intelligence** refers to the use of flexible reasoning to draw inferences, solve problems and understand the relationships between concepts. Theorists suggest that mathematical experts tend to make their major contributions early in adulthood because of their fluid intelligence. **Crystallised intelligence** refers to the accumulation of knowledge that comes with life experience and education (Ding et al., 2019).

Another type of intelligence that tends to become more important during the adult years is **practical intelligence**. This is the kind of common-sense thinking that allows a person to successfully negotiate their daily activities (Hoffnung et al., 2019). It has been noted, for example, that some people who are unable to read and write are still able to lead successful lives because they have organised themselves so that these skills are not a priority. It has been demonstrated that individuals living with an intellectual disability can develop the practical skills necessary to cope with their lives in a highly successful fashion, despite gaps in both fluid and crystallised intelligence.

HEALTH IN ADULTHOOD

It is in middle adulthood that the effects of lifestyle first begin to have a significant impact on physical health. Diet, smoking, exercise (or lack of it), alcohol consumption, risk-taking, stress and repetitive activity begin to cause permanent changes in the body and its functions. The onset of problems varies greatly, and it is in the later years that the impacts become most dramatic. Change in behaviours (lifestyle factors) during the young adult period often delays the onset of these problems, and even prevents their occurrence.

The current lack of symptoms and poor health literacy regarding the later impacts of lifestyle factors can make it difficult to persuade young adults that changes are necessary. In addition, early adulthood is a busy time for the establishment of family, work and societal

---

The role of cognition in health is explored in detail in Chapter 7.

Mind (psyche) and body (soma) connections are explored in Chapter 10.

Fluid intelligence
The use of flexible reasoning to draw inferences, solve problems and understand the relationships between concepts.

Crystallised intelligence
The accumulation of knowledge that comes with life experience and education.

Practical intelligence
Common-sense thinking that enables a person to successfully negotiate their daily activities.

The role of health literacy in affecting behaviour choices is explored in Chapter 15.

connections, so people often place a low priority on healthy habits due to a lack of time or priorities. It is common for this low priority to continue and become habitual, and consequences are not evident at this time.

AGEING

There are four accepted main reasons why some people live to be very old but others do not. Reasons include good genes, good overall health throughout life, good psychological resilience and good luck. This statement matches the views of researchers about the determinants of development overall.

The links between physical, social and cognitive development become more significant as people age, emphasising the mind–body connections. It is now recognised that a person's intelligence does not necessarily decrease with age but as a result of health status in general. The healthier and more active an individual is in their middle years, the healthier they are likely to be in their later years. It is important to remember that health should be considered holistically; we have discussed the biopsychosocial model of health which considers the biological, psychological and sociological domains in terms of health and well-being (Jones et al., 2019).

We will now discuss four widely accepted **theories of ageing**: the wear and tear theory, free radical theory, errors in copying theory and obsolescence theory.

Theories of ageing
Varying approaches to explaining the causal impacts of ageing within the human body.

Wear and tear theory

In one model of the wear and tear theory, the human body wears out merely by being lived in and exposed to environmental stressors (Jones et al., 2019). The body is seen as a biological machine that wears out with time and use. Even young people experience health problems of wear and tear. Professional athletes usually reach their peak during their 20s–30s, then often retire. The commonly cited reason is that the body can no longer maintain the schedule and stress of elite-level training and competition. Even if there are no specific sites of damage, such as scar tissue from repeated injury, it may take longer to recover from each contest.

Popular treatments for reducing the effects of ageing through wear and tear include pharmaceuticals (including alternative and complementary approaches) that are advertised to replace or restore tissue. Examples include collagen and glucosamine supplements. Another model of wear and tear theory is based on the idea that the body wears out due to the gradual accumulation of toxins (Jones et al., 2019). This includes environmental exposure to substances such as heavy metals and chemical compounds that the body cannot dispose of through normal processes.

Free radical theory

An active area of ageing research is the free radical theory. This theory focuses on the accumulation of oxidates in the body leading to damage of the cells (Ziada et al., 2020). This oxidative stress or load contributes to body fragility, and therefore it would be beneficial to health to improve the body's resilience to fragility through dietary intake (e.g. increasing antioxidants) (Vina, 2019). Many natural or near-natural products are advertised as containing antioxidants. These include tea, red wine, dark chocolate, fruit and vegetables. The implication is that these products will prevent disease or slow ageing (Healthline, 2021).

Additional treatments, such as dietary supplements, are being manufactured to contain antioxidants, specifically with the intention of slowing or reversing the effects of ageing.

Errors in copying theory

One of the basic processes of life is that cells regularly replicate (copy) themselves to replace the loss of the original. Copying is error-prone, and some cells will eventually fail to replicate correctly. If sufficient numbers of cells fail to replicate this may lead to defects (altered pathology) or, in more dramatic circumstances, to "error catastrophe" (Voit & Meyer-Ortmanns, 2019, p. 43045). The errors in copying theory suggests that copies are not exact and have errors. Incorrectly copied cells may not produce noticeable issues or may cause entire body systems to eventually fail. Early in life, most copies are quite accurate. Errors in copying cells gradually increase as a person ages, leading to further errors in subsequent copies and poorer repair by other cells. The theory is logical if we consider the mathematical basis that the longer a person lives, the more likely a copy of a cell will be faulty.

Another element of the errors in copying theory is related to the wear and tear theory: it suggests that exposure to environmental influences will increase the risk of faulty copies (somatic mutation theory). The range of environmental influences is large, ranging from sunlight and industrial pollution to ordinary food or cooking processes, and includes the heavy metals and chemicals already mentioned among accumulated wastes. Cancers represent a special case of errors in copying, where the faulty cells reproduce themselves vigorously at the expense of accurately reproducing cells.

Obsolescence theories

Several researchers suggest that the body has an internal program, determined by genes or cells, that sets a limit to how long it can work efficiently. The simplest version of this theory is that the body has an internal clock built into the nervous, endocrine or immune system that simply runs down and fails. This leads to degenerative diseases due to the inability of cells to regenerate. A recent variation of this theory, related to errors in copying, concerns telomeres. Telomeres are repetitive segments on the ends of DNA strands that protect the important information coded in the strand from being lost (Razgonova et al., 2020). The theory states that, with each replication, some of the telomere material is lost. Eventually, enough is lost that the core information is affected. Contemporary research indicates that telomere length is a key feature of human ageing, with stress as a contributing factor (Razgonova et al., 2020).

Stress and coping are discussed in Chapters 12 and 13.

Another consideration is that social change within the individual's environment, such as compulsory retirement and reliance on a pension, can place a degree of stress on the individual. Stress is a compounding factor for impacts of ageing.

Other theorists have suggested that people's disengagement from wider society as they age can contribute to cognitive disengagement and continual decline (Hamm et al., 2020). **Disengagement theory** suggests that ageing individuals tend to modify their amount of interaction with the society around them to suit their capabilities. This suggests that those who are physically fit, mentally alert and financially secure tend to maintain a high level of social engagement into their 80s or even later. This behaviour is linked with motivation and sense of self-worth.

Disengagement theory
The idea that ageing individuals tend to modify their amount of interaction with the society around them to suit their capabilities.

As age increases, the probability that disease will cause significant loss of function also increases. Most people over 75 experience impairment in sight, hearing and mobility, resulting from the continuation of physical changes that began in young adulthood. Atherosclerosis, loss of bone density and the development of cancers are further examples of impairments due to physical changes and disease processes. Among the very old, fragility is a significant problem.

As the population ages, there is an increased number of older Australian adults living with dementia. In 2021, the prevalence of dementia in Australia was approximately 472 000 individuals, with a projected cohort experiencing this condition increasing to 1 076 000 by 2058 (Dementia Australia, 2020). The cost of providing care for this population is estimated to be approximately $A47.8 billion by 2050 (Standfield et al., 2018). While dementia is not an inevitable part of ageing and may affect younger people as well, it is a growing burden on Australian health care.

Behaviours associated with chronic conditions are discussed in Chapter 5.

Based on ABS statistics from 2016, dementia has become the second-highest cause of death in Australia overall. It is the leading cause of death for Australian women, exceeding heart disease (Dementia Australia, 2020). Although research has not yet found cures for dementia-causing diseases, such as Alzheimer's disease, there have been many advancements in management including improvements in brain scans for detection and monitoring, medication trials, health promotion campaigns and better education for service providers who deliver front-line care.

Alzheimer's disease
A significant impairment of cognitive ability, memory or problem-solving ability resulting from abnormalities of cells in the cerebral cortex.

There are several types of dementia, the best-known of which is **Alzheimer's disease** that results from abnormalities of cells in the cerebral cortex. Alzheimer's disease accounts for 70% of individuals living with dementia, or three in every 10 Australians aged over 85 (Dementia Australia, 2020). While the onset of Alzheimer's disease may be subtle, the first symptoms include problems with short-term memory, such as an inability to remember names or where things have been put. This is followed by more general memory problems (e.g. forgetting recent events) and increasing confusion (Dementia Australia, 2020). Personality may seem to change, as individuals become frustrated and anxious about their coping abilities. Finally, impairment is so drastic that the individual becomes totally dependent on others for eating, dressing and the usual activities of daily living.

Elderly clients may be slow to understand or respond to instructions, not because of loss of mental abilities but due to a slowness in processing time and difficulty in assessing the instructions. The frail aged, and those living with dementia, may be fearful when admitted to residential health care settings. These fears may result from uncertainty about the environment, about the stresses that will be placed on them, or about the loss of personal dignity involved in daily care procedures. It is important that health professionals keep quality of care and not speed of treatment in mind when working with all patients, but this is particularly true with older people. Early planning for individuals experiencing dementia is essential to reduce unnecessary stress on the individual and their family as their condition deteriorates.

3.2 CASE STUDY

PATTIE AND HENRY'S GOLDEN YEARS

Pattie (aged 75) and Henry (73) have lived all their lives in Maurice Hills, an affluent suburb in the city of Julian Cove. Pattie has been a home-maker since she married her childhood sweetheart Henry. The couple recently celebrated their 50th wedding anniversary. Henry had a distinguished career in the police service and held the rank of police inspector until he retired three years ago. The couple owns a six-bedroom home and are looking forward to their older son Ben (a police prosecutor), his wife Mary (a nurse) and their sons Tom (15) and Chris (13) coming to live in the main house while Pattie and Henry downsize to the self-contained parent retreat by the pool. Pattie and Henry have been avid travellers, enjoying adventures over the past 10 years in their mobile home and they have planned some longer trips in the coming months. Both have active roles in the golf club and Pattie is on the fundraising committee. They are well known in the community and often entertain at home.

Recently, Henry has noticed some changes in Pattie's behaviours. Last week, Pattie was unable to tell the taxi driver her address after attending her weekly hairdresser appointment. Pattie is also becoming short-tempered with other people on the golf committee and is not her usual organised self. Three times in the last month, Henry has heard the kettle whistling on the stove and come into the kitchen, finding Pattie looking confused and saying she couldn't remember what she was doing. Henry has tried to take on more of the cooking and household activities to reduce the demands on his wife, but this only seems to have made matters worse. At times Pattie is reduced to tears as she cannot do the things she once did.

1   What factor(s) might place Pattie at risk for Alzheimer's disease?
2   What type of memory might be affected, based on the above information?
3   What might be the impact on Ben, his wife and sons?
4   What advantages or protective factors might exist for the family unit?

Death and grieving

In the absence of illness, disease or disability, the senior stages of the lifespan pass uneventfully for most people, with some physical deterioration but without major mental challenges. As seniors age, their social network reduces as friends and family pass away. Connections with children and grandchildren are often reduced due to the geographical dispersity in Australia and relocation for education, career and work. The loss of a partner is a stressful event for the surviving person. This can all contribute to a sense of isolation. Older people may reflect on their own mortality as more of their friends die.

Generally, it is reported that older people are not afraid of dying but view death as familiar. Where an individual or their spouse/partner is living with a health condition that is life-limiting (e.g. Parkinson's disease, Alzheimer's disease) or carries a significant burden of pain (e.g. osteoarthritis, lordosis, some cancers), death may appear a welcome end to the daily pain and difficulties of existence. There may be a reconnection with spiritual or religious practices that provide comfort in the later years.

For older people, their quality of life (QoL) at the senior stage of the lifespan is often a priority over longevity. Seniors approaching end of life stages (EoL) may refuse treatments that offer them a short extension of life on the grounds that the loss of dignity, awareness or personal control is not worth the small gain of time (Chuang et al., 2020). Debates have arisen within the political, legal and health care systems regarding issues of assisted suicide and voluntary euthanasia, and there are often inconsistencies between the older person's wishes and family members' perspectives (Chuang et al., 2020). In Australia, each state and territory has its own legislation on these practices.

People can make their EoL wishes known in advance through legal avenues such as **advance health care directives (living will)**, do not resuscitate orders, power of attorney and pre-planning their funeral. These actions are **anticipatory decision-making directives**. They enable the individual to exert more control over the process of EoL (dying). The common elements of a living will are statements that the individual wishes to receive adequate pain relief to avoid suffering, even if that hastens death, and that the person wishes to be allowed to die and not be kept alive by artificial means or heroic measures. There are legal implications for these processes and in some situations the individual's wishes and instructions may be disregarded. This falls into the field of medico-legal practitioners and the Office of the Public Guardian, who may be called to make decisions in complex situations.

Advance health care directive (living will)
A statement signed by an individual about the treatment they will accept when they are dying.

Anticipatory decision-making
Advance planning by an individual regarding a significant future event. Directives provide guidance for family members and others regarding the decision-maker's preferences and wishes.

The five stages of dying

It has long been recognised that dying is a process rather than a point in time. One of the first health professionals to offer a theory of dying was psychiatrist Elisabeth Kübler-Ross (1969). After lengthy experience working with dying patients, Kübler-Ross described it a five-stage process.

1 *Denial.* In this stage, the person's reaction is described as 'Not me!' The person simply refuses to accept the information. They may continue with life activities as if they had been told nothing. This can be frustrating for health professionals and often for families, but has a protective effect for the individual. Even though their denial may appear irrational, it can provide them with time to take actions that will enable them a better adjustment later.

2 *Anger.* The person has accepted the validity of their situation but experiences anger over the perceived unfairness of it. The typical reaction is 'Why me?' Their anger may have any number of targets: themselves, others who may have exposed them to risk, parents for passing on a genetic vulnerability, health professionals or their god.

3 *Bargaining.* Having now recognised that the outcome cannot be changed, the person tries to bargain about the details. The typical reaction is 'Not now'. They may try to negotiate a reprieve from the doctor if they promise to change their behaviour. They may make promises to their god in exchange for a little more time or a miracle.

4 *Depression.* In this stage, the person recognises the reality of the end of their life and experiences the sadness of it. They may withdraw into clinical depression but are more likely to experience an appropriate and transient sadness. It is likely that they will begin to make plans for their death, change their life activities and disengage from many people and events.

5   *Acceptance.* By this, Kübler-Ross meant far more than simply admitting that death is inevitable. She described a complex pattern of withdrawal from life. The dying person begins to say goodbye to things and people, and progressively cuts off contact with others until they reach a point where they prefer to be with only a few close people, usually family. They also withdraw from activity, spending more and more time in sleep. They may experience a loss of sensation, and even severe pain may fade away. At the very last stages, they often want to be alone with a spouse or child, and may prefer to avoid talking in favour of simply holding hands or being in the same room. In Kübler-Ross's view, this is a positive stage in that it allows the individual to die in comfort and with dignity.

GRIEVING

Kübler-Ross's theory has been criticised for suggesting that all the stages occur for every person, that they occur in a fixed order and that once past a stage the individual does not return to it. The model is only one of several theories to explore and explain the grief process. A further criticism of grief models is that they are based on family systems that are entrenched within Western society and may lack cultural considerations (Dorrian et al., 2017).

Figure 3.1 depicts a more general grieving model. The advantages of this model are that it can be used to describe the experience of those who experience grief as a sense of loss over previous good health (e.g. someone diagnosed with a life-impacting but not life-limiting condition such as diabetes) as well as those are at the end of their lifespan, with disease present or not. A further criticism of grief theories in general is that they only promote negativity, and that by encouraging an individual's acceptance of their condition they may be reducing survival by decreasing motivation and the 'fighting spirit'.

FIGURE 3.1 The grieving cycle

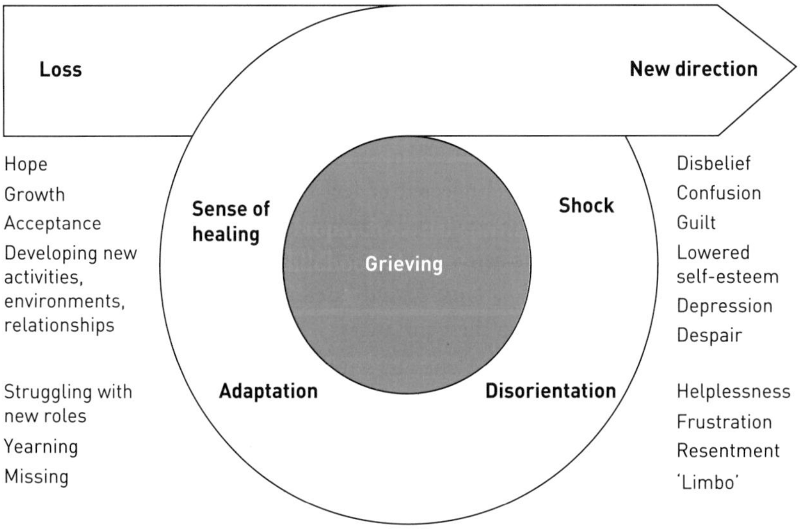

Adapted from LoCicero (1991)

It needs to be highlighted that grief can be related to loss, and is not limited to death. Grieving can take place at any time a person experiences a significant loss throughout their lifetime. This could include loss of another through death, divorce or moving away; loss of function through amputation, stroke or ageing; loss of activities due to disability or barriers; and loss of self through any of the above, plus dementia or impending death. Those who are grieving may seem so miserable that we have an urge to prevent or stop the process; however, the work of grieving needs to be done before recovery can be complete. Expressions of grief can vary between and even within cultures. Open expressions of grief may be encouraged in one culture, whereas in other cultures the name of the deceased person cannot be mentioned. The duration of mourning is also shaped by tradition and culture (Dorrian et al., 2017).

Anticipatory grieving
Grieving that takes place before an expected loss has occurred.

It is possible for grieving to take place before the loss has occurred. This **anticipatory grieving** (Berman et al., 2021) is common where the impending loss is known ahead of time. If the period of time before the actual loss is long enough, grieving may well be complete almost as soon as the loss is ultimately experienced. Sometimes outsiders are amazed by how little grief seems to be experienced or displayed by the surviving partner of an elderly couple. This does not mean a lack of feeling for the lost partner, but simply that there has already been sufficient time for grieving to take place. The surviving partner may feel that everything that needed to be said was said, and that with their partner's suffering over, there is no grieving left to do. It must be emphasised that grief is a uniquely personal experience.

Morbid grief
Grieving that is too intense or inappropriate to the loss.

Grieving can cause problems if it continues for too long without change or a sense of being adapted, if it is too intense or if it is inappropriate to the loss. This type of grief is known as dysfunctional **morbid grief** or as complicated grief, and is usually an indicator of other psychological issues. Grief can produce problems if it is blocked, prevented, postponed or denied.

Grieving can also produce problems if the people involved get out of sync with one another; that is, if they are experiencing different stages of grieving. Imagine, for example, a case in which doctors inform an elderly father that he has only six months to live. He and his partner will begin the process of grieving. Their middle-aged child who lives some distance away may only arrive in time for the parents' final stages of grieving. They may be angry, bargaining or depressed at a time when the parents have achieved adaptation and acceptance. The adult child may feel rejected or feel that the parents are indifferent to the seriousness of the situation. If the adult child then tries (appropriately to their own stage of grieving) to get doctors to take heroic measures to save the dying parent, this may cause more friction between child and parents. As indicated above, there is often a lack of consensus on the approach to be taken in these instances.

In the same way, an individual with Alzheimer's disease may lose so much of their memories, thoughts and personal characteristics as a result of their dementia that their partner regards them as 'lost' long before they die. In this case, the partner may have completed grieving for the person and continue taking care of the body, which, as the partner sees it, is all that remains. When death finally occurs, the major feeling may be relief.

3.3 CASE STUDY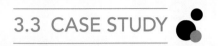

PATTIE AND HENRY (CONT.)

Soon after Ben and his family come to live with Pattie and Henry, a long consultation was arranged with the family doctor. Specialists were consulted and second opinions obtained; the conclusive diagnosis was that Pattie has Alzheimer's disease. Pattie was well enough to understand the condition as explained by medical professionals and at first she denied there was anything wrong. Her condition progressed and Henry decided to cancel their planned holiday as he felt he could not manage his wife's needs as she became more unpredictable. Henry has become sullen and often says "We led good lives and waited for retirement to finally enjoy ourselves. It's like a curse". Pattie wants to remain in her home in her later years and the family arranges for community nurses and other supports to provide her with quality of life in her declining years. Pattie says that under no circumstances does she want to end her days in a hospital on a ventilator surrounded by strangers. While she is able to make decisions for herself, she requests that the family help her plan for her final send-off.

1   Which stages of grief can be identified in this scenario?
2   What actions can Pattie take so her wishes will be known and acted upon?
3   How might anticipatory grief be experienced by the family?

CHAPTER SUMMARY

- Important themes of adulthood revolve around responsibility towards family, work and society.
- Lifestyle choices of earlier adult stages of the lifespan begin to emerge towards the end of middle adulthood and into the senior years.
- The individual's QoL and EoL factors are often prioritised differently from those of family members.
- Ageing brings life changes as a result of societal expectations.
- Healthy older people live a life that is very similar to that of the middle aged.
- Death and dying are important issues at the end of life and legal processes can be important preplanning tools.

Learn more
Access additional resources to broaden your understanding of this chapter. See the Guided Tour for access details.

FURTHER READING

ACRC [Aged Care Royal Commission] (2021) *Final Report*.
https://agedcare.royalcommission.gov.au/publications/final-report
Hayslip B, Patrick J & Hollis-Sawyer L (2020) *Adult Development and Aging: Growth, Longevity and Challenges*. Sage.
Higley E (2019) *Defining Young Adulthood*. DNP Qualifying Manuscripts no. 17.
https://repository.usfca.edu/dnp_qualifying/17
Werth S & Brownlow C (2018) *Work and Identity*. Springer.

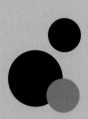

4 Reactions to Illness

Introduction

Reactions to illness vary considerably. For most people, minor aches, pains and other illness symptoms are an inescapable, and even an expected aspect of daily living. An individual's response to symptoms of illness can range from ignoring the symptom to immediately seeking professional emergency medical care. In between these extremes are self-care responses ranging from relatively passive (getting more rest, increasing hydration) to active behaviour (losing weight, stopping smoking). This chapter explores factors that influence individuals' reactions to illness. These reactions can be influenced by the illness itself, the situation and the person. Following your reading of Chapters 2 and 3, you can appreciate that individual responses to illness will differ according to the person's stage of development. There has been increasing interest in the factors that appear to be involved in the individual's decision to seek medical care, including symptom severity, cultural and family background, social networks, psychological distress, illness beliefs, locus of control, learning history, personality factors and availability and affordability of care services. Although some of these factors remain constant, others are subject to change. Variability of the different factors creates challenges in building a consistent picture of who regularly uses medical services and perhaps unnecessarily accesses services such as an emergency department when they are not experiencing an emergent issue. Additionally, it is difficult to identify those people who are seldom seen by health professionals, even though their condition warrants diagnosis and intervention.

Typical reactions to illness are very similar to reactions to any other stressful life event, whether it is a loss or a pleasant experience. These typical reactions can be examined under four headings.

1   *Physical responses.* These are changes in bodily states and processes. Physical responses include loss of or change in appetite, sleep problems and tiredness. These may result directly from the illness or underlying disease process (e.g. an increase in body temperature, a rash appearing on the skin).

2   *Emotional responses.* Emotional responses could include sadness, anxiety, anger, irritability or relief and happiness. In some cases, when the individual sees that blame can be assigned for their illness, specific emotional reactions are common. If the blame for an individual's situation rests with themselves (e.g. a smoker who develops lung cancer), that person may experience feelings of guilt. Where the blame can be seen to rest with another (e.g. lung cancer resulting from exposure to pollutants in the workplace), anger is common. Like physical reactions, emotional reactions may result directly from illness processes or indirectly.

3   *Cognitive responses.* These are responses relating to thinking and judging. Cognitive responses include preoccupation with symptoms, perceptions of self-image, and memories. These kinds of reactions are often overlooked because the physical and emotional ones are more obvious to the individual and others.

Loss of **self-esteem** is common in many health conditions and may interfere with many aspects of the individual's life. Men who experience getting or maintaining an erection as a result of a medical condition associated with ageing, for example, may feel that they have become less 'manly' or that they will have difficulty in establishing and maintaining an intimate relationship. Like physical and emotional reactions, cognitive reactions may have direct or indirect causes. A direct cause relating to cognition is a

Self-esteem
An individual's perception that they are a good and worthy person.

urinary tract infection that could potentially cause confusion in an elderly person. An indirect cause that alters cognition may be preoccupation about the condition and subsequent anxiety and rumination.

4   *Behavioural responses.* Behavioural responses to illness could include changes in habits, restlessness, withdrawal from people, and help and information seeking. Many such changes are seen as normal in the initial stages of an illness but regarded as abnormal if they continue. Behavioural responses could range from something as simple as beginning to take vitamins to a complete lifestyle change (e.g. eliminating gluten or following a prescriptive diet). A substantial part of the behavioural reaction consists of an attempt to cope with the stress of a situation.

The more serious the illness symptoms, the more likely we are to expect and accept these reactions from individuals. In a similar way, the more serious the illness, the longer we will see these reactions as being normal and appropriate. Remember that illness is subjective and felt by the individual experiencing the situation, whereas disease is a state of altered pathology that is identified by a qualified and independent observer.

If an illness is chronic (it occurs regularly or repeatedly over a period of time or is permanent), we will expect and accept some persistence of the reactions. Chapter 2 included a further category of altered health, classified as disability. Persistence of reactions is particularly true for people living with visible disabilities. An individual who is unable to mobilise without a wheelchair as a result of injury may be forever exempt from a range of activities. The situation where disabilities are invisible (e.g. intellectual disability) do not always receive the same acceptance of reactions (Howie et al., 2021).

Stress is discussed in Chapter 12.

Disability is discussed further in Chapter 14.

PAUSE & REFLECT

Think back to the last time you were ill (you experienced symptoms indicating reduced health).

What kind of physical, emotional, cognitive and behavioural reactions did you experience?

What reactions did you observe in the people around you?

4.1 CASE STUDY

ROHIT'S CHANGED HEALTH STATUS

This case study considers how people react to the experience of changes to their health and examines the factors that influence these reactions.

Rohit is a widower aged 60, has recently retired and lives on a boat in a marina. He has two children who are married and have young families of their own. They live in different states of Australia. Sailing has been Rohit's lifelong passion and in retirement he plans to take long trips around Australia. He recently bought a new boat that he can sail solo in the open ocean and has been preparing for his first lengthy voyage.

Rohit has enjoyed reasonably good health for most of his life. Recently, he noticed that he was urinating more frequently, feeling lethargic, always seemed thirsty and was putting on weight. Rohit did not feel it necessary to inform his children of his concerns and thought perhaps he was worrying over nothing. He did not want to make a fuss; however, he did briefly mention his symptoms to a trusted friend, Mike. Having some knowledge about men's health, Mike encouraged him to get a check-up, indicating that prostate cancer and diabetes were considerations in light of his symptoms and stage of the lifespan.

Rohit was diagnosed with adult-onset diabetes and placed on medication to manage his disease. He was in total disbelief as he had led a healthy life and was very active. He sought a second opinion, which confirmed the diagnosis. Rohit became withdrawn. He told Mike that he was updating his will and planned to sell his boat. Reflecting on his past, Rohit began to feel that his life and his plans for grand voyages were totally wasted. He felt he no longer had any control over his life.

Fortunately, Mike was supportive and encouraged Rohit to contact a community diabetes service. He even accompanied Rohit to his appointments. After several sessions with the diabetes educator, Rohit realised that he could manage his condition and his lifestyle would need only minor modifications.

1   What might have happened if Rohit had not spoken to Mike or acted on his advice?
2   Would the grief cycle (Chapter 3) apply to Rohit?
3   Can you identify the loss Rohit may be experiencing?
4   What kinds of reactions did Rohit exhibit during this event?

Illness behaviour

Illness behaviour is the process by which an individual goes from being a well person to being an unwell person. The focus is on the nature of the individual's response to their experience of being unwell. Changes in our health are almost inevitable. Sudden and unexpected changes are stressful events which contribute to the type of reactions we display. Support from those around us can be a critical factor in developing coping skills. People may feel in control of their health; conversely, they may feel that the universe is conspiring against them and they have no control at all. This links to the concept of locus of control. A person's information- and help-seeking behaviours link to their capabilities, environments and motivations.

People may have a sense that their health is not quite right yet choose to ignore symptoms in the initial stages, in the hope they will disappear. Next, they may seek advice from people whom they trust. These early disclosures are most commonly made to friends who may or may not have correct medical knowledge or provide appropriate advice (health literacy). This response of seeking information and help can be thought of as a coping response to the stress of an alteration in health.

Illness behaviour
The process by which an individual transitions from being a well person to an unwell person.

Locus of control is discussed in Chapter 13.

Capabilities and environments are discussed in Chapter 14.

ARE MY SYMPTOMS NORMAL?

People may delay acting on symptoms of illness if they do not consider them to be serious. This is a process of normalisation. An example could be the increased urination experienced by Rohit in Case Study 4.1. This change was annoying, and Rohit may have taken actions such as reducing his fluid intake to ease the problem. The same situation might arise for someone experiencing a headache. Rarely would someone seek a doctor's appointment for a minor headache; instead, the learnt behaviour may be to purchase an over-the-counter analgesic. A headache is usually considered as a nuisance factor and can be 'explained away' by normalising it (e.g. caused by too much screen time, not eating, not drinking enough water). Once a problem is rectified by time, lifestyle change or medication the matter is not considered further; the event has been normalised and is soon forgotten. A chronic symptom, such as low-grade back pain, may be accepted as a normal part of ageing or as a response to a regular activity such as sports or gardening. On some occasions the individual experiencing the symptom might compare themselves to others; for example, a middle-aged woman experiencing hot flushes. Non-professional people, such as family and friends, may be consulted to see if they think that the symptom is real ('Is it just me, or is it hot in here?') or serious ('Do you ever have headaches on one side of your head?'). Normalising occurs when a friend says 'We've all been through this. Not much you can do but it does get better'. The woman was seeking validation of her symptoms and a way to rationalise or normalise them. She was reassured that the symptom was not significant and was common for all women at that stage of the lifespan. It should be noted that menopausal symptoms can have significant and far-reaching impact on the individual and their family, and should not be readily dismissed as that may lead to maladaptive coping and poor health outcomes (Hashemipoor et al., 2019).

SHOULD I SEE A PROFESSIONAL NOW?

In Australia, a registered health practitioner is someone who has completed an accredited tertiary program leading to registration, such as doctors, nurses, psychologists, dentists, occupational therapists, physiotherapists and chiropractors. Some individuals will consult alternate and complementary therapists such as massage therapists, herbalists, naturopaths, reiki or faith healers. Regardless of the practitioner involved, the general process of becoming a 'patient' follows the same path. The question of when to consult must be settled.

Five common triggers for the decision to seek professional help have been identified.

1   *Perceived interference of symptoms with work, recreation or activities of daily living.* The person feels they cannot work or do things they need to do because of the symptoms.

2   *Perceived interference with social activities or personal relationships.* The person may be well enough to do the things they have to do, such as going to work, but feel too tired or ill to do things they would like to do, or that others would like them to do.

3   *Occurrence of a personal crisis (e.g. divorce or bereavement) that disturbs usual coping and emotional well-being.* A symptom that would normally be tolerated if there was not the additional stress of an unusual or unexpected event.

4   *The symptom has been persistent or passed a self-imposed deadline.* Often, the length of this deadline is affected by symptom severity. We will tolerate low levels of symptoms (e.g. pain and lethargy) that do not appear to mean anything major much longer than we will tolerate severe or worrying symptoms (e.g. significant pain that interferes with sleep, unusual bleeding, blurred vision).

5   *Pressure from others to seek help (sanctioning).* Family and friends are often the catalyst for people to consult health professionals. They may be more concerned about interference with activities of daily living, duration or meaning of a symptom than the individual who actually experiences the symptom.

WHAT CAN THE PROFESSIONAL PROVIDE?

Usually, health professionals can relieve symptoms by means of treatment, reducing anxiety about the symptom through explanation and reassurance, or validation of the disease as indicated by the symptoms. Prior experience with professionals is very important in deciding what they can provide and if this service is useful to the person. If the individual has previously been disappointed with outcomes or side effects of treatment, or even the kind of treatment they received, they may look for a different approach such as a naturopathy, osteopathy or religion. This links to expectancy theory and motivation.

Expectancy theory is discussed in Chapter 7.

PAUSE & REFLECT

What factors might lead someone to consult a naturopath rather than a general practitioner?

Motivation is discussed in Chapter 8.

4.2 CASE STUDY

ROBERT'S BACK PAIN

Robert thought he sprained some back muscles while gardening a few days ago. His back pain has continued and is now disturbing his sleep. Robert has not joined his friends on their usual morning run for the past few days. One morning he spoke to a pharmacist about his pain and current use of ibuprofen, rather than visit a doctor for a diagnosis. He did consider going to the doctor for reassurance and to stop family members from worrying and nagging, even though he was not overly worried himself.

Later on the day he visited the pharmacy, Robert began to experience excruciating pain in his groin. He made several visits to the bathroom but was unable to urinate. He took the maximum dose of pain relief as discussed with the pharmacist, but was unable to find a comfortable position and resorted to pacing while he waited for the medicine to take effect. However, the pain continued and in fact increased. Robert recognised the need for help and was frightened as he remembered his father had a similar experience with pain, which led to surgery. His first thought was to phone his brother Peter, but he remembered that Peter was at work. As the pain was unbearable, Robert decided to phone 000. He described his situation and gave his address. Paramedics arrived within 15 minutes, administered narcotic-based medication for pain and transferred Robert to hospital for an emergency admission with a suspected diagnosis of nephritis due to a possible kidney stone (renal calculi) creating a blockage in his ureter. The emergency doctor told Robert that if the stone did not pass via urination in the next eight hours, surgical intervention would be required. The recovery period post-surgery would be approximately two weeks.

1 Robert was able to recall his father's experience with sudden pain. How might his situation be different from that of someone who had not known anyone who had had a similar experience?

2 Were there elements of normalisation of the situation?

3 Why did Robert choose to speak with a pharmacist rather than a doctor?

4 What was the main reason Robert sought urgent and immediate help?

Points to consider

Robert's status suddenly changed from being a well person to becoming a patient due to assessment by the ambulance service and admission to hospital. If he needs surgery, he will miss work and may worry about lack of sick leave and/or loss of income. Robert will be granted the rights of the sick role—from family, friends, hospital and employer—even if the kidney stone passes naturally and he does not require surgery. In Robert's case, his entitlement to the sick role is very clear.

The sick role

Sick role
A social agreement involving a balance of rights and obligations granted to an individual who is regarded by others as sick.

In looking at what it means for the individual to be sick, sociologist Talcott Parsons (1951) described the **sick role** as a social agreement involving a balance of rights and obligations. The rights include:

- being excused from normal roles and responsibilities;

- being regarded as not personally responsible for being sick (which means that the individual has a real problem and cannot be expected to get better simply by willpower or by deciding to do so) (Cheshire et al., 2021).

The obligations include:

- having the intent to get better (recover);

- cooperating with appropriately qualified and competent interventions (Cheshire et al., 2021).

Parsons believed that the sick role was present in every culture and always included these rights and obligations. Obviously, different beliefs about the causes of symptoms (e.g. germs, the evil eye, curses, spells, witchcraft or manifestations) will affect what is meant by terms such as 'not personally responsible' and 'technically competent help'.

The significance of culture is further discussed in Chapter 14.

The decision about who deserves the sick role is often loaded with moral judgments. Consider the adult who continues to smoke tobacco or consume alcohol in a risky way despite knowing that these behaviours are likely to have adverse effects. If advertising promotes the use of a product, then conversely promoting the negative effects should also encourage the person to cease the behaviour; however, this is not the case (Dorrian et al., 2017). The person who smokes, drinks heavily or binge drinks may continue these behaviours even after the adverse effects are known due to addiction, inadequate coping and motivation or other environmental factors. Should the person who commences or continues smoking and drinking be considered responsible for health consequences, given they are aware of the harmful effects and yet did not act upon this knowledge? Should they be granted the same rights as those who do not smoke? Premiums for health and life insurance are often higher for smokers. People with other lifestyle-associated diseases or risk factors may be declined health and life insurance. Automobile accidents can happen to anyone but are far more likely to happen to at-risk drivers, including drink drivers, texting drivers and drivers who speed. Should we blame people in these categories in the same way that we tend to blame smokers? The debates over treatment of HIV/AIDS, genital herpes and alcoholism often revolve around value judgments and risk-taking behaviour, yet debates about treatment of obesity-related disorders such as heart disease seldom do. A contemporary debate has arisen regarding access to treatment for COVID-19 for those who have not been immunised.

Risky behaviour is discussed in Chapter 7.

As public awareness of the risks associated with obesity changes, so too are attitudes changing. We tend to agree that genetic predisposition is not something a person can be blamed for, but what about failing to take appropriate action to reduce the genetic risk? These arguments have a great deal to do with our responsibility-oriented culture. In many other cultures, these issues are never considered at all.

Eating disorders are discussed in Chapter 9.

Abnormal illness behaviour

When a continuing reaction towards illness on the individual's part is judged by others as disproportionate to general expectations, their behaviour may be considered an overreaction and therefore abnormal. The point at which it is considered abnormal will depend on who is doing the judging, the nature of the illness, the age and gender of the sick person and their responsibilities. Abnormal illness behaviours are also called non-rational behaviours (Dorrian et al., 2017).

Pilowsky (1978) identified a pattern of behaviour he called **abnormal illness behaviour**. While his work focused on pain and psychiatric responses, it paved the way for researchers to explore abnormal responses to illness and disease. It should be highlighted that abnormal illness behaviour is distinct from abnormal behaviour. Pilowsky defined abnormal illness behaviour as persistent maladaptive perception regarding an individual's changed health status.

Abnormal illness behaviour
The persistence of inappropriate or maladaptive modes of perceiving, evaluating or acting in relation to health after the person has received an appropriate explanation of the nature and management of the illness from a professional.

Earlier we looked at the sick role as including the obligation of an individual experiencing the illness or disease to make all efforts to recover (e.g. by following medical advice). Abnormal illness behaviour could relate to requesting the rights of the sick role when they are not actually needed, or avoiding the obligations. These behaviours are seen as maladaptive responses. Behaviours that we have observed during our formative years and into adulthood inform our personal responses towards illness and disease. This situation is linked to classical conditioning and learnt behaviours.

4.3 CASE STUDY

ERIKA

Erika is 45 and works as a cleaner for the local motel on a casual basis. She has a history of headaches which she manages by resting in bed with a cup of tea. Her mother Mavis and her aunts also frequently experienced these headaches; it appears to be a family pattern. Erika has been to numerous doctors and has had extensive testing, but no cause has been found. She has been prescribed medication to take as a preventive measure and additional medication to take at the onset of symptoms during an acute event. Erika does not like to take the medication and prefers to rely on herbal teas to address her illness. Erika's partner and children (aged 14 and 16) do the cooking and cleaning when she is not able to manage these tasks. Erika is served her meals in bed and has a bell to ring when she needs something. She adopted this behaviour from her mother. Her partner says that Erika has behaved this way since the children started school.

1   What aspects of the sick role are evident?

2   What obligations would be reasonably expected?

3   Why might there be a lack of motivation to recover from these acute episodes?

4   Does this fit with the definition of abnormal illness behaviour?

We have mentioned the biopsychosocial model of health and noted that one criticism relates to the assumption that an individual has control over their circumstances. We have also mentioned that the early signs of illness originate from the individual's perception of something being not quite right. These situations have an underlying assumption that an individual understands and is aware of how they are behaving and perceived by others. Abnormal illness behaviour may be deliberate (as identified to some degree by Erika) but, frequently, abnormal illness behaviours are not conscious acts. To some extent, the diagnosis of abnormal illness behaviour will involve value judgments by the professional or the person's family, friends or associates. Additionally, stage of life and cultural differences contribute to what is judged to be inappropriate and maladaptive behaviour.

Illness may also serve as a trigger for psychological challenges such as depression, anxiety, adjustment disorders, substance abuse, dysfunctional family functioning, social or occupational problems and even psychosis (severe mental illness). Although a life event or crisis may trigger consultation with a health professional, if the person is already predisposed to the development of psychological symptoms, a physical illness may trigger that psychological disorder or make it worse.

Factors affecting reactions to illness

The illness, the situation and the person are all factors that can affect reactions to illness.

THE ILLNESS OR DISEASE

The nature of an illness or disease can affect how people react to it. Severe illnesses and significant diseases are likely to cause greater reactions. Cancers, even those that are slow in developing, easily treated or present a low risk of disability or death, often produce very strong reactions due to images portrayed in mainstream society. Another, more dramatic, example is that of a flesh-eating virus that combines rapid onset, horrific physical damage and low probability of cure to inevitably produce a fearful impact. Conditions that are known to produce long-term effects (diabetes, epilepsy) or affect many areas of life (spinal injury, Alzheimer's disease) also tend to produce greater reactions. Even the recommended treatments may affect how people react. Chemotherapy for leukaemia, for example, may result in the loss of all hair: this is a highly visible indication of the individual's condition, even though the condition itself may have few obvious external signs. The attitudes of others to an ill person's condition may further isolate that person, as fear of contracting the condition is common. We only have to recall the situation of COVID-19 to highlight this point.

THE SITUATION

The size and accessibility of the individual's social support network, their financial and work situation and access to health care can affect how they react to an illness. Other situational factors can include where they live and concurrent stresses in their lives. Reactions to a condition will be quite different if, for example, the individual is temporarily unable to participate in a favourite activity, rather than being forced to give up that activity forever. Loss of social status or income due to an illness or disease can produce strong and prolonged reactions. The importance of social support to an individual's health and well-being is well recognised. Those who have a greater social network to call on, or who have people who are willing to provide very high levels of support, find coping with health challenges much easier in general than those who must rely on their own resources.

Social support is discussed in detail in Chapters 13 and 14.

THE PERSON

The effects of a particular behaviour on health will not be the same for every person. Personal characteristics that influence the impact of a health behaviour include vulnerabilities (things that make the impact greater) and capabilities (things that lessen the impact).

Vulnerability and capability

GENETIC PREDISPOSITIONS

Vulnerability
A characteristic or behaviour of the individual that increases the impact of a negative event.

Capability
A characteristic or behaviour of the individual that protects against a negative event.

Each person inherits **vulnerabilities** and **capabilities** as part of their genetic make-up. A person's internal structure and function can predispose them towards either developing or resisting specific health problems. Examples include heart disease and risk factors (high cholesterol, high blood pressure), cancers, diabetes and mental health conditions, where research has established genetic components (De Rosa et al., 2018). Some genetic predispositions are primarily found within specific families (Huntington's chorea), specific populations (thalassaemia, haemophilia) or are widely distributed.

Whether a specific genetic predisposition results in disease or illness depends on the type of predisposition. Inheriting a faulty chromosome from a parent means that a person will develop the condition, regardless of any behavioural or environmental factors. Haemophilia, for example, is an X chromosome recessive disorder, and if a male with haemophilia produces a daughter she will become an obligate (carrier of haemophilia). Other combinations of genes will either preclude or increase the chances of offspring inheriting the condition (Bernard et al., 2018). Other events, such as a first mutation in the genetic sequence, produce a particular situational influence (a novel gene mutation).

In some cases, the genetic predisposition is development of a risk factor rather than a disease. An individual may, for example, be predisposed to produce moderately high levels of cholesterol. This is not in itself a disease and is largely symptomless in the early stages but it is a risk factor for atherosclerosis, which in turn produces symptoms of heart disease. The mere predisposition to high levels of cholesterol does not mean that the individual will inevitably have symptoms. Factors that occur later in life, such as diet, exercise, smoking and alcohol use, will have a large influence.

Psychological traits
Thought patterns such as feelings and emotions that produce a behaviour (action). They are uniquely formed by each individual.

Genetic predispositions may influence **psychological traits** as well as physical ones. Individuals are born with differences in temperament: some may be excitable, others quiet and steady. While it may be possible to trace these **behavioural predispositions** back to biological causes, it is often more useful to consider them at the level of behaviour. Certain styles of dealing with stress run in families. Stress produces a hormone known as cortisol. Individuals who have high stress levels produce higher amounts of circulating cortisol. Studies have linked high cortisol levels with obesity and weight management issues, which then carry further risk of cardiac events and other comorbidities later in life (Ajibewa et al., 2021).

Behavioural predispositions
Actions that have been learnt by the individual as a response to situations.

Some theorists suggest that complex patterns of behaviour, such as addiction or substance dependence, may run in families. Situational, environmental and behavioural characteristics can all contribute to addiction in some individuals, but not others (Howe et al., 2019). These findings raise doubt about the influence of a person's genetic make-up on their risk of addictive behaviours such as smoking, misuse of alcohol or gambling.

IN UTERO ENVIRONMENT

Development of a human being from the time of conception is called the gestational or in utero period. The terms refer to the environment inside the uterus, where the foetus develops. The influence of events, both negative and positive, during this gestational stage of development is profound.

Exposure to certain chemicals or events may cause major damage to the developing foetus. While medical science has developed many medications with noted benefits, all medications carry a risk of side effects that can range from mild to severe for the foetus. One of the most significant and publicised examples of tragic side effects is that of a medication containing the drug thalidomide. Thalidomide is a tranquilliser that became popular for its benefits in reducing severe morning sickness and it was regularly prescribed for pregnant women in the late 1950s and early 1960s (Hoffnung et al., 2019). The use of thalidomide, particularly during the first trimester of gestation (when morning sickness is usually most severe), resulted in major birth defects, including stunted or deformed or missing arms and legs, and brain damage. Many of these deformities were not realised until birth, as medical technology and routine antenatal screening tools such as ultrasound and other diagnostic technology were not yet developed. The medication was withdrawn for the purpose of managing morning sickness, but was later approved for use in treating some cancers and Hansen's disease (leprosy, a serious bacterial skin infection) (Hoffnung et al., 2019). Following the thalidomide tragedy, research focused on developing greater understanding of the in utero environment and subsequent impacts as the infant progressed into adulthood.

Other health influences on the developing foetus produce different consequences. For example, foetal alcohol spectrum disorder (FASD) occurs when the developing foetus has been exposed prenatally (prior to conception) and antenatally (in utero) to high levels of alcohol consumed by the mother (Dorrian et al., 2017). There are no established 'safe' levels of alcohol consumption during pregnancy, and women are advised not to drink (DoH, 2019a). FASD causes thiamine deficiency and can produce in utero growth restriction, low birthweight, dysmorphic features (altered facial structure including cleft lip and palate), central nervous system deficits, sub-optimal brain development and behavioural abnormalities (Kloss et al., 2018; Hoffnung et al., 2019; Dorrian et al., 2017). The link between congenital abnormalities and a mother's and/or biological father's use of alcohol, tobacco and other substances prior to conception is an area of emerging research (Kloss et al., 2018).

PERINATAL EVENTS

Perinatal events occur around the time of birth and during the first few weeks of life. They can include problems associated with birth itself, such as arising from a prolonged lack of oxygen during passage through the birth canal. Medication given to the mother to relieve pain during labour may influence the baby's alertness, heart or respiratory activity. Mostly, these medication effects are of short duration or easily reversed after birth. The baby could also experience physical damage from forceps, vacuum extraction or other equipment used during the delivery. Environmental exposure to certain events, such as infections or excessive light and heat, may also have adverse effects.

A child's survival and advantageous start in life has been linked to exclusive and sustained breastfeeding (WHO, 2021b). Children who are breastfed inherit maternal antibodies that contribute to protection against some diseases in the early days of life by boosting immune capabilities. WHO (2021b) indicates that children who are breastfed rank higher in intelligence tests and have reduced risk for weight issues, obesity and diabetes later in life. A significant amount of research has identified that continued breastfeeding reduces the risk of asthma (El-Heneidy et al., 2018).

Some mothers are not able to breastfeed for physical, psychological or social reasons. In these instances, health professionals in consultation with the mother must choose the most suitable formula substitution. Mothers who are not able to breastfeed need support rather than experiencing judgmental behaviours.

PAUSE & REFLECT

What range of factors do you think may hinder breastfeeding?
What are some physical and psychological benefits of breastfeeding, for mother and baby?

Prematurity is another perinatal source of vulnerability. Any baby born earlier than 37 weeks' gestation (a full-term pregnancy is 40 weeks' duration) is exposed to influences that it may not be physically ready to face. The earlier a baby is born, the more health and developmental difficulties it may face. Around 26 000 babies are born prematurely each year in Australia (APBPA, 2015). Premature babies often suffer immaturity of the lungs and the part of the brain that regulates temperature. If the digestive system is not fully ready, feeding may produce problems. These situations contribute to systemic organ challenges that can persist for long periods of childhood and even through the entire lifespan. An example of a disease status linked to prematurity is asthma. Children born prematurely have a 36% increased risk of developing this respiratory disease (Zhang et al., 2018). Asthma remains a health priority in Australia. It carries a considerable burden of disease due to physical constraints on the individual living with the condition, social and economic disadvantage, and a substantial impact on health care resources (DoH, 2019c).

EARLY LIFE EVENTS

In the early stages of life, the child is vulnerable to a variety of events that may predispose them to immediate harm and/or later problems in life. In addition to injuries and infections, a major category concerns relationships. Postnatal depression in the mother may prevent close bonding between mother and baby, predisposing the child to anxiety or other psychological problems that may not be identified until many years later. Mothers living with disability may have additional challenges in coping with the skills or stresses of caring for a baby. A child with a disability presents additional challenges that impact on a parent's capacity.

Impacts of disability are discussed in Chapter 14.

Childhood adversity can take the forms of abuse and neglect which present not only immediate threats to the baby but also long-term threats to cognitive functioning (Loxton et al., 2019). Deprivation of adequate food and shelter places the child at immediate risk of survival. Non-supportive or non-stimulating environments and emotional neglect place a child at risk of developmental delay. Good, trustworthy caregiving provides a child with opportunities to develop relationships and cognitive skills. Conversely, being a target of sexual abuse and domestic violence, or witnessing these events, poses significant consequences not only during the events but throughout all stages of the lifespan (Loxton et al., 2019).

Domestic violence and trauma are discussed in Chapter 12.

PERSONALITY TRAITS

Our vulnerabilities and capabilities are often linked to personality clusters. There have been many attempts to link personality traits to risk and protective factors for health. However, there is no single agreed definition of personality. In normal conversational terms, 'personality' refers to persistent impressions that an individual makes on others (their social stimulus value), which is very difficult to pin down because people will have different experiences with the individual. Some may see a person only at work, some only during leisure times and some, particularly health professionals, only when the individual is sick. Another problem is defining 'persistent', as people may act and respond differently according to circumstances.

One of the oldest attempts to link personality and health involved defining a personality trait called neuroticism (N type), linked to the responsiveness of the autonomic nervous system (Eysenck, 1976). The N type described people who tended to develop neurotic symptoms under even relatively mild stress. But judgments about the mildness of stress are made by an observer and do not take account of the individual's appraisal of the situation.

The most familiar theory attempting to link health and personality is the type A (coronary prone) behaviour pattern (Friedman & Rosenman, 1974). This theory proposes that individuals who show a pattern of competitive achievement, an exaggerated sense of time urgency and aggressiveness and hostility are at greatly increased risk of heart attack. Individuals are classed as type A if they show high levels of these characteristics in an interview or on a questionnaire, and type B if they show the opposite. Friedman and Rosenman (1974) suggested that these types were stable attributes of the individual that persisted over much of the lifespan. An individual could be measured at one point in time and is then assumed to stay true to type.

Type A personality traits are frequently associated with cardiac issues, and this was a popular field of research in the 1980s. Type A individuals often display a pattern of frequent high levels of emotional and/or physiological **arousal** in response to a variety of stimuli. This pattern of hyper-reactivity could lead to physical responses such as surges of adrenaline and periods of hypertension.

Arousal
The activation of the sympathetic nervous system, which produces visceral changes and provides energy for behaviour.

A type D personality (the distressed personality) often exhibits excessive worry and a sense of doom and gloom (negative affect). Health links include glycaemic (blood sugar) dysregulation, inactivity (resulting in weight gain), psychological and social challenges and increased inflammatory responses (Jandackova et al., 2017). While similar correlations were found between type A and type D individuals, type D personality displayed the highest risk overall for cardiac events (Steca et al., 2016).

In general, research attempting to link personality to illness, such as anxiety with type A, cardiac disease with type D and cancer with type C, is hampered by a number of constraints. First, there tends to be a lack of evidence about the stability of personality characteristics. Gradual changes in the type A behaviour pattern have been noted, particularly where the person's situation changes. In many cases, studies may examine the effects of long-term (or even fairly short-term) situations that are not typical ways of coping for that person. Coping strategies can be learnt and lifestyle changes implemented over time by that person.

Second, it is difficult to demonstrate cause and effect. It is very rare to characterise personality types in a large sample to show that the personality pre-dated the illness or disease. In some cases, the opposite is true—people with an illness or disease are found to have similar personality characteristics. In others, the illness and the personality characteristic may result from some common catastrophe.

Third, for personality to produce illness it must logically be through the mechanism of biochemical or physiological change. In most cases, links between personality types and bodily responses are unreliable. Many factors need to be considered when establishing such correlations.

4.4 CASE STUDY

MAYA AND ANXIETY

Maya is 68 and her friends say that she has become increasingly anxious as she has aged. For a long time, Maya has known that she often becomes breathless when exposed to animal hair, going outside on a cold day, working in the garden or is under stress. She is constantly worried about getting influenza, as this complicates her asthma management. Maya has seen a doctor who prescribed medication to use during an episode. She also has support from the respiratory nurse practitioner who provided education following her diagnosis with asthma.

Maya understands the importance of having her medication on hand and being able to easily fill her prescription and obtain emergency supplies. Her local pharmacy is vitally important to her. Maya does not venture out without her medication and tries to limit her outings during winter. She describes her medication as "an easy-to-use puffer that fits perfectly into my handbag and brings me fast relief with just one or two puffs".

1 What are some of Maya's vulnerabilities and how may they affect her asthma?
2 What are some of Maya's capabilities and how might they produce a positive impact?
3 What factors in her earlier life may have contributed to her asthma?
4 What triggers are present for Maya and what strategies does she use to manage them?
5 How might the concept of motivation relate to this scenario?

Behavioural strategies

Jones (1991) argued that behaviours are a response or strategy—an action on the part of the individual to challenges in the environment—and not simply a personality characteristic. The choice of strategy (action) may be maintained by the success that it produces. Behaviours that require less effort on the part of the individual yet produce a favourable outcome are more likely to be continued (Dorrian et al., 2017; Schreiber, 2016). Behaviours that do not lead to success are likely to be abandoned.

Individuals select a variety of behavioural strategies for dealing with the environment. These may be selected at any stage in life but tend to show a certain consistency from early life stages. Some strategies produce physical responses. When the sympathetic nervous system is activated, there is an increase in the number of circulating platelets (cell fragments that are used to patch damage in blood vessels) in the bloodstream. While this is protective in that it helps to deal with injuries to vessel walls, long-term continuation may increase the likelihood of atherosclerosis and heart disease.

Other people may choose to deal with the environment by adopting arousal reduction strategies, such as drinking or drug use, that put them at risk of organ damage and dependency problems if taken at risky levels or for prolonged periods. Disassociating or creating withdrawal responses to a harmful environment is another strategy. For example, a child who was severely abused or neglected early in life may adopt withdrawal as a strategy. This may allow the child to keep their resources for the task of simply maintaining life. This **conservation withdrawal** is a coping strategy and may literally be a lifesaver in the face of extreme events, but if it is used frequently it can result in severely disturbed coping in later life. Similar responses may occur in the presence of domestic violence and other situations where survival is threatened.

As with conservation withdrawal, any strategy can be viewed as either protective or harmful to the individual's health or well-being in some way, especially if it is carried to an extreme, used for long periods or is the only strategy. Since the early work of Heath (1964), numerous authors have suggested that individuals need to use a variety of coping strategies if they are to maximise their health and well-being. We need to be able to exert effort when effort will yield results, and withdraw from uncontrollable situations when effort will be wasted. Arousal reduction strategies are very useful, particularly if the stimulus causing arousal is not controllable. Arousal reduction based on control of the ability to relax or decrease impact, is especially useful.

In general, negative emotional states (e.g. anxiety, depression, hostility) are associated with negative health outcomes. Psychological and physiological factors explain some of this association. Behaviours also need to be included in the explanation, as individuals who are frequently anxious, depressed or angry may not live a healthy lifestyle or adopt healthy coping strategies (Tyrer et al., 2021). Some examples of health challenges are anxious and depressed people having difficulty getting adequate sleep, and angry people having difficulty maintaining relationships with others. Anti-social ways of addressing these situations may include self-treatment with alcohol, cigarettes, prescription or illegal drugs, and even with food.

A pessimistic style may be stable during adult life and predict a variety of negative health outcomes, including depression and physical illness. This is partially because a pessimistic style may become a self-fulfilling prophecy. If we appraise outcomes as likely to be bad, we are more likely to view them as bad, no matter how a more objective observer might see them. Again, this is more usefully understood as a strategic choice than as a fixed personality characteristic. Interventions including cognitive behavioural therapy have been demonstrated to significantly improve the lifestyle of many individuals in these situations (Tyrer et al., 2021). It also needs to be considered that continual changes in personality can occur during adulthood (Hoffnung et al., 2019).

CAPABILITIES AND COPING STRATEGIES

Just as with vulnerabilities, people have more or less stable capabilities and coping strategies. Dispositional **optimism** is a tendency to expect that outcomes in life will generally be good ones, which may affect the health of the individual in a number of ways. People might choose to minimise the significance of minor symptoms, or expect that others will provide support and therefore be more willing to ask for it. Positive attitudes informed by optimistic

Conservation withdrawal
An extreme pattern of withdrawal from interaction with a neglectful or abusive environment by an individual in order to preserve life.

The use of strategies to deal with stress is discussed in Chapter 13.

Eating disorders are discussed in Chapter 9.

Optimism
A tendency to expect that outcomes will generally be good.

traits in our core values, beliefs and modelled behaviours can contribute to recovery even in the presence of a chronic condition where return to pre-illness or pre-disease status is unlikely (White et al., 2018).

This suggests that a significant advantage of being optimistic lies in what it leads the individual to do. While an optimistic style is often productive, it is not wise to adopt an unrealistically optimistic approach, particularly where life-and-death decisions are concerned. A critical and objective evaluation of all the issues is likely to be more successful and can protect the individual from making poor guesses about the amount of risk that they face. We might admire the optimism of an elderly individual who decides to try bungy jumping, but if their bone density is low as a result of osteoporosis this may be a very dangerous decision for their health.

Hardiness
A behaviour pattern of commitment, a belief in the individual's ability to control events and a willingness to tackle challenges in the face of high levels of stress.

Another proposed capability is **hardiness** (Kobasa, 1979). Those who face many stressors but stay healthy were found to have a particular approach to life, including commitment, a belief in their ability to control events and a willingness to tackle challenges. These do not have to be fixed qualities but may be strategies applied as needed.

Beliefs about control appear to be particularly important to health outcomes. As we discuss in Chapter 12, beliefs influence an individual's appraisal of situations and have a significant role in how stressful those situations are seen to be. Behavioural capabilities may include a predisposition to make stable relationships, which has been found to be protective of health in a variety of ways.

Illness perceptions

Every individual will have a personal view or theory regarding their health. This is created from their unique experiences including symptoms, information from the external environment (e.g. what they have been told by others, what they have read or seen in social media) and previous experience with altered health. Views and theories will differ from person to person with the same illness, as the above factors vary between them. This set of **illness perceptions** will be more important to how the individual reacts than objective facts about the illness.

Illness perceptions
An individual's views or theories about their illness, based on bodily experiences such as symptoms, information from the external environment and previous experience with illness.

The individual uses their perceptions (their ideas) to guide their coping, including judgments about the seriousness of their condition, and decisions such as whether to take medication and perhaps elect or decline further investigations and interventions. It is useful at this point to know something about the basic processes that are covered by the term 'perception', and how perception works.

PERCEPTION

During our interactions with the world around us, we collect information about the nature of that world. For example, we use our senses to locate objects and identify them, listen and respond to the communications of others, and experience textures. Most of us assume that the information we get from our five senses (sight, hearing, smell, taste and touch) is a true and complete representation of the world. But is it? How often, for example, have you unsuccessfully searched a room for a set of lost keys, only to have someone else point out that they were in plain sight all the time? Have you noticed that, in the middle of a noisy crowd, if someone mentions your name you can isolate that one voice from among all others and track what it says?

In order to understand our interaction with the world, it is necessary to consider the related processes of sensation (the response of receptor organs to stimuli from the environment) and perception (the conscious experience of objects and events). The study of sensation usually takes place in a psychology, physiology or anatomy laboratory where the structures are fairly constant and the processes are straightforward and observable.

The study of perception is more complex. Although physiological and biochemical processes are part of the explanation of what is perceived, higher mental processes such as memory and cognition are needed to complete the picture.

In the medical context, perceptions raise problems or provide information. A dramatic experience-based illusion is phantom limb syndrome. This syndrome was first theorised in 1552 by French surgeon Ambroise Paré (Rugnetta, 2020). Some amputees experience a wide range of sensations including perceptions of movement, touch and, most distressingly, pain. These experiences relate to neuroplasticity, where the brain's neurons modify the connections and a pain phenomenon is created (Rugnetta, 2020). Although it is obvious to both patient and doctor that such events cannot be taking place in the missing limb, the fact that they are experienced as real must be accepted and the symptoms may require treatment. In recent times, phantom limb syndrome is being researched in connection with phantom breast syndrome that occurs after some mastectomy surgeries (Coates & Jha, 2019).

When a patient's perceptions vary from those of others around them, this may be a clue as to whether the problem is sensory (involving damage to the receptor) or perceptual. A blow to the back of the head, where the visual area of the cortex performs the task of integrating the two separate images from the eyes into one, may result in double vision. In anorexia nervosa, sufferers become so obsessed with their weight and body image that they may literally starve themselves to death. Although others see them as emaciated, they perceive themselves as too fat.

Perception and body image linked to eating disorders are discussed in Chapter 9.

BASIC PERCEPTUAL PROCESSES

One of the more remarkable properties of perception is that it serves to make sense of an enormously complex amount of sensory input. We are able to identify objects when their colour has been changed, when we see them from a new angle or even when they are reduced to a pattern of disconnected dots. This observation that we are able to perceive more than just the basic sensory stimuli led to the scientific study of how we perceive form. This work was begun by German researchers who used the term 'gestalt' (a meaningful grouping or whole). The Gestalt School was interested in the rules the brain uses to organise sensory input.

At the most basic level, some of the incoming stimuli are perceived to belong to objects; others are perceived not to. Stimuli perceived to belong to an object are referred to as the 'figure' and the others as the 'ground'. Note that what is a figure in one instance may be a ground in another; for example, pebbles may be the ground when we are searching for a shoe on the beach, but the figure when we find one or two pebbles in the shoe. During cricket matches, a sight screen is placed behind the bowler so that the batter can have a plain ground for the figure of the ball instead of having to pick the ball out of a background of spectators. Figure–ground relationships occur in other senses as well, such as when you are able to pick a single voice out of a crowd and track what it is saying. If you hear a significant word from another voice, you can switch your attention to make that voice the figure. The ability to make figure–ground discriminations appears to be innate. Studies of people who were blind from birth but had their sight restored in adulthood can discriminate figure from ground immediately. Long before they can identify objects by name or purpose without touching them, they can tell what a figure is and is not. This relates to **perceptual constancy**.

Perceptual constancy
The tendency to see objects as unchanged in spite of changes in sensory input.

Not all of our perceptual processes are innate, and even innate ones can be modified by **learning**. Cultural differences are a good example. In some cultures, the environment contains objects (designed from different shapes) that become familiar to individuals existing in that world. Some of the most impressive illusions are based on distortions from our expectations; for example, that walls are shaped as rectangles. In some places in Africa, round houses are the standard form, and cultures have few rectangular artefacts. This is an example of an individual's perceptual environment. In the same way, desert-dwelling peoples, including some First Peoples in Australia, can focus on detail at the horizon and are therefore less prone to illusions caused by context. Culture has a strong effect on how we perceive health and illness.

Learning
A change in understanding and/or behaviour that results from experience with the environment.

Culture is discussed in Chapter 14.

EXPECTATION AND PERCEPTION

Optical illusions are based on images that either give only partial information or provide misleading elements. Perceptual processes normally operate smoothly and consistently in interpreting the world. We are able to navigate without too many accidents, reinterpreting and remapping where problems arise. We expect that the world will make sense, that objects will remain constant and that sensory data and external events will correspond. Occasionally, we make mistakes because the cues we receive do not fit the reality of the objects we perceive. You may have walked into a familiar room in the dark, reached confidently for the light switch and found that your hand was not touching the switch. What happened was that you used your expectations about the switch's location and came up with an answer that was not quite right.

This situation relates to a perceptual set, which is a tendency to expect to see a particular thing or combination of things. A perceptual set may be the result of learning in a particular context. When a friend from the US first arrived in Australia, he frequently injured himself on doorknobs because the average Australian doorknob is a good deal higher than the average US doorknob. As there is almost certainly nothing innate about expectations regarding the heights of doorknobs, this must have resulted from learning.

PERSON PERCEPTION

The perception of other people involves many of the same processes as the perception of objects and is subject to many of the same errors. We use three main processes for inference about others, processes that are quite similar to perceptual constancies or sets. We assume constancy over time, across the characteristics of an individual and across categories of similar individuals. The first expectation we bring to person perception is when we meet someone for the first time, we tend to assume they are being their usual self. If that person is drunk, we may assume they have a drinking problem. This process is called temporal extension. It involves interpreting the past and future on a sample of behaviour and explains why first impressions are so strong. A second, or third or 20th contact can never completely erase the first. Gradually, if enough contradictory evidence is obtained, those expectations will change. There are a number of assumptions of the temporal extension model, and specific attention has recently focused on the influence of the individual's environment (Dishop, 2020).

The second expectation is that an individual will be consistent within themselves. This may not always hold true (Dishop, 2020). People change throughout their lifespan or in connection with an environment, such as the workplace. This assumption of individual consistency will lead us to assume that someone with an unusual haircut will be unusual in other ways, or that someone who can perform mathematical wonders will be intelligent.

The third process is stereotyping. In this, a member of a category of people is assumed to share all of the characteristics, including goals and objectives, of that category's stereotype (Dishop, 2020). Such assumptions include the ideas that fat people are jolly, people with red hair have quick tempers or health science students have no leisure interests. However, goals between individuals are not consistent even within a similar group (Dishop, 2020). For example, people may study medicine because of the employment opportunities, for the prestige, for the attractive salary or for an altruistic motivation such as wanting to help people.

It is easy to reject stereotyping as prejudice, and to maintain that everyone should be treated as an individual and on their own merits. However, much of our behaviour is based on dealing with categories of people—waiters, pedestrians, women or men, Americans or First Peoples—and having knowledge of appropriate ways to deal with the categories is very useful. Imagine how complex life would be if drivers had to treat each pedestrian as if they had no common patterns of behaviour, such as where they would cross the road or whether they would look first. Stereotyping inevitably leads to a breakdown of communication to the extent that these perceptions are inaccurate, and may even lead to disaster where it is used to justify discriminatory behaviour. This can influence an individual's access to appropriate treatment when they are ill.

4.5 CASE STUDY

SANDI AND BREAST CANCER

This case study considers how a younger woman may react to the experience of a serious health condition.

Sandi is a 32-year-old mother of two children, Sam (6) and Kristie (2). Her partner Abdul is a contract builder. Sandi is a partner in the family business: she schedules appointments for Abdul, orders materials and does the accounting. Working from home suits Sandi, especially while the children are so young. Sandi breastfed both her children and stopped night-time feeds with Kristie 12 months ago. From time to time, Sandi was aware of lumps in her breasts. Recently, when Sandi discovered a lump in her left breast, she thought it would pass. When it was still there three weeks later, she decided to see her doctor.

Sandi thought the lump was not normal and sought medical attention relatively quickly, but she did not consider the potential seriousness of her illness. Her GP quickly referred Sandi for a mammogram and a cell biopsy of the lump. She was told that the results indicated cancer and that surgery was recommended for removal of the tumour and associated lymph nodes under her arm. These events occurred quickly.

After Sandi was discharged from hospital she said, "I no longer felt like a woman. I lost my breast. I did not feel attractive anymore. When you see your mastectomy scar, it starts under your arm and goes right across your chest. There's no way you can hide that, it's there. Every time you look in the mirror you are reminded of the breast cancer."

Sandi felt angry that her happy life had been taken away. She was also distressed by the scarring to her body. At her life stage she was enjoying her family responsibilities. She was disadvantaged by the fact she had to attend medical consultations and outpatient treatments by herself without a support person, because her husband and other family members were either working and/or caring for the couple's children.

Sandi found herself emotionally supporting others in the family, "My close family, including my mother, found it very difficult to accept the diagnosis and I found I was counselling them. That was demanding because I had to set aside my own emotions in order to cope with other people's grief. I lost a lot of weight from the stress. I stopped doing activities like swimming because I really didn't want my kids to be seeing my body like this."

1   How might Sandi have reacted differently to the thought of something being wrong when she first discovered the lump in her breast? What perceptions might she have had at this time?

2   How would the speed of the diagnosis have affected Sandi's ability to cope with this event?

3   How did Sandi react to the recommended treatment?

4   In what ways did Sandi's life stage influence her responses to the breast cancer treatments?

5   How might Sandi's grief reactions about her illness differ from those of a person in their 70s?

6   What are some of Sandi's capabilities? How might they affect her ability to complete her treatment and move forward?

CHAPTER SUMMARY

Learn more
Access additional resources to broaden your understanding of this chapter. See the Guided Tour for access details.

- Individuals who identify that they are ill—that something is not right with them—may experience physical, cognitive, emotional and behavioural reactions.

- The process by which a well person comes to think of themselves as unwell is called illness behaviour. This can be thought of as a series of decisions about the individual's experience that may lead them to take on the sick role.

- Taking on the sick role involves accepting two obligations (to desire to get well and to cooperate with appropriate experts) in return for being granted two rights (being excused from normal responsibilities and not being blamed for being ill). If the sick role is accepted for too long, the person may be regarded as showing abnormal illness behaviour.

- Reactions to illness are influenced by characteristics of the illness, the individual and the situation. Each person has a particular set of vulnerabilities and capabilities that may result from genetic factors, which either predispose the individual to the development of future problems or protect the individual from them.

- Genetic predispositions do not guarantee a particular set of health outcomes, as these can be modified by exposure to the environment. This can happen during development in the uterus (in utero factors), around the time of birth (perinatal factors) and throughout the lifespan.

- Vulnerabilities and capabilities can include strategies that are adopted for dealing with life situations, some of which appear to have negative effects (hyper-reactivity, negative emotions) while others appear to have positive effects on health (optimism, hardiness, positive emotions).

- Illness perceptions arise from the individual's experience and guide their behaviour with regard to the illness. These perceptions follow the same principles as other perceptual processes, involving innate and learnt components. As with perceptual illusions, they may not accurately reflect reality.

FURTHER READING

Abrahams H (2007) *Supporting Women after Domestic Violence: Loss, Trauma and Recovery.* Jessica Kingsley Publications.

Hassed C (2011) The essence of mental health and mindfulness. *TLN Journal* 18(2), 36–9. https://search.informit.org/doi/10.3316/aeipt.194045

Kirmayer LJ & Looper KJ (2006) Abnormal illness behaviour: Physiological, psychological and social dimensions of coping with distress. *Current Opinions in Psychiatry* 19(1), 54–60. doi: 10.1097/01. yco.0000194810.76096.f2. PMID: 16612180

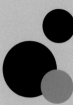

5 Understanding Reactions to Chronic Conditions

CHAPTER OBJECTIVES

By the end of this chapter, you should be able to:

» define and give examples of chronic conditions

» discuss the prevalence of different chronic conditions

» outline the emotional, physical and social challenges faced by individuals who have a chronic condition

» describe common reactions to living with a chronic condition

» explain factors that may influence positive coping

» apply self-care models to explain varying ways of managing a chronic condition

» describe practical interventions and care programs for people with chronic conditions

KEYWORDS

» acceptance

» affective support

» chronic condition

» cognitive responses

» collaborative model

» compassion fatigue

» complicated/chronic grief

» controllability

» disability

» efficacy beliefs

» helplessness

» incidence

» instrumental support

» medical model

» multimorbidity

» optimism

» perceived benefit

» prevalence

» psychosocial interventions

» self-agency model

» self-care

Chronic conditions

Chronic conditions are permanent, incurable and irreversible. While such conditions do not cause death, they do require ongoing attention and care. The prognosis for many chronic conditions may be unclear and treatment and/or management prolonged. Increasingly, people with chronic conditions experience **multimorbidity** which is two or more chronic conditions at the same time (AIHW, 2020b). Multimorbidity is associated with complex health needs and poor quality of life. For health service providers, multimorbidity requires ongoing management and coordination of specialised care across different sections of the health system.

Common chronic conditions in Australia include arthritis, asthma, back pain and problems, cancer, cardiovascular diseases (selected heart, stroke and vascular diseases; excluding hypertension), chronic obstructive pulmonary disease, diabetes, chronic kidney disease, mental and behavioural conditions (including mood disorders, alcohol and drug problems and dementia) and osteoporosis (ABS, 2018a). These 10 selected conditions are regularly monitored by the Australian government. Chronic conditions (e.g. some forms of cancer) may be life-threatening, some (e.g. dementia and vision impairment) may require help with daily activities over a long period of time and some are painful—but all demand adaptive behaviours on the part of the individual. Other chronic conditions are ambiguous, with vague symptoms that are difficult to diagnose. These include interstitial cystitis, chronic fatigue syndrome, fibromyalgia, irritable bowel syndrome, Crohn's disease and coeliac disease. These conditions require people to be persistent in their attempts to obtain an accurate diagnosis, leading to frustration and uncertainty which add to the emotional burden of living with a chronic condition.

Chronic conditions can also cause **disability**, depending on the extent of impact on daily life. It is important to understand that disability is neither inability nor sickness, as almost everyone will have at least one disability at some point in their life (AIHW, 2020b). The general public, governments and health professionals may have different views about how 'disability' is perceived, labelled and discussed. Negative perceptions by health professionals may marginalise individuals with disabling conditions and create obstacles and barriers to the access and provision of services. In fact, disability is as much about environmental obstacles and challenges as it is a medical condition.

Chronic condition
A medical condition that is permanent, incurable and irreversible.

Multimorbidity
The presence of two or more chronic conditions in a person at the same time.

Disability is also discussed in Chapter 14.

Disability
A chronic condition of the body, mind or senses that results in a limitation, restriction or impairment in performing activities of daily living.

PAUSE & REFLECT

What are your personal beliefs about individuals with a disability?

The words used about people influence attitudes. Previously, it was acceptable to describe individuals with a mental or physical disability as 'retarded' or 'handicapped'. These terms are no longer acceptable because they imply that the person is somehow completely incapable. Even the term 'disabled' should not be used because it suggests that the whole individual is disabled and has no abilities. Although less fluent, the terms 'person with a disability' and 'person living with a disability' are more accurate and less limiting.

Prevalence of chronic conditions

Prevalence
The number of existing and new cases of a specific disease present in a particular population at a certain time.

As discussed in Chapter 1, **prevalence** is the number of existing and new cases of a specific disease present in a given population at a certain time. Chronic conditions account for the bulk of health care expenditure and mortality in Australia (AIHW, 2020b). Individuals living with chronic conditions form a large health care consumer group. According to the National Health Survey 2017–18, over 47% of the population (more than 11 million people) were estimated to have one or more of the 10 selected chronic conditions in 2017–18 (ABS, 2018a). Mental health or behavioural conditions were the most reported (20% or 4.8 million) chronic condition for both males and females.

Incidence
The rate at which new cases of a specific disease occur in a particular population during a specified period.

Incidence (the rate at which new cases occur in a population during a specified period) of disability tends to increase with age. While 7.6% of children aged 0–14 years have a disability, around 50% of Australians aged 65 and over had a disability in 2017–18 (ABS, 2019b). Disability is not inevitable in older age but it does become more common. Conditions such as dementia, back pain and arthritis are leading causes that severely limit activities of daily living (AIHW, 2020b). Ageing can also accelerate the level of impairment associated with a chronic condition.

Most chronic conditions of childhood, unlike those of adults, are not preventable by lifestyle changes. Surprisingly, at least 10% of adolescents live with a chronic condition. Some conditions are characterised by increasing incidence (e.g. type 1 diabetes) or improving survival rates (e.g. cystic fibrosis), while other conditions such as cancer or mental health conditions are concerning because the outcomes are poorer for adolescents than for adults. Young people with chronic conditions are doubly disadvantaged. In a scoping review, DiFusco et al. (2019) reported that adolescents with chronic cardiac conditions engaged in risky behaviours (e.g. alcohol and drug use) as often or more often than their healthy peers, but had the potential for greater adverse health outcomes from these behaviours. For young males, the risk of disability lies more frequently in injury from accidents, whereas in the middle years of adulthood the risk factors tend to be work-related injury or conditions such as arthritis, cardiovascular disease, hearing problems and mental health conditions (AIHW, 2020b).

Gender may be associated with certain chronic conditions. Arthritis is a group of conditions characterised by inflammation of the joints causing pain, stiffness, disability and deformity (AIHW, 2020b). Worldwide, osteoarthritis (degenerative disease of the joints) is the most common musculoskeletal disorder. It affects 2.2 million Australians, with females more affected than males (AIHW, 2020b). Similarly, osteoporosis (low bone density) is a disease that mainly affects postmenopausal women. Although it is preventable, osteoporosis is a silent disease because symptoms often do not become evident until there is a major incident, such as a fracture. Women across all age groups are also more likely to be diagnosed with depression. This is not to say that gender is predictive of certain chronic conditions developing. Rather, this relationship is more likely to reflect that women live longer (85.4 years) than men (81.5 years) and so proportionally there are more women with degenerative conditions such as dementia or arthritis. Similarly, it is well known that women are more likely to express their distress and seek professional help than are men, and so are more likely to be diagnosed with symptoms of depression or any other condition.

Impact on daily life

Living with a chronic condition or acquired disability can have disruptive effects on many areas of functioning, and requires positive and persistent coping strategies. The sense of loss may be more debilitating than the condition itself. People with a chronic condition may not require acute medical interventions beyond the primary diagnosis and treatment, but this does not mean that they are free to live an unrestricted life. Chronic conditions affect work, social life, relationships and recreational activities, as well as interactions with family, friends and the community. Individuals are faced with managing their condition every day. Some chronic conditions limit movement and the person may require daily assistance with activities such as hygiene, walking or communication. Much of this assistance is provided by informal sources such as family, friends and neighbours (AIHW, 2020b). Individuals not only live with the physical symptoms of their condition (pain for arthritis sufferers) but may also endure ongoing fatigue, depression and sleep disturbances. They also often suffer financial stress from treatment costs and loss of income.

5.1 CASE STUDY

BEN AND MULTIPLE SCLEROSIS

This case study explores the experience of living with a chronic condition.

Ben is a divorced 42-year-old mechanic who owns a busy mechanical repair outfit. He has two teenage children and has custody every second weekend. Recently, Ben experienced tingling in the fourth and fifth fingers of his left hand and began to feel uncoordinated when working on a motor. It was as if he had lost feeling in his hands. He went to his doctor, who identified some minor neurological changes (intermittent tingling and slight loss of strength). The doctor thought there was nothing to worry about and the symptoms disappeared after six weeks. When the symptoms reappeared the following year, Ben was referred to a neurologist for a comprehensive assessment. The MRI revealed abnormal changes in his brain and spine. A detailed history identified that symptoms had been evident for the past five years. Ben was diagnosed with multiple sclerosis (MS) and began intramuscular injections every second day. These need to continue even when he has no symptoms.

1   What might be Ben's immediate reaction to his diagnosis and treatment?
2   Which areas of Ben's life might be affected by the symptoms of his condition?

MS is a chronic and highly disabling condition. The myelin thickness (covering) around nerves is reduced; this results in muscle weakness, balance problems and spasticity (MSAustralia, 2021). Although MS usually affects young women, 30% of sufferers are men. For three in four (77%) people with a disability, their main form of disability (i.e. their main condition or the one causing the most problems) is physical. This includes diseases of the nervous system (6.7%), such as cerebral palsy and MS (ABS, 2019b). The degree of disability depends on which nerve myelin is affected and the course of the disease: relapsing, remitting or progressive. Fatigue is one of the symptoms most frequently reported. Therapy for MS involves supportive care, management of symptoms, and disease-modifying drugs that may delay progression and reduce the number of exacerbation (deteriorating) episodes.

Psychological responses to a chronic condition vary, but it is common for individuals to feel helpless, anxious and depressed. At times they may feel resentful that this is happening to them. As the condition continues, the person may feel inferior to others, guilty for being a burden on their family, fearful of the future, discouraged by the continuing decline in their health and lonely because of social isolation.

Feelings of anxiety may be associated with a lack of knowledge about the condition and its long-term implications. While some conditions have a relatively stable course, others involve cycles of exacerbation and remission, with all the associated fluctuations of emotion. Responses may be akin to mourning, since the individual experiences several losses—including loss of bodily functions—and a wide range of social limitations. As discussed in Chapter 3, stages of mourning include shock, denial, emotional confusion, attempted resolution and acceptance or closure. Individuals are unlikely to progress through these stages in a neat, linear fashion; stages tend to overlap, occur in parallel and recur.

Complicated/chronic grief
Unresolved grief characterised by an impaired ability to recall personal life details, as well as imagine and plan for the future.

Living with debilitating chronic conditions may lead to **complicated or chronic grief**. MacCallum and Bryant (2011) observed that individuals experiencing chronic grief had difficulty recalling positive personal life details and imagining future events. The ability to picture the future is important for effective planning of day-to-day activities, evaluating future outcomes, judging likelihood of success and deciding on a particular course of action. Imagining specific details of events in the future can affect whether or not a person takes action. For example, individuals who develop specific plans about where and when they intend to start a particular health-related behaviour (e.g. going for a 7am walk in the park) are more likely to do it. Individuals living with a chronic condition are faced with many new and challenging situations. Difficulty imagining specific future events may impact not only on day-to-day tasks, but also on the degree to which these individuals are able to develop new roles and aspects of their identity.

The broader issues of coping with stress are addressed in Chapter 13.

Positive emotions also play a role in living with a chronic condition. Humour, hope and courage have been found to be positive coping factors for individuals learning to live with a chronic condition. In one Irish study, patients with diabetes often used humour during consultations as a coping and communication strategy (Schöpf et al., 2017). For others, reflecting on a sense of purpose and meaning of the experience was helpful.

Individuals with a physical disability because of their chronic condition also suffer other life stressors and limitations, including poor employment prospects and low income. Many pay for in-home care, or their family may need to pay for respite care. A physical disability may isolate a person, making it difficult to form friendships and intimate relationships, which in turn can contribute to emotional issues such as depression (Holland et al., 2016). Some people who are socially isolated and dependent on others can be at increased risk of abuse from carers, particularly family members under stress (Santos et al., 2021).

Chronic conditions also have ramifications for family or other carers. Consider, for example, the roles and responsibilities of parents not only caring for a child with a chronic condition, but also managing the child's developing understanding of their illness (as discussed in Chapter 2). An Australian study by an author of this text revealed that parents' attitudes often define the situation, including whether they focus on illness and vulnerability or on normalcy and capability (Creedy et al., 2005). Parents of children with a chronic condition carry out many tasks to manage the condition, such as administering medication, developing a consistent parenting philosophy and having a family routine that is as normal as possible and allows some fun. Finally, there are future implications and expectations about the impact on the child and the family. A picture emerges of what it might be like to care for a child with a chronic condition or disability, including how parents can shape the child's identity as someone who is sick or someone who copes, and the demands on parents to be knowledgeable and capable about treatments, and work together to have an integrated care strategy. Other issues include how the child's condition might dictate or dominate family life, and the parents' concern for the child's future. At the other end of the age spectrum, the burden of caring for ageing parents is increasingly falling on their middle-aged children.

Having a close relative or friend involved in care can have positive implications for the person's experience of living with the condition, in terms of both following treatment advice and engaging in other health-promoting behaviours. However, providing care for someone with a chronic condition can take a toll on family and other caregivers. Those providing long-term care for individuals with a chronic condition can suffer **compassion fatigue**, which is one cost of caring for an individual who is not going to recover completely (Lynch et al., 2018). Compassion fatigue is a deep physical, emotional and spiritual exhaustion related to repeated exposure to another's suffering and can lead to depression, anxiety and burnout.

Compassion fatigue
A deep physical, emotional and spiritual exhaustion related to repeated exposure to another's suffering.

PAUSE & REFLECT

Imagine that you have just been diagnosed with a chronic condition such as diabetes, asthma or epilepsy.

How would you feel?

Would one type of chronic condition be better or worse than another? Why?

5.2 CASE STUDY

BEN (CONT.)

Initially, Ben found it difficult to think of himself as sick, and he was resentful about the need to have injections every second day. A year after his diagnosis, the symptoms reappeared for three weeks. This episode unsettled Ben. The reality of his condition became obvious to him in a way that he had not thought about before. He was worried about his future: his health, his business, his ability to care for his children, and how his new partner Li Mei would cope with being in a relationship with 'an invalid'. These thoughts kept going around in his mind and contributed to sleeplessness and, subsequently, depression.

His doctor prescribed antidepressant medication, but after a week Ben didn't feel any different and stopped taking it. His schedule of injections was changed to weekly to reduce the likelihood of drug fatigue. Ben's brother, who is also a mechanic, agreed to join the business and now manages the repairs. Ben continues to be involved by doing minor work and managing the financial aspects. He can cope with routine tasks but becomes frustrated easily and has difficulty with problem-solving due to changes to the frontal lobe of his brain. He wonders how he will cope when he has another episode.

1   What other day-to-day difficulties might Ben and the people in his life face?
2   How might Ben's children respond to changes in him? What might they understand about his condition?

Variations in individual coping

Individual differences in vulnerability are discussed in Chapter 4.

The discussion of cognition and health continues in Chapter 7.

Cognitive responses
How a person views their condition.

Helplessness
A negative and maladaptive response to a condition that has long-term adverse implications for psychological and physical health.

Acceptance
A more neutral or middle-of-the-road reaction to a condition that diminishes the negative meaning of the condition and decreases negative thinking.

Perceived benefit
A positive response to a condition that adds optimistic meaning through increased positive thinking.

Psychological responses and problems associated with chronic conditions are not always similar. It is incorrect to assume that all people living with chronic conditions or disabilities experience or cope with a particular condition in the same way. Individuals may respond with either problem-focused coping or emotion-focused coping, or both. Whether individuals cope well with their condition relies on a range of factors, including the type of condition, how they rate their health, the way they think about their condition, their belief in their ability to cope (their optimism) and the controllability of their condition.

For example, a diagnosis of HIV/AIDS has a profound psychological impact, with complex stressors and multiple symptoms along with potential discrimination and loss of social support. Cancer is a particularly frightening diagnosis as it often requires a person to face the possibility of death and an unpleasant and difficult treatment regime that has debilitating side effects. As identified in the case study of Ben, MS is a progressive disease that produces a wide range of symptoms that the person cannot predict or regulate. MS affects several life domains, including physical well-being, work, family, relationships and sexual functioning.

Cognitive responses, or the way a person views their condition, have received considerable attention in research. Research has shown that people's views about their health can range from excellent to poor, even when they have the same chronic condition. When faced with the long-term stress of a chronic condition, individuals can react in favourable and unfavourable ways. These responses represent reliable and stable patterns and can be classified into three common cognitive evaluations of what is an inherently life-changing situation (Crielaard et al., 2021).

The first type of response is **helplessness**, which emphasises negative aspects, and pictures the condition as unmanageable, uncontrollable and unpredictable. This cognitive pattern is associated with increased functional disability. The second type of response is **acceptance**, a more neutral or middle-of-the-road reaction that diminishes the negative meaning of the condition and the amount of negative thinking. It consists of accepting the condition and learning to tolerate or live with it. **Perceived benefit** is the third response. It adds optimistic meaning to the condition and increases the likelihood of positive thinking and coping. Individuals who think this way may see the condition as an opportunity to reassess their life and priorities, such as spending more time with their family or slowing down at work. Acceptance and other adaptive thoughts are associated with less focus on disease-related activity, fewer physical complaints and more positive mood (Burian et al., 2021).

Efficacy beliefs play a key role in coping. Fear remains high if the person does not believe the recommended treatment is effective (response efficacy) and if they do not believe they can carry out the treatment (self-efficacy). In a study of young people with type 1 (insulin-dependent) diabetes, Lee et al. (2019) found that many participants reported high anxiety about the future and had low perceived control of their condition. Rather than taking action to manage the condition and address threats to their physical well-being, they tried to reduce their fear in unhelpful ways (e.g. smoking marijuana, drinking alcohol, taking tranquillisers and other drugs, or distracting themselves).

Optimism is another factor that determines how well or poorly individuals cope. There are three types of optimistic beliefs: positive outcome expectancies (an expectation that things will turn out well), efficacy expectancies (the belief that demanding situations can be managed) and optimistic bias (a tendency to unrealistically expect that only positive things will happen). A systematic review of 21 studies with 3769 participants investigated the role of cognitive, emotional and behavioural factors on pain and disability following shoulder surgery. De Baets et al. (2019) found outcome expectations and self-efficacy predicted pain and disability, and optimism helped to moderate pain catastrophising and disability. These findings suggest that individuals with positive outcome and efficacy expectancies are more likely to adapt and take positive action to cope.

Controllability is also associated with coping and can be both actual and perceived. If the individual believes they can control symptoms, they are more likely to adjust, enjoy life and avoid depression. However, some diseases are more manageable than others. Controllability of MS, for example, is low, whereas type 2 diabetes can be controlled through diet, exercise and insulin. A person with type 2 diabetes, therefore, is likely to perceive high levels of control over their condition and frequently demonstrate this.

Perceptions of control can be influenced by the unique characteristics of specific conditions. Asthma and epilepsy, for example, can have dramatic and severe episodes interspersed with periods of relative symptom-free health. Epilepsy, however, is associated with a lower quality of life in young people, partly because a seizure is more dramatic and unpredictable than an asthma attack.

Models of self-care

Self-regulation, first introduced by Leventhal et al. (1980), is a useful theoretical perspective for understanding how a person manages their chronic condition. **Self-care** or self-regulation in the context of a chronic condition relates to the action taken by a person to improve their health and limit the negative effects of the condition. A review of literature on the concept of self-care (LeBlanc & Jacelon, 2018) concluded that self-care is a person's capacity, disposition and activity when managing their multiple chronic conditions. These features (capacity, disposition, action) influence one another and are hierarchical and continuous (LeBlanc & Jacelon, 2018). There is good evidence that self-regulation has many benefits, including improved health status and better quality of life. Individuals who can regulate their thoughts and feelings are more likely to proactively approach problems and develop certain thoughts and beliefs that guide how they respond to their condition in order to manage it.

Efficacy beliefs
A person's belief that they can carry out required treatments and that the treatments will be effective.

Optimism
A tendency to expect that outcomes will generally be good.

Controllability
The level of control over a condition. It can be both actual and perceived.

Self-care
A person's capacity, disposition and activity when managing their chronic condition.

Self-regulation is modified by feedback such as blood glucose levels in the case of diabetes or peak flow measures of lung capacity for a person with asthma. These measures provide immediate feedback to a person about how well they are managing their condition, and motivate them to keep up the good work or make some changes in their lives. Coping strategies may include short-term and immediate action to manage the physical symptoms, such as taking preventive medicine to avoid serious asthma attacks, or long-term action such as maintaining a low-dust environment in the home. Coping also includes learning how to engage with the health system for care, obtain support from health care services and organisations, and seek out information.

Other self-care behaviours, such as diet and exercise, require persistence before longer-term impact is observed. Since this feedback is not immediate, individuals are less likely to carry out this aspect of regulating their condition. There are many models of self-care or self-management for chronic conditions. We discuss three: the medical model, the collaborative model and the self-agency model.

Medical model
A model that is prescriptive and focused on patients' compliance with or adherence to medical management instructions.

The **medical model** for managing a chronic condition is prescriptive. It focuses on patients' compliance with or adherence to medical management instructions about medication and testing routines as directed by health care practitioners (in most cases, the general practitioner). In this model the individual is objectified as the patient, the health practitioner is the authority, and the person isn't given much credence. The doctor manages the disease process, with the patient compelled to trust the doctor's medical knowledge. The focus is on medical criteria. Little thought is given to how the condition affects other aspects of day-to-day life and how to cope with that.

Collaborative model
A model in which patients are active participants, in partnership with health care providers, in regulating and managing their chronic condition.

A less paternalistic model of care sees the person as an active participant in regulating and managing the chronic condition. This **collaborative model** of self-management is a partnership between the person and health care providers that draws on a combination of biomedical knowledge and patient experience. This model is often reflected in services offered by community-based clinics, where people can learn about a range of strategies to manage their day-to-day life as well as medical management involving medication and monitoring (Shulman et al., 2021). A variation of this model is supported self-care, which aims to empower individuals, views the person as the expert, and ultimately reduces demand on health care resources. The role of health professionals in this model is to identify the person's existing strengths and skills and work towards using those abilities more effectively. Increasingly, programs based on this model reveal high levels of patient satisfaction and reduced health care costs (Shulman et al., 2021).

Self-agency model
A model in which individuals take charge of their condition, identify their responses and manage their lives accordingly.

The **self-agency model** requires individuals to take charge of their condition, identify their responses to the condition and manage their lives to create order, control and discipline. Although individuals with a chronic condition are usually required to regularly take medication and follow the recommended regime of care, this model also involves self-monitoring and developing lifestyle habits to accommodate the condition. People may exhibit strategic cheating or non-compliance. It is possible for a person with diabetes, say, to be less strict with their diet and medication in a well-thought-out fashion, such as when they need to make compromises in their diet for work or a social event. In the self-agency model, individuals choose when to call upon professional health expertise. People who have lived with their condition for a long time often develop a great deal of expertise about managing their lives and their condition. The knowledge and skills of the health care providers are added to their own. The power of self-agency was recognised in one study in which older adults with higher self-agency

Part IV of this book looks at other aspects of agency.

were more likely to be independent and report fewer depressive symptoms than those with less agency (Isik et al., 2020).

PAUSE & REFLECT

There are different models of self-care.

What factors could determine whether individuals with a chronic condition, and health care practitioners, prefer one model over another?

5.3 CASE STUDY

BEN (CONT.)

One of Ben's friends looked up MS on the internet and gave him a lot of information about it. Some of it was very confusing and technical, especially regarding exacerbations of the condition. Ben and Li Mei went back to his doctor to try to get a clear, simple explanation of the long-term consequences of MS. The doctor spoke about the condition and suggested that Ben and Li Mei attend the MS clinic at the local hospital, as well as book in for an information session there.

Over dinner on the weekend, Ben's teenage daughter said that she had been reading about people with MS. Hayley had not realised that MS affects a lot of people around the world. Later, Hayley told her mother that she had noticed some physical changes in her dad, and he sometimes became angry over little things that would not have bothered him before. She was worried about him and wondered what she could do to help.

By going to the information session, Ben and Li Mei started to get some understanding of what having MS really meant. Ben was struggling with the regular injections and found it hard to cope with functional changes to his hands and balance, as well as his mood swings. He sometimes felt quite well and wondered if the injections were really necessary and if the doctor's dire warnings about what might happen to him were just scaremongering. Ben believed that his MS isn't that bad. Surely nothing really serious would happen to him?

1   How might Li Mei benefit from going to the clinic?
2   How would you describe Ben's coping at this stage?
3   What sort of support does Hayley need right now? How can she best support her dad?

Practical care and interventions

By definition, chronic conditions do not have a cure. Therefore, health professionals try to help the person to adapt, be resilient and obtain the best quality of life they can. Helping people with a chronic condition requires a shift in thinking from acute-care models to flexible, long-term approaches. Rehabilitation and other health interventions focus not only on physical health, but on helping the person to engage or re-engage with day-to-day life and broader society in the form of work, community groups and so on.

The aim of interventions for those with chronic conditions or a disability is to achieve a satisfying, hopeful life in which contributions can be made and valued. This requires the support of people who will support and believe in the person. Life-long coping requires persistence and patience since there will be many small gains and just as many setbacks. People with chronic conditions need a range of different supports. One study of people with cancer found that **affective (emotional) support** (e.g. family and friends communicating positive feelings and providing constructive feedback and advice) was more useful than **instrumental support** (e.g. physical assistance or checking up on the person) (Linn et al., 2019). Affective support is known to help reduce symptoms of depression and help individuals to adapt. Instrumental support does not have such positive effects, even though individuals recognise that they often need physical help with their condition.

Health care providers working with people with chronic conditions are usually part of a multidisciplinary team of nurses, physicians, psychologists or other mental health workers, pharmacists, occupational or physical therapists, and members of the clergy or other spiritual support people. This multidisciplinary approach can be illustrated in the care of a child with cerebral palsy. Cerebral palsy results from damage to the brain prior to or during birth. There are physical consequences (e.g. muscular impairment) that affect physical coordination, speech and movement. As the child grows, there are risks of secondary physical problems such as bronchitis, and emotional problems such as depression and anxiety. An integrated disciplinary approach involving doctors, nurses, psychologists, dieticians and physiotherapists is required because the condition adversely affects mobility, self-care and learning, and limits social roles and participation in education, work and relationships.

Affective support
The act of communicating feelings and providing constructive feedback and advice.

Instrumental support
The act of giving tangible assistance and practical aid.

HEALTH PROMOTION

The concept of health has traditionally been defined as the absence of disease (as discussed in Chapter 1), making it difficult to conceive that people with a disability might otherwise be healthy. The health of individuals with a chronic condition varies as much as it does among people without any such condition. Health is a dynamic entity that oscillates from good to poor throughout life. Someone with a spinal cord injury who eats well, exercises and maintains the right weight could be considered at the higher end of the health continuum, whereas another individual with the same disability might eat poorly, be overweight and sedentary, and thus be at the lower end of the scale.

Health promotion strategies are discussed in Chapter 16.

Health promotion and disease prevention are crucial for people with chronic conditions, not only to improve wellness and functioning but also to prevent secondary conditions such as obesity and osteoporosis. However, people with disabilities may experience difficulty accessing general health monitoring and screening services. Due to changing building codes, clinics need to easily accommodate people with wheelchairs, and enable patients to stand or manoeuvre themselves to access standard equipment such as mammogram machines or examination tables. People with a disability may need longer appointment times and more help from additional staff during examinations. During adolescence, a young woman with a chronic condition may not be interested in long-term disease prevention for conditions such as osteoporosis or diabetes; however, education at this stage is vital to take preventive action as these conditions are more likely to appear earlier in women with disabilities (Sharifi et al., 2019).

PSYCHOSOCIAL INTERVENTIONS

Psychosocial interventions aim to address the psychological and social consequences of living with a chronic condition. Emotional support and information will help reduce the initial confusion and shock associated with diagnosis, and, in the longer term, help individuals and their families to avoid negative emotional symptoms. Accurate information improves patients' coping because they are able to develop a realistic view of their capabilities. Psychosocial interventions also need to focus on practical aspects of living with, and managing, the chronic condition. In the case of asthma, for example, understanding factors that trigger an attack, treating symptoms quickly and staying calm and optimistic means fewer attacks, fewer visits to hospital outpatient departments, fewer days off work and better overall quality of life.

Attention should also be given to challenging false beliefs and reframing possible negative thoughts about the condition as an unmanageable or uncontrollable burden. Psychosocial interventions aim to strengthen individual self-efficacy beliefs regarding coping with adversity, and to encourage more positive reappraisal. A systematic review of 33 studies found that people who are positive and optimistic about their condition are more likely to rate their health as better and have lower health care costs than those with less positive views (Finkelstein-Fox et al., 2020). Providing people with HIV access to support groups and education about stress management and coping skills, for example, means they can stay focused on engaging with life, suffer less distress and depression, and cope better with treatment (Finkelstein-Fox et al., 2020). Provision of psychosocial interventions has also been associated with increased satisfaction with treatment, closer adherence to the treatment plan and better quality of life than might otherwise be possible.

> **Psychosocial interventions**
> Psychological, social and educational strategies that aim to minimise the adverse emotional and social impact of a condition on an individual and their family.

5.4 CASE STUDY

BEN (CONT.)

Three years have passed and Ben is recovering from a recent episode in which he experienced severe muscle spasms. He often gets tired, and has needed to make substantial changes to his work and home routines. As the disease has progressed, Ben has experienced symptoms including muscle spasms, sensitivity to heat and sexual problems. By mid-afternoon he feels exhausted and is unable to concentrate. He tries to avoid heat as his symptoms seem worse after a hot shower or when he is close to a hot car engine at work. During this last episode, Ben felt light-headed and as though everything was spinning. His doctor later explained that these symptoms are caused by damage to the nerve pathways that coordinate vision and other inputs into the brain that are needed to maintain balance. Ben has vision problems with blurring in one eye.

He has suffered other depressive episodes and, with Li Mei's encouragement, he is taking his prescribed antidepressant medication. Ben and Li Mei are attending sessions at the MS clinic at the local hospital every month. At the sessions, Ben met other men with MS and they have formed a men's support group. He also learnt some useful tips on coping with fatigue and maintaining a good level of physical well-being. His business is still operating with the help of his brother.

1   What else might Ben be able to do to improve his situation?

2   What are some of the physical and psychosocial issues Ben will face as he gets older?

PAUSE & REFLECT

Negative beliefs and attitudes make it more difficult for individuals to adjust to their condition.

What might be some of the challenges to developing positive beliefs and attitudes?

Psychosocial interventions should also be offered to the family in order to promote coping and build capacity. An Australian study of young women with cancer found that family members played an essential role in providing emotional support, but also struggled to adapt to their changing circumstances (Coyne et al., 2012). Families who have a member with a life-threatening condition often need help to deal with conflict, and learn how to avoid overprotective or oversolicitous behaviours that may disempower the person they are trying to support.

There is considerable research that shows that providing psychosocial interventions to people with chronic conditions can be effective. Interventions include stress management, relaxation training, cognitive reframing and enhancing self-efficacy beliefs. Such interventions improve individuals' ability to monitor their condition, take corrective and preventive action, and reduce the distress, anxiety and depression that may accompany their condition.

5.5 CASE STUDY

ALINTA AND OSTEOARTHRITIS

Alinta is 62 years old and lives in a small rural community in South Australia. She was diagnosed with osteoarthritis five years ago, but recognises that she had signs of arthritis many years earlier. Her joints have become stiffer and harder to move and she notices grating sounds when she moves. On a usual day, Alinta finds it hard to move when she first wakes up in the morning. The stiffness usually lasts for 30 minutes or so. It improves as she goes about her daily activities that 'warm up' her knee and ankle joints. However, later in the day, the pain gets worse when she is more active and feels better when she is resting. On some days, the pain is still present when she is resting. Overall, the pain is persistent, even at night.

Alinta worked as an enrolled nurse for 20 years and realises that the physical tasks played a role in the development of her arthritis. She receives a disability pension through her superannuation fund. Her mother, who died seven years ago at the age of 74, also had arthritis. Alinta is divorced, and her children are married and have families of their own to care for. Although Alinta knows that her children do care, the discomfort and pain of arthritis is invisible to anyone who doesn't have it, and they cannot appreciate the restrictions it places on her. If she says "I can't" or "My legs hurt" or "I'm having one of my bad days", she knows her children and grandchildren understand but still are disappointed or impatient.

Alinta was upset after finally being diagnosed with arthritis. Within three years she needed to resign from work due to incapacity. She realised that she needed to accept her diagnosis and started thinking about how to adapt her life.

Alinta knows that osteoarthritis cannot be cured, and that it will most likely get worse over time. However, she is trying her best to stay positive and control her symptoms. She reminds herself: "It just helps to put this in its place. You have arthritis—it does not have you." She knows that she will eventually need to have both knee joints replaced, and that this major surgery will be performed in Adelaide. She will need to find accommodation in the city and have a lot of help during her post-operative recovery and rehabilitation. Meanwhile, she has engaged in a range of things that cannot make the arthritis go away but can help delay surgery. Alinta was 22 kg overweight but has lost 16 kg to reduce wear and tear on her hip, knee and ankle joints. She takes over-the-counter pain medication and her doctor recommended nonsteroidal anti-inflammatory drugs (e.g. aspirin or ibuprofen). If the pain is continually present, Alinta has corticosteroids injected into the joint to reduce swelling and pain.

Alinta lives an hour from the closest hospital, and finds that driving for that long while in pain drains all her energy before she even arrives. However, she continues to do volunteer work on the days when the pain is not too bad. She helps to make craft for the Red Cross. She said, "Coming out of the spin cycle of dwelling on the pain and letting it dominate my thoughts helps me cope."

1 What might Alinta's reaction be to her initial diagnosis and treatment?
2 What are some positive and negative effects of family attitudes on the person with a chronic condition?
3 How could Alinta be assisted in coming to terms with her condition?
4 How would you describe Alinta's response to her condition? Has her response changed over time?
5 What might be some warning signs for Alinta and her family that she is depressed?
6 What other activities could someone like Alinta be involved with?

> **Points to consider**
>
> The challenges and problems associated with chronic conditions are felt more strongly by those living in rural areas, due to social isolation. There are also fewer health care resources for rural residents, and they may have to travel long distances to obtain treatment. The lack of local support groups may contribute to feelings of isolation. Access to the internet can address some of these restrictions.

Learn more
Access additional resources to broaden your understanding of this chapter. See the Guided Tour for access details.

CHAPTER SUMMARY

- Chronic conditions such as asthma, epilepsy and diabetes are long-term, irreversible and require ongoing management.
- Individuals with chronic condition(s) have to make many adjustments to the physical, emotional, social and financial challenges of their situation. The extent to which such individuals can engage in day-to-day life varies; however, it is incorrect to assume that they are not able to carry out most activities.
- Comorbid chronic conditions are prevalent, particularly among older people. This prevalence is expected to increase and will place a heavy burden on health care systems and informal carers.
- The onset of a chronic condition or acquired disability can signify many life changes, including grief and loss, ongoing emotional ups and downs, and the need to deal with the usual demands of daily life, along with the extra challenges imposed by the condition. Other factors include financial stress and impact on family and friends.
- Cognitions play a significant role in how well individuals cope. Responses include feelings of helplessness, acceptance and positive benefits. Self-efficacy beliefs and optimism contribute to positive coping.
- Self-regulation and self-care are essential for understanding and managing chronic conditions.
- Different models of self-care may marginalise the individual's role (medical model), see it as a partnership (collaborative model) or place the individual actively at the centre of care (self-agency model).
- Care implications are long-term. They involve managing physical symptoms and, just as importantly, promoting overall quality of life through diet and exercise, avoiding secondary conditions, and managing negative emotions and cognitions through stress relief, reframing, promoting efficacy, and optimism.

FURTHER READING

Hughes S, Lewis S, Willis K, Rogers A, Wyke S & Smith L (2020) How do facilitators of group programmes for long-term conditions conceptualise self-management support? *Chronic Illness* 16(2), 104–18.

Lynch S, Shuster G & Lobo M (2018) The family caregiver experience: Examining the positive and negative aspects of compassion satisfaction and compassion fatigue as caregiving outcomes. *Aging & Mental Health* 22(11), 1424–31.

Marrie R (2017) Comorbidity in multiple sclerosis: Implications for patient care. *Nature Reviews Neurology* 13(6), 375–82.

Shulman R, Arora R, Geist R, Ali A, Ma J, Mansfield E, Martel S, Sandercock J & Versloot J (2021) Integrated community collaborative care for seniors with depression/anxiety and any physical illness. *Canadian Geriatrics Journal* 24(3), 251–7.

PART II
HEALTHY AND RISKY BEHAVIOUR

» Chapter 6: Understanding Health Behaviour 90

» Chapter 7: Thinking about Health Behaviour: Cognition and Health 113

» Chapter 8: How to Change Health Behaviour 137

» Chapter 9: A Complex Example: Activity, Eating and Body 160

HOW COVID-19 HIGHLIGHTS THE RELATION OF HEALTH AND BEHAVIOUR

Following the beginnings of the COVID-19 pandemic in early 2020, the influence of individual behaviour on health was constantly in the news. The various responses taken by nations, institutions and individuals provided a worldwide experiment into how individual health behaviour could—and more importantly whether it should—be a concern of society:

> Never in our history has our collective destiny and our collective health depended so completely on our individual behaviours (UK Prime Minister Boris Johnson, 23/09/2020).

In some parts of the world, nations saw the virus as a threat requiring immediate and dramatic action by the whole population. New Zealand, for example, introduced nationwide constraints on individual behaviour including lockdown on social activities. Schools, businesses, government and social interaction were banned and social isolation was made a public health response. In other nations, such as Brazil, leaders denied the existence of the pandemic until the number of deaths made it impossible to ignore. Even when the risks of the pandemic were recognised, many places viewed the disruption produced by public health measures such as lockdowns as too great a risk to other societal values, such as economic sustainability, or even personal freedom. Responses were affected by the various ways in which public health is organised and administered; for example, in Australia and the US each state has a separate and varied public health system, with different areas and levels of authority.

The complexities of the COVID-19 pandemic response are too great to tackle here, so looking at one central question is the clearest way to begin. Why do some people choose *not* to wear facemasks, *not* use hand hygiene and *not* avoid social contact where those behaviours are required or strongly recommended as ways to protect their own health and that of others?

Why does unhealthy behaviour continue?

The media is full of information about health. Information about the risks of smoking has to be included on the packaging of tobacco products. Almost every issue of every popular magazine discusses weight in one way or another. Information about COVID-19 precautions and restrictions was included in all media during the worst of the pandemic. So, why do people still continue to do things that are bad for them? And, more importantly, why does it seem to be so hard to do things that are good for you? In Chapter 6, health and risky behaviours are discussed, and concepts from learning and memory are used to help understand these behaviours.

A critical part of the answer to these questions relates to agency; that is, what or who is responsible for those things happening. In the case of experimental animals in the laboratory, such as Pavlov's dogs or Skinner's rats, the experimenter has control over the stimuli that trigger behaviour—and/or the costs and gains of those behaviours—which makes the experimenter the agent for change.

For health behaviour, the agents are complex. Usually, we believe that it is the individual who needs to become the agent for their own change. Not surprisingly, whether this happens is dependent on what the individual is thinking (their cognitions). A very simple statement of this part of the equation comes from Bandura (1998, p. 624): "Unless people believe they can produce desired effects by their actions, they have little incentive to act." People also need to believe that action will make a difference. These outcome expectations can come from a number of sources. This may be the most important lesson to be learnt from the COVID-19 pandemic— that media, political parties, religious authorities and scientists are competing to present expectations that may differ dramatically, and individuals choose which sets of expectations to adopt. Chapter 7 deals with cognitions, particularly beliefs about health and the influence they can have on health behaviours.

An understanding of how behaviours are acquired, and why they continue, provides a basis for thinking about how to modify them. Chapter 8 examines the principles of behaviour change, attempting to link the two previous chapters to solutions. The control of the stimuli that trigger behaviour, and the reinforcements that support those behaviours and keep them occurring, are discussed along with the impact of cognitions on how health behaviour can be modified.

A significant modifiable influence on health is overweight and obesity. However, issues associated with the direct health risks of obesity are complex and involve much more than how many kilojoules an individual consumes. Other issues (e.g. habits, beliefs, culture, self-image and self-esteem) also need to be considered if we are to understand weight as a health issue. Chapter 9 is devoted to a detailed consideration of this one critical area of health behaviour.

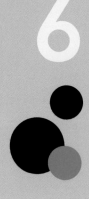

6 Understanding Health Behaviour

The relationship between behaviour and health

Chapter 4 looked at the effects of health, illness and disease on behaviour. This chapter looks at the other side of the coin: the effects of behaviour on health, illness and disease. Due to extraordinary progress in biomedical sciences and public health, patterns of health and illness have changed enormously over the last century. Even during the COVID-19 pandemic, infectious diseases (e.g. gastroenteritis, poliomyelitis, influenza, sexually transmitted infections, diseases of childhood) were not the main killers in developed countries. Chronic conditions such as heart disease, cancer and cerebrovascular disease (stroke) are now the major killers in all high-income countries and many middle- and low-income countries. These are known as **lifestyle diseases** because they are linked to lifestyle factors such as overweight and obesity, insufficient physical activity, tobacco smoking and alcohol use (AIHW, 2018a).

Lifestyle diseases
Diseases in which behaviours of the individual over a prolonged period influence the development or course of disease, such as heart disease, many cancers and stroke.

PAUSE & REFLECT

Review the section 'Measurement of health and illness' in Chapter 1.

How do we know that lifestyle diseases are the major causes of disability and death?

Prevention of illness and reduction of suffering are no longer simply matters of medical science producing a vaccine, or a doctor providing treatment of physical symptoms. A large proportion of the morbidity and mortality associated with lifestyle diseases is preventable. The US Burden of Disease Collaborators (2018) estimates that nearly half of the disease burden in the US is related to modifiable behaviours. Access Economics (2008) estimated that 20–25% of diabetes, cerebrovascular disease, osteoarthritis and cancer is caused by obesity. In fact, overweight and obesity have passed smoking as the number-one modifiable risk behaviour in developed countries (although AIHW (2021d) still nominates smoking in Australia). Chapter 9 has been devoted to weight and the related issues of diet and exercise. Modification of eating habits, alcohol consumption, exercise, leisure pursuits, sexual behaviour and even minor habits (e.g. slouching or nail-biting) could also improve quality of life, extend life expectancy and reduce the risk of ill health.

The influence of gender on health is discussed in detail in Chapter 14.

Risky behaviours

A number of behaviours produce a risk to the health of the individual. In some of these, the risk is a direct result of behaviour (e.g. smoking damages tissue), while others are more indirect in their effects (e.g. driving while angry increases the risk of accidents and has a subsequent health impact). Important **risky behaviours** include cigarette smoking, alcohol and problem drinking, illegal drugs, unsafe sexual behaviour and dangerous activities. These are now discussed in more detail.

Risky behaviours
Behaviours that increase the individual's chance of ill health.

CIGARETTE SMOKING

Approximately 12% of adult Australians were smokers in 2019 (AIHW, 2020e) which reflects a continuing downward trend. The proportion of adults who smoke at all has decreased by more than half since 1989–90 (AIHW, 2020e), and the number of cigarettes smoked each day has also decreased. Smoking is difficult to eliminate in existing smokers because the nicotine in tobacco is highly addictive. In addition, cigarette manufacturing and sales make large contributions to the economy and taxation revenue of governments, so the process of controlling smoking by regulation has been difficult and slow. However, a large number of harmful substances in tobacco smoke adversely affect the cardiovascular and respiratory systems and are risk factors in many illnesses.

Restriction of areas/spaces where smoking can take place has progressed worldwide. In many countries, smoking is prohibited in public buildings, indoor spaces such as restaurants and hotels, outdoor spaces where people are close together, and even cars when children are present. Although the main aim of such restrictions is to reduce passive exposure to second-hand smoke, the effects of making smoking appear to be antisocial impact on smokers as well. In most developed countries, cigarette packages must contain health warnings, and even graphic pictures of health problems associated with smoking. In 2012, the Australian government became the first in the world to require that all cigarettes be sold in standard plain packaging. A number of other countries have followed suit, despite tobacco companies claiming that this is restraint of trade.

6.1 CASE STUDY

JAMES AND SMOKING

This case study looks at a risky behaviour and examines the reasons for its development and maintenance.

James is 40 years old and smokes 25–30 cigarettes a day. His father was a smoker and died at age 57 from a heart attack; his mother does not smoke. James had his first cigarette at 12, when he and a friend obtained cigarettes from an older brother. By the time James was 15, he was smoking regularly on the way to and from school with this same friend. At first, he just smoked because his friends and the 'cool kids' did. However, he quickly learnt to enjoy the experience of smoking, finding that he could use cigarettes to calm himself when he was tense or wake him up when he was tired. Even though he realised smoking was bad for him, when he tried to do without cigarettes he felt irritable and restless.

1   Why might James have been attracted to smoking in the first place?
2   Why does James' experience of the positive aspects of smoking (peer pressure, pleasure, regulation of mood) appear to outweigh the negatives (coughing, financial costs, knowing that smoking was a factor in his father's early death from heart disease)?

Cigarette smoking has become less common, but vaping has increased and is a controversial behaviour. There are claims that vaping is less harmful or is a good way to quit smoking, but other information suggests that it may produce its own health risks (LFA, n.d.). The risks of passive vaping are not at all clear at the moment.

Do you think restrictions on vaping should mirror those on smoking?

ALCOHOL AND PROBLEM DRINKING

Although there is evidence that moderate alcohol consumption—one to two standard drinks a day—has some health protective effects, overuse and abuse of alcohol have major negative impacts on health, partly as a result of direct effects on bodily tissue that give rise to liver, kidney, gastrointestinal and nervous system problems. Problems also occur as a result of indirect effects on the behaviour of drinkers, such as accidents, violence and other unhealthy habits that tend to go with alcohol abuse, such as smoking (WHO, 2018). While direct effects take time to occur, indirect consequences of alcohol's effects on the drinker occur even in new drinkers. Binge drinking and associated accidents and violence are big risks for young drinkers, such as university students. While it appears that the proportion of the Australian population who drink regularly is decreasing, evidence regarding risky levels of drinking is less clear.

Read a discussion paper by Creedy and colleagues (2020a) on how care by a known midwife throughout pregnancy, birth and postpartum can help women make healthy decisions about drinking and prevent foetal alcohol spectrum disorders.

To what extent do you think health professionals could be effective in preventing alcohol misuse?

ILLEGAL DRUGS

Although fewer people use illegal drugs than tobacco and alcohol, the level of health risk and likelihood of associated consequences are quite high. Illicit drugs include marijuana, cocaine, opiates (e.g. heroin), amphetamines and designer drugs such as ice and ecstasy. Like alcohol and tobacco, these have direct physical risks and indirect behavioural risks. Although the use of illegal drugs is decreasing slightly among adults (AIHW, 2020e), this may have been affected by limitations placed on over-the-counter medications containing codeine, which is a base ingredient in some drugs.

A major problem with the use of these substances is that many people mix them with other drugs such as alcohol or prescription drugs, which can greatly increase the risks. Even mixing these drugs with energy drinks containing high levels of caffeine, taurine and/or guarana can be dangerous, because the combination can lead to overexertion and dehydration. Some people mistakenly believe that because these energy drink ingredients are legal and natural, they pose no risk. However, all of them—on their own or in combination—have been linked to physical and psychological problems (particularly when used to excess) and even to death (Nuss et al., 2021). With repeated use, all of the mentioned illegal drugs pose some risk of addiction or psychological dependence.

OTHER ADDICTIVE BEHAVIOURS

It is not only drugs that present a potential for addiction. Gambling addiction is such a significant problem in Australia that all states now have some sort of gambling healthline for affected individuals. Much of the attention on problem gambling has been aimed at harm reduction rather than attempting to stop people from gambling (Hing et al., 2019). The harms from problem gambling include financial hardship, relationship conflict and breakdown, emotional and psychological stress, physical health impacts, cultural harm, impaired work and study performance, and criminal activity (Langham et al., 2016).

Another type of addictive behaviour raising community concern is internet addiction (Kuss & Lopez-Fernandez, 2016). Issues include online gaming, social media use, pornography and gambling. Although much of the attention in internet addiction has been on young people, the addiction can occur to people of any age.

These are complex topics, and will not be dealt with here. Chapter 8 includes discussion of opponent-process theory and its application to addiction.

RISKY SEXUAL BEHAVIOUR

Unsafe sex
Having sex without using devices such as condoms to protect against pregnancy and STIs, and/or not finding out about a partner's sexual history.

The two most obvious risks of unsafe sexual behaviour are unwanted pregnancy and sexually transmitted infections (STIs). **Unsafe sex** includes not using devices such as condoms to protect against pregnancy and STIs, and not finding out about a partner's sexual history.

The most dangerous STIs have changed with advances in biomedical science and changes in behaviour. Many STIs, such as syphilis and gonorrhoea, can be easily cured if detected early and treated. Other STIs, such as genital herpes, have become more important health issues because they are not curable. Some, such as HIV and chlamydia, are important because symptoms are often silent, so the carrier does not realise they are infected or that they can pass it on to others.

The major change in risk associated with an STI has been the development and distribution of a vaccine against human papillomavirus (HPV), due to a strong link between HPV and later development of cervical cancer. The vaccination program has led to a major reduction in cervical cancer rates around the world (Lei et al., 2020).

DANGEROUS ACTIVITIES

A number of activities expose individuals to a higher than normal risk of injury. Soft tissue injuries (e.g. bruising and muscle strains, broken bones, tendon and cartilage damage) are not uncommon in sports such as football, tennis and skiing. Some sports (e.g. boxing) have very much higher risks. Indeed, there are several sports that the medical profession believes have risks that are so high that they should be banned. Boxing is at the top of the list. Steps can be taken to make some of these activities less dangerous; for example, proper equipment and training are important. The wearing of crash helmets and protective clothing by cyclists and motorcyclists has greatly reduced serious injuries and deaths.

The major causes of premature death for young adults are traffic accidents, suicide and homicide (ABS, 2021a). If we include injury, traffic accidents are by far the leading preventable cause of death and injury from five to 29 years of age. The combination of a willingness to take risks and the circumstances under which young people are likely to drive—at night, in groups, when tired or after consuming alcohol or other drugs—often leads to the most serious accidents.

The next section looks at behaviours that either reduce risk or actively encourage health.

PAUSE & REFLECT

What other examples of risky behaviours with regard to health can you think of?
Do you have any risky behaviours?

Health behaviours and risk-reduction behaviours

Two types of behaviour are directly related to improving a person's state of health and well-being. **Health behaviours** are those that promote health, such as eating the right foods, getting enough sleep, relaxing and exercising sensibly. **Risk-reduction behaviours** refer to actions that reduce the occurrence of unhealthy behaviours such as smoking, drinking alcohol in excess and unsafe driving. COVID-19 brought a dramatic focus on risk-reduction behaviours, with mask-wearing, hand hygiene and social distancing all aimed at reducing infection rates both for those who practise the behaviours and those to whom the infection may be spread. A by-product of these behaviours has been a reduction in the rates of other infectious conditions, such as influenza and the common cold (Dadras et al., 2021).

> **Health behaviours**
> Behaviours that are carried out specifically to promote the health of the individual.

> **Risk-reduction behaviours**
> The avoidance of unhealthy behaviours specifically to protect the health of the individual.

Sometimes risk-reduction behaviours are categorised as preventive behaviours, but as many of them involve simply avoiding the risky behaviour in the first place the term 'risk reduction' is preferred here. Many direct associations have been demonstrated between health behaviours, risk-reduction behaviours and health outcomes, not just in terms of the targeted problems but also in terms of the sense of overall well-being and ability to cope with other life events. A good example of risk-reduction behaviour is exercise (Kramer, 2020). The physical and mental health benefits of exercise are well known and will be considered in more detail in Chapter 9.

A risk-reduction behaviour that is frequently overlooked is sleep (Worley, 2018). Research has been conducted into how much sleep is needed to ensure maximum alertness and performance across various age groups (Chaput et al., 2018). The recommendation for young adults and those in their middle years is seven to nine hours. It has been found that young adults in particular are likely to put sleeping at or near the bottom of their list of priorities. Secondary and tertiary students frequently prioritise study, social life and part-time work over sleep. One common pattern that can have serious negative effects is trying to make up for lack of sleep by having a long sleep at some other time, such as sleeping all day on a weekend.

Overall, getting adequate sleep on a regular basis is associated with better grades and higher productivity (Okano et al., 2019). Recommendations include regular sleep patterns (going to sleep and waking at the same time), not eating large meals or exercising close to bedtime, limiting use of social media and other computer activities close to bedtime, avoiding stimulants such as coffee, tea and cola during the evening, and complete avoidance of energy drinks. Use of sleep aid medication is a short-term response to serious sleep difficulties, and may cause rebound effects when stopped. Behavioural interventions for serious sleep problems, such as cognitive behaviour therapy, are not only more effective but don't have side-effects (Worley, 2018). Sleep apnoea and other sleep problems linked to physical issues require more intensive medical management.

Road rage has received a lot of media attention in recent years. The risks associated with driving are greatly increased if individuals are in a competitive and aggressive state of mind. This state of mind leads them to take unnecessary chances, then blame other drivers for any behaviour that affects them as a result. Such behaviour leads to anger. The biggest risk of driving while angry is not that an individual may actually get out of their car and murder someone, but that their judgment while behind the wheel is impaired, resulting in dangerous behaviour. Angry people are much more likely to put themselves in situations where the margin for error is small, which results in both a greater likelihood of accidents and a greater chance that those accidents will be serious. A risk-reduction strategy might involve dealing with the connection between anger and driving. For example, as individuals often drive aggressively when they are late or under time pressure, changing a driver's approach to time management could lessen their tendency towards road rage.

Alcohol and anger were formerly believed, incorrectly, to be the underlying impetus for relationship abuse, also known as domestic and family violence. However, we now know that while substance abuse might make the extent of abuse worse, it does not cause violence. The abuser tends to abuse only their partner and/or their children. Their abuse is not generalised to others in different contexts such as work or sport; it is based on their sense of entitlement and belief they have the right to control their family members. People who assault their partners while under the influence of alcohol or drugs generally engage in a pattern of coercive and controlling behaviours even while sober because they believe they have a right to control their partners. Therefore, domestic violence programs need to focus on issues of power and control. Traditional interventions such as couples counselling, family therapy and misinformed mediation practices are inappropriate for domestic violence situations where there is a power imbalance. Australian research with women about domestic violence revealed that many women did not want to leave the relationship but wanted their partners' behaviour to change (Creedy et al., 2020b).

HABITS

Habit
An activity that has become automatic through prolonged practice.

When a behaviour is practised regularly it becomes a **habit**, is more likely to occur and becomes automatic (i.e. it occurs without awareness). Habits are learnt and remembered. Even minor habits can influence health and well-being. Snacking while we watch television, for example, can have disastrous effects on an otherwise healthy diet. Chairs in school and university classrooms tend to be designed to be stackable or indestructible rather than to encourage good posture. As a result, they may encourage slouching for comfort, which leads in the short term to back, neck or joint pain. If bad posture becomes a habit, it can lead to chronic pain, or affect joint health or the operation of the digestive system. Biting fingernails can lead to infections and even loss of sensation or function. To understand habits and begin to think about their modification, some understanding of basic concepts of learning and memory is necessary.

The basis of learning and memory: The changing brain

Until recently, it was believed that the number of cells in the brain was fixed fairly early in life, and that its structure then remained fairly constant throughout life. Research in a variety of areas has made it clear that the brain is much more changeable than was formerly understood (Doidge, 2008).

The basic neural processes that allow us to throw a ball, remember what we had for breakfast or walk without falling over seem so automatic that we rarely consider how remarkable they really are. However, if we were to lose some of our abilities—perhaps as a result of damage received in an accident—it would seem an enormous loss. Imagine the difficulties experienced by someone who suffers from dementia, gradually losing more and more of the basic information that allows them to function in the situations they encounter. It is little wonder that those sufferers often experience frustration, anger and anxiety. But how does the biological machine that each of us occupies accomplish enormously complex mental tasks? And equally important, what can be learnt from the structure and function of the nervous system that will help with the understanding of human behaviour?

Interconnectedness of the nervous system

The nervous system can accomplish so much—from movement, to thought, to emotion—largely because of its incredibly high level of interconnectedness. Each of the billions of individual neurons may have between 1000 and 10 000 synapses and be connected to up to 50 000 other neurons. In such a structure, any one neuron is unlikely to exert very strong control over any other neuron all by itself. Each time a neuron fires, it communicates widely and often not very deeply. However, neurons are not spread randomly into a sort of homogeneous pudding of cells. They often run in common patterns because they are physically close to one another and going in the same direction. They may form bundles that run from one location to (or at least in the general direction of) another. These bundles are nerves, and the information they transmit depends not on the individual neuron but on the preponderance of action of many neurons.

The way in which a particular neuron responds to information from other neurons can be seen as having parallels with the process of voting at an election. The total sum of the information received determines the rate of firing of the neuron. Imagine the behaviour of a television quiz show contestant when the presenter asks, "Would you like to continue or stop now?" At this point, people in the audience *always* start shouting advice. Some will shout "Yes" and some "No", some will shout totally incomprehensible or irrelevant things, some will say nothing at all. Although the contestant already prefers stopping or continuing, this audience advice will have an effect—particularly if it is unanimous. If everyone in the room shouts "No", it is likely to make the contestant hesitant to say "Yes" no matter how much they want to. In a similar way, the neuron responds to the preponderance of incoming information—excitatory (yes) minus inhibitory (no)—by varying its firing rate. The television contestant is also likely to be most influenced by those who yell loudest, or they may look to family or friends in the audience for advice. Similarly, the neuron responds more strongly to strong input, which may come from particularly excited neurons or from neurons with which it has a large number of synapses all giving the same information. Each time the neuron fires it has to pause, although this time is measured in microseconds, as the rate of firing can be quite high. This allows the neuron to build up its resources for another firing. This is a gradual process, and during this time the neuron will only respond if the input is strong. The stronger the input, the closer the neuron will come to firing at its maximum possible rate.

The influence of one neuron on another does not cease as soon as firing takes place, because the message is carried by neurotransmitters that remain in the gap between the neurons (the **synaptic cleft**) for greater or lesser periods of time. These may influence neurons after the incoming neuron has stopped signalling, and it takes time for the receiving neuron to free up its receptors by breaking down or releasing the neurotransmitters. Less normal events may occur as well. As an extreme example, heroin or other drugs introduced into the body can block receptor sites that are intended for neurotransmitters, and so interfere with normal transmission. Substances may be introduced that break down a neurotransmitter before it can lock into receptor sites, thereby reducing the amount of that neurotransmitter in the synaptic cleft. Other substances may prevent the breakdown or re-uptake of a neurotransmitter and thereby increase the amount present. These principles underlie a great deal of the drug treatment for conditions as divergent as high blood pressure, depression, cancer and impotence. As shown in the following sections on learning and memory, firing changes the neuron. Information is permanently stored through actual physical change in the structure and interconnections of the neuron. The effect of all this action is that the influence of information spreads widely. It becomes associated with other information— and the more similar the information, the more closely associated it becomes.

Particular input tends to be dealt with primarily in certain locations because of the structure of the nervous system, but because of the high degree of interconnectedness it is also communicated to other brain locations. Following damage to the preferred location, this communication can allow another—usually neighbouring—area to take over a function, although this may take a great deal of retraining. This **neuroplasticity** suggests that functions within the brain that are lost through injury or illness are not gone for good, but can be recovered through appropriate retraining. This notion that functions can be replaced through training forms the core topic of Doidge's best-selling book, *The Brain that Changes Itself* (2008). However, it also highlights that the basis for all learning and memory lies in physical changes to the brain.

Because the brain is a constantly developing organ, the earlier in life that damage occurs, the more rapidly functions can be transferred to nearby areas. For example, children who lack the usual number of cells in the language areas of the brain, perhaps because of developmental problems or injury, may develop language in a normal way and at the usual times, using other brain areas. For adults, relearning language skills after damage may be a very slow process because it involves retraining rather than the initial training of brain cells. Special treatment procedures have been developed that offer hope that this retraining can be sped up and can reach a wider range of lost functions than previously believed (Doidge, 2016).

Synaptic cleft
The tiny space between two nerve cells, across which they communicate using neurotransmitters.

Neuroplasticity
The brain's ability to reorganise itself by forming new neural connections throughout life.

6.2 CASE STUDY

JAMES (CONT.)

Clearly, James had learnt a great deal about smoking before he ever had a cigarette himself. From observing his father, he learnt that smoking is something that adult males do, and that a person that he is close to and admires does. He also learnt a lot about smoking—though not about its disadvantages—from movies and television, and from observing others around him. His friends contributed to his knowledge about smoking and his attitudes towards it. They also changed the availability of cigarettes. All these sources indirectly taught James how he should feel about the bodily effects that resulted from smoking. He had to learn that the bodily effects were pleasant—as most people feel ill the first time they inhale cigarette smoke. As he continues to smoke, he begins to associate other experiences (e.g. parties and time with friends) with smoking.

1   Learning about smoking from parents and friends is just one of the factors that contribute to smoking in young people. Could there be other forms of learning involved in James' smoking?

2   How do experiences of one kind (in this case, smoking) become associated with experiences of a completely different kind, like socialising, drinking alcohol or taking breaks?

Learning

Why do some people develop an irrational fear of flying? Why do you get very hungry exactly at the end of your 1pm class? How do we gain the skills that allow us to survive in a complex environment? Why do we do things that we know very well are bad for us? All of these responses depend on **learning**. Learning is such a basic process that it is hard to come up with a good working definition. Probably the clearest way to think about learning is that it is a change in behaviour that results from a person's experience with the environment. This would exclude the instance of a child who could not roll over at three months of age being able to do so at four months (the result of maturation), or of a rat working harder to get food when it is hungry than when it is not (the result of change in internal state over time). However, if someone threatens to hit a person if they don't shut up, and as a result that person does shut up, that is learning. It is perhaps easiest to understand the nature of learning by looking at some of the simplest models of learning.

Learning
A change in understanding and/or behaviour that results from experience with the environment.

CLASSICAL CONDITIONING

Probably the most famous experiments in psychology are those involving Pavlov's dogs (Pavlov, 1927). What is generally remembered about this, and parodied in cartoons, is that Pavlov taught his dogs to salivate at the ringing of a bell. However, what is most important is that, through experience, an already existing response to the presentation of food (salivating) became connected to a previously irrelevant stimulus (bell ringing). This kind of learning is called **classical conditioning**.

Classical conditioning
A learning process through experience where an already existing response to the presentation of food (e.g. salivating) becomes connected to a previously irrelevant stimulus (e.g. bell ringing).

Stimulus
Any change in physical energy that activates a receptor, and activates or alerts an organism.

For classical conditioning to take place, there must be an unconditioned response (UR) that reliably follows an unconditioned **stimulus** (US) whenever it occurs. Examples of stimulus–response pairs that fit this model are reflexes such as blinking your eye (UR) when air is puffed into it (US), or the leg jerk (UR) that follows the knee being tapped by a hammer (US). Learning occurs when an irrelevant stimulus is paired with the US; that is, they are presented at roughly the same time. Any initially irrelevant stimulus will do. It is not the nature of the stimulus that matters, only its pairing with the US. After this pairing has occurred a few times, the irrelevant stimulus will have become a conditioned stimulus (CS). If the CS is then presented without the US, it will produce a response that looks like the UR. This response is called the conditioned response (CR). Although it looks like the UR, it will be weaker, and if the CS is presented repeatedly without the US, the CR will gradually fade away or extinguish.

Phobia
A strong, persistent and irrational fear of some object, person or event.

We can see how a **phobia** might develop through classical conditioning. A child will quite typically react with distress (UR) when startled (US). Suppose the child meets a strange dog (CS) and, not being afraid of it, begins to play with it. Worried about the child's safety, the child's parent suddenly shouts at the dog (US), startling the child and producing distress (UR); the dog runs off. If this sequence is repeated, the child will begin to show distress (CR) to the presence of strange dogs (CS).

One characteristic of classically conditioned responses is that they generalise to other stimuli that are similar to the CS. The strength of the response to a new stimulus will be directly related to how similar it is to the original CS. In this case, the child's conditioned fear of dogs could generalise to all small furry animals.

Stimulus generalisation
The principle that a conditioned response will tend to occur in the presence of stimuli similar to the original conditioned stimulus.

PAUSE & REFLECT

When an individual, such as a member of a sporting team, acts badly, we may think that other members of the team will do the same.

How can **stimulus generalisation** help to understand this process?

Why does the phobia not extinguish over time? If the child was placed in a situation where encountering strange dogs was unavoidable and a parent was not present to produce the UR of fear by producing the US of screaming, then the phobia probably would extinguish. Phobias are frequently maintained by avoidance behaviour. Each time the child has an opportunity to interact with strange dogs, it is likely to choose instead to avoid them. This avoidance learning represents another kind of learning, called operant conditioning.

OPERANT CONDITIONING

Classical conditioning on its own could hardly explain all learning, especially the learning of complex or novel behaviours. A different kind of conditioning occurs in trial-and-error learning situations. Suppose a hungry rat is placed in a new enclosure. It will scramble around doing a variety of things until it discovers food or is removed from the enclosure. In fact, the hungrier the rat gets, the more vigorously it will scramble around and the greater the variety of things it will do. If it finds some food, the behaviours that occurred at about that same time will be learnt; that is, they will become more likely to occur in future when the rat is hungry. Over repeated trials, any random behaviours—those that actually had nothing to do with the food—will be likely to stop occurring (extinguish). The only behaviours that will really stick will be those that operate to produce the desired outcome (operant conditioning). The rat's behaviour will become more precise and faster as the correct responses are stamped in and the incorrect ones are stamped out. These behaviours become habits and may occur automatically. This describes a fairly typical study in operant conditioning as developed by Skinner (1938), who created much of the theory surrounding our current understanding of operant conditioning.

Originally, discussions of operant conditioning used common language terms (e.g. reward) to describe what was happening, but these can prove to be confusing. What is rewarding to one rat (e.g. a food pellet) might not interest another, and its effect on a given rat when it is hungry is quite different from the effect when the rat has just eaten. The concepts become clearer if events are described in terms of their effects on behaviour. Positive **reinforcement** is when the occurrence of a consequence or outcome in conjunction with a particular behaviour makes that behaviour more likely in future (such an outcome might be food, money or sex). The consequence is called a positive reinforcer or a positive reinforcement. **Punishment** is when the occurrence of a consequence makes a behaviour less likely (e.g. an electric shock or a bad grade). Putting an end to a pleasant state (e.g. turning off the television or being awakened from a nap by being yelled at) is also punishment because it reduces the likelihood of the target behaviour.

Note that the termination of an unpleasant state (e.g. ending an electric shock or allowing the individual to avoid it) can also serve to increase the likelihood of a behaviour. To emphasise its special characteristics, this is sometimes called negative reinforcement. Note that it is reinforcement because it increases the likelihood of a behaviour. Don't allow the word 'negative' to lead you to confuse it with punishment.

When the behaviour to be learnt is complex, **shaping** can be used whereby incremental steps towards the desired behaviour are reinforced. Parents often use shaping to teach their children things such as writing their name. At first, the child is praised for holding the pencil properly, then for scribbles that look like writing, then for individual letters, then for groups of letters, and so on until they are actually writing. Most of what we learn is complex behaviour that probably results from shaping arising from our experiences with the environment.

Learning without reinforcement or punishment is discussed later in the chapter.

PUNISHMENT

The impact of punishment on behaviour is more complex than positive reinforcement (Walters & Grusec, 1977). Treatment approaches based on punishment of unwanted behaviour—**aversive conditioning**—frequently produce unexpected outcomes. One treatment for alcoholics involves the taking of a substance (Anatabuse) that makes the patient violently ill if they subsequently drink alcohol. The expected result is that an aversion to the taste of alcohol should be classically conditioned, but the actual result tends to be a very high drop-out rate from therapy unless the patient is highly supported by family and friends. One way of viewing this is that patients find it easier to acquire an aversion to the treatment than to alcohol. This is an example of **avoidance learning**. When the individual avoids a punishment, the behaviour that leads to avoidance gets reinforced.

Another drawback of punishment is that it may generalise; that is, its effects may spread to similar stimuli so that desirable behaviours disappear along with the undesirable. If a child is punished for being noisy in class, that child may withdraw into not only quiet but

Reinforcement
A consequence or outcome that, in conjunction with a behaviour, makes that behaviour more likely in future. Reinforcement can be positive or negative.

Punishment
A consequence or outcome that, in conjunction with a behaviour, makes that behaviour less likely in future.

Shaping
Teaching a complex behaviour by reinforcing, one at a time, the series of steps that make up the behaviour.

Aversive conditioning
The use of punishment to decrease the occurrence of unwanted behaviour.

Avoidance learning
The learning of a response, such as fear, that will allow the individual to escape punishment. It is reinforced by a reduction in the level of fear experienced.

also passive behaviour. The child is no longer disruptive, but they may also no longer ask questions about things they have not understood. The loss of positive interaction with the teacher and other children may handicap the child's learning. Punishment also generalises to the punisher, so that the child may come to dislike the teacher, the class or school in general.

Reinforcement works in two ways. The right behaviour is stamped in and the wrong behaviour, which is not reinforced, extinguishes. Punishment stamps out the wrong behaviour but it provides no information about the right behaviour, which may therefore extinguish. Because of this, aversive conditioning needs to be paired with reinforcement of the right behaviour. Treatment for alcoholics is likely to be more effective if adaptive behaviours are taught and reinforced, as well as drinking being punished. Alcoholics Anonymous, as an example, encourages alcoholics to call for the company of a sober mentor when they are tempted to drink. This act reinforces non-drinking behaviour and puts the focus on interpersonal rather than internal events. The elimination of aggressive behaviour by punishment usually works best when accompanied by training in appropriate assertive behaviour, using positive reinforcement, as a better alternative.

LEARNING WITHOUT REINFORCEMENT

Learning is based on the development of associations between stimuli and responses. Conditioning theories account for much of this development, but not everything that fits the definition of learning can be explained in conditioning terms. Can you recall the slogan from a particular commercial? Can you sing the words of a song you don't like? It is hard to see how you could have been reinforced for acquisition of these behaviours.

It is easier to account for events such as these if we consider the complex mental activity going on inside us. We have elaborate mental networks of expectations about the workings of the world, sometimes termed schemas. These schemas can be affected by conditioning, but other things affect them as well. If we place a non-hungry rat in a maze, it will explore (possibly out of curiosity). If we then place the same rat in the same maze when it is hungry, we will see clear evidence that it has learnt something about the arrangement of the maze from its previous experience, which the rat only calls into play now that it is hungry. This latent learning (Tolman, 1932) indicates that schemas can develop or change without reinforcement, because they might be useful at some future time.

Learning by observation is an example of this. Bandura (1977b) proposed that reinforcement is more important in getting an individual to display a behaviour, than its initial learning. In a famous study on the learning of aggression (Bandura et al., 1963), children were shown films of adults behaving in unusually aggressive ways towards toys. When the children were put into a room with the same toys, they did not tend to show aggressive behaviour unless they were angered. Only then did the children imitate, in detail, the specific acts of aggression that they had seen modelled. Observation of the behaviour had added the new behaviour to their repertoire of aggressive behaviour, so that it was there when needed. It appears that a lot of aggressive behaviour is learnt in this fashion.

It seems paradoxical that people who are abused in childhood are more likely than other people to grow up to abuse their own children. It is expected that they should know how bad child abuse is, and avoid it. It appears that, by observing the people who abused them, they learnt a strategy for behaving towards children. When they in turn experience anger and frustration towards their own children, they may act out this latent learning.

Certain characteristics of an observed behaviour may make it more likely to be learnt by observation. Seeing someone else being reinforced for a behaviour is likely to make that behaviour appear to be worth learning (vicarious reinforcement). Behaviours may be acquired if they are novel enough to be interesting in themselves. Children in particular like to learn things that produce spectacular effects. For example, learning 'rude' words is interesting because adults respond to them in interesting ways.

A major way in which we learn by observation is through the use of language. Although we may never have seen a particular gadget or piece of flat-pack furniture before, by reading the instructions we can obtain information about the correct behaviour; that is, what we have to do to make the gadget work or to assemble the furniture. Imagine the wear and tear on patients if health professionals had to learn about their professions solely through conditioning of randomly occurring behaviours!

PAUSE & REFLECT

How would theories of learning explain why people continue to carry out risky health behaviours? For example, why would someone drive if they think they may have had too much to drink?

LEARNING TO BE SICK

The earlier description of how a person can acquire a phobia illustrates one way in which someone can learn to be sick. There is a variety of others. When an individual experiences temporary tissue damage (e.g. a sprained ankle), they will very quickly learn what causes pain and avoid those triggers. This is useful because it gives the damaged tissue time to recover. However, it is possible to over-learn avoidance. For example, a young person has been in an accident and received significant back injuries. While these injuries are healing, the person may develop powerful avoidance learning. Sitting up may cause extreme pain, so the person learns to lie still. Eventually, the muscles may begin to atrophy through disuse. The person may have learnt avoidance so well that they have great difficulty in allowing themselves to move normally even when recovered. They may move awkwardly, thereby increasing the likelihood of re-injury. This can occur even if the person has not become phobic about movement through their experiences of pain, but just because they have learnt habits of restricted movement.

Sometimes being ill has **secondary gains**. If an individual's family and friends have learnt that that person is likely to injure themselves if they lift heavy weights, they will tend to move things for that person or avoid asking them to help with strenuous activities. The person with pain described above, for example, may be excused from doing some things they would otherwise have been asked to do (a right of the sick role). Complaints of pain tend to result in increased caring behaviours from others. The bringing of pain relievers, expressions of sympathy, praise for the sufferer's courage and even pillow-plumping can all follow from complaining of pain and reinforce the complaining behaviour.

Treatment of chronic pain usually involves staff and families setting up routines that do not reinforce complaining, but reinforce testing the limits of movement. Medication, because it relieves or prevents the onset of pain, is also a reinforcer in chronic pain, and patients often become conditioned to certain dosages and times of medication even if pain

Secondary gain
A gain or advantage received by an individual as a result of being ill.

Pain is such an important part of health and behaviour that Chapter 11 is devoted to it.

is not present. This is another kind of avoidance learning: the medication prevents the pain occurring, so if medication is missed its absence becomes anxiety-provoking. Ultimately, the patient is taking the medication as much for anxiety relief as for pain relief. The kinds of learning just described for pain can occur with almost any other symptom, including nausea, itching and tiredness.

A more severe kind of learning to be sick can occur when an individual cannot avoid unpleasant events that they would like to avoid. Early studies of escape by animals from electric shock sometimes showed that when shock could not be avoided or escaped (or when the animal was unable to find out how to avoid or escape it) a pattern called **learned helplessness** occurred (Seligman & Maier, 1967). In this pattern, distress increases to a point where behaviour is impaired. Learning is retarded, and the animal may quit trying to learn. The stimuli that signal the beginning of shock result in giving-up behaviour such as freezing, whining, shivering or apathy. Researchers found some disturbing similarities between the ways in which the animals behaved and ways in which some people behave. A person who is regularly abused by their partner may come to simply accept the abuse without making any attempt to escape. As a result of experience, they have learnt a helpless pattern of behaviour. Even where avoidance or escape appear to an observer to be easy, they are not attempted. In other cases, the helplessness may be more subtle. The reasons why a person would stay in an abusive relationship are of course far more complex than this; they include financial uncertainty, children, belief systems and many other factors.

Learned helplessness
Distress to the point where behaviour is impaired or the individual gives up in the face of punishment that cannot be controlled.

The key elements in this kind of learning are helplessness and hopelessness: the individual gives up on behaviour and sometimes shows a pattern of withdrawal from the outside world. It has been suggested that in situations where action is hopeless, this withdrawal protects the person by conserving resources. Conservation withdrawal has been observed in children who have been severely abused or neglected, and in prisoners of war. The similarities to the psychiatric disorder of depression are strong enough that learned helplessness is considered to be one of the pathways to depression.

Depression is discussed in Chapter 10.

6.3 CASE STUDY

JAMES (CONT.)

Learning without reinforcement could have played a part in James' smoking. He observed his father, some of his friends and characters in films smoking and learnt it as a possible behaviour. He would have learnt a great deal about where and when to smoke, how to hold a cigarette, how to light up and how to blow out the smoke. James might have also learnt through vicarious reinforcement, such as hearing people say things like "That tastes good" or "I needed that". Tobacco companies formerly poured a great deal of money into films to have the principal characters smoke, particularly if those characters were attractive, strong or sexy. They were trying to increase learning and memory effects with regard to cigarettes. It is vital to decrease these processes by banning depictions of smoking from popular entertainment.

James will have stored memories about how cigarettes and smokers look and behave from his observation of others. He will have semantic memories (e.g. what smoking-related terms such as "Have you got a light?" mean), procedural memories (e.g. how to light a cigarette on a windy day) and his own episodic memories about smoking (e.g. how it feels, times when he has tried to quit, information that he has received from other people).

1   How does memory affect James' behaviour?

2   How do all these memory processes fit together?

Memory

This section considers how experience is retained once learning has taken place. As with learning, **memory** has a significant impact on how people behave. What we remember about our experiences in terms of being well and being ill are very important in determining how we will react, what we expect to happen and how we will respond to attempts to modify our health.

An elderly patient suffering from dementia—a global deterioration of intellectual functioning resulting from damage to brain tissue—may be able to recall every detail of their childhood home but not remember the name of the nurse who takes care of them or what they did five minutes ago. A friend may remember a story about you that you are certain never actually occurred. Memory is amazing in its ability to hold millions of bits of information, and the ease with which information may be lost or altered. No computer memory can match the flexibility or usefulness of the human memory—or its inaccuracy.

Memory consists of three related processes: sensory memory, short-term memory and long-term memory (see Figure 6.1). Each operates in a different way and serves different functions, but all three have things in common. Some authors have suggested that there is also medium-term memory, which is used for things that are likely to be needed not far into the future. The need for a process different from long-term memory to explain this is not clear, and there does not seem to be a good theory of how the two types of memory would differ. The discussion that follows looks at the three best established types.

Memory
Processes (including sensory, short-term and long-term memory) by which experience is retained within the organism.

FIGURE 6.1 Types of memory

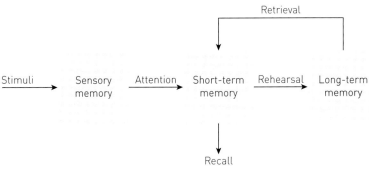

SENSORY MEMORY

Look at the room around you for a moment, then close your eyes and try to remember every detail about the wall to your left. You will probably be surprised at how much you can recall. However, if you now try to remember the detail of the right-hand wall, most of what you remembered about the left will have gone. In the same way, if you hear a bell ring or feel something touch your skin, there will be a momentary lingering—a few seconds of that sensation. For that time the impression will be quite detailed, but it will not be possible to hold onto it for long, particularly if something else happens that involves the same sense, such as another sound or touch. It appears that we have a separate sensory store for each of the five senses. This sensory memory seems to serve the function of allowing us time to search for information while allowing us to get rid of the detail that we don't need. If we had to keep all of the detail that we sense from moment to moment, it would overload the storage capacity within the receptor system (including parts of the nervous system and sense organs), which is constantly being overwritten by new information. Once we identify information that is needed, we can focus our conscious attention on it.

PAUSE & REFLECT

How good is your memory for pain? Can you really remember the sensory memory or do you have only long-term memories about the experience?

What might be the result if you had a really good memory for the sensory experience of pain?

SHORT-TERM MEMORY

The information that we focus on then moves into short-term memory. This is our working memory, and it decays after a short time. When you look up an email address or website, for example, it comes into your awareness and stays as long as you actively think about it; that is, long enough to enter the information. If something distracts you, you will probably need to go back to the source of the information. Repetition enables you to extend the time over which you keep something in short-term memory, but if you do not repeat the information it will fade in about half a minute. The capacity of short-term memory appears to be surprisingly constant between people. Regardless of individual characteristics such as sex, age or intelligence, we all seem to be able to hold about seven (plus or minus two) separate pieces of information at a time (Miller, 1956).

This makes it hard to understand how we manage a task such as reading, in which we need to retain whole sentences made up of lots of letters. We do this by gathering information into larger units, a process called 'chunking'. Instead of remembering individual letters, we remember whole words. Since the rules of language are fairly regular, we can omit remembering words such as 'the' or 'of' and fill them in later. In conversation or reading, and particularly in sending SMSs, we can chunk at the level of ideas as well. If something holds our attention, we read at a high rate, balancing 7 ± 2 ideas in short-term memory at a time. If we are less interested or the information is unfamiliar or difficult, we may have to read seven words at a time, making progress much slower.

Although the physiological basis of short-term memory is not absolutely clear, it is generally believed that impulses circulate around complex loops of neurons. If this circulation of impulses is interrupted by input that interferes with it, or by an injury such as a blow to the head, the information is lost. Without short-term operating memory, it would be very difficult to carry on our normal activities. For example, we use short-term memory to store information about goals while we carry out actions, store the topic of a sentence while we get from the beginning to the end of it, and store information about a procedure while we are actually carrying it out.

LONG-TERM MEMORY

The third storage level is long-term memory, our library of reference material. It can hold massive amounts of information indefinitely. In general, information is stored into long-term memory by rehearsal but important things may be recorded on one trial, which probably results from the fact that important things are related to already present memories and are therefore rehearsed without particular awareness of the fact. Long-term memory capacity is amazing. The process that allows us to remember massive amounts of information indefinitely is structural change in the neurons in the brain. As groups of neurons are affected by information, the interconnections between them are modified. Some connections are strengthened, involving actual physical growth, while others are weakened. Eventually, the changes become stable and we have a long-term memory.

It is useful to classify the kinds of things that we put into long-term memory. We remember how things are done, such as how to tie a shoelace or use a mobile phone. These procedural memories become so well established that we can carry out the procedures automatically, without remembering the individual steps in the process. Another kind of memory relates to the meanings of things (semantic memories). We hold memory of the words in our language, symbols and other codes that we use regularly, so that we can use them as soon as they are needed. We only have to think about retrieving meanings when we find an item that we do not recognise or where the meaning is not readily clear. Episodic memories are individual memories about experiences in our lives: our record of where we have been, what we have done, who we have met and even who we are.

THE ORGANISATION OF MEMORY

The concept of neuroplasticity offers some useful suggestions about how memory may be stored. We know that the brain is producing new neurons all the time, although only in small numbers. It appears that these new neurons are produced in central areas of the brain (the midbrain) and migrate into the cortex. There they may help to form new memories by linking up with other neurons. Although new neurons might be handy when we are learning new things, they do not appear to be necessary, and may not even be particularly helpful in some cases. As we rehearse information to move it into long-term storage, we tend to cause the retrieval of existing related memories, which suggests that new information does not create entirely new circuits. Instead, it produces loops of neurons that interconnect with existing ones. The new is added to the old and is coded in related ways. This will not only make the new information easier to retrieve the next time it is needed, but may also affect retrieval of the old. As the old loops are fired by the related information, they may become more firmly implanted. In this way, having similar experiences brings order to the memory traces and they become stronger and easier to retrieve. Most of us have the experience of recognising a face that we have seen before, but being unable to retrieve any memory of where or in what context. At this stage, the face is coded as a face only. Repeated experience with the person connects more and more information to the memory of the face, until seeing even a similar face may call up memories that are linked to the original face.

How does the organisation of memory help to explain the loss of recent memories but retention of old memories in a patient with brain damage?

MEASURING MEMORY

Remembering consists of more than just recalling total pieces of information and there are several ways that memory can be measured. While it is true that we often test for memory by asking people (e.g. students) to recall information, there are other, more subtle forms of measurement. Even when information cannot be recalled on demand, an individual may still be able to recognise it. Recognition forms the basis of multiple-choice questions. The individual is not asked to reconstruct the memory, only to recognise what they have seen before. Information may still be retained even when we cannot be sure that we recognise it. An even more subtle measure of memory is how long it takes someone to relearn material to which they have previously been exposed. If a person learnt a poem last year in three hours and cannot now recall or even recognise it, they could nevertheless relearn it in less than three hours.

FORGETTING

Since long-term memory involves physical change in the arrangement and operation of neurons, it may seem surprising that memory is not more perfect. We do forget, and often find it difficult to recall things as basic as the name of a friend or our own telephone number. How well we remember depends on how efficiently information has been coded for storage and retrieval.

No matter how we search for evidence of remembering, it is clear that some information is lost, even things that we once knew very well. Poems, dates of historical events or mathematical formulae that once got us through examinations will prove to be irretrievable for most people; even the face of our first great love can vanish. Psychologists have suggested three basic theories of forgetting. The oldest is decay theory, which suggests that memory traces simply fade away over time. For sensory memory and short-term memory, this seems to be the case. Problems occur with decay theory when we try to extend it to long-term memory. Why do some memories persist, others fade gradually, and some seem to disappear all at once? Why are procedural memories (e.g. how to ride a bicycle) resistant to fading even over a period of many years? What is it that decays? Is it neurons?

The second proposed cause of forgetting is interference: memories interfere with one another. Earlier events may interfere with the remembering of later events, but the opposite can happen as well.

The third proposal, known as motivated forgetting, suggests that we forget because we want to; that is, we repress memories that make us feel anxious or uncomfortable. It suggests that we still keep the memory in our unconscious but just do not retrieve it, and that we may choose not to store something in our memory at all.

Many people are able to recall extremely detailed episodic memories from their past, often during sleep or under the influence of hypnosis. A surgeon named Penfield (1969) reported that, during surgery, stimulation of certain brain areas would produce episodic memories. This suggests that everything we experience is stored away intact and that we may be able to unlock absolute truths about the past by reaching this memory. However, it is not uncommon to find that these complete and detailed memories are contradicted by the memories of other people, or by objective information (Loftus & Loftus, 1980). We appear to flesh out our memories by adding plausible detail—a process called **confabulation**—without being aware that we are doing so. We may combine several similar events into one. If we are asked to remember our sixth birthday party, we may retrieve a jumble of memories from a number of childhood birthday parties and fit them together to make one coherent scene. In the most extreme cases, people claim to remember past lives. This is most probably a mixture of details remembered from their current lives, history books and the media, and fitted with other material into a plausible confabulation. Keep in mind that there are likely to be reasons for it occurring and that people are not generally aware of those reasons, or even that they are confabulating.

Although much can be done to improve the accuracy of memory, it will always remain fragile. When the basic structures involved in memory fail to function properly, problems inevitably arise. One of the symptoms of dementia is that the process of moving information from short-term to long-term storage becomes faulty. Patients have no trouble remembering the distant past, but the recent past becomes murky. Because this is an unpleasant experience, confabulation may fill the gaps.

Confabulation
The addition of plausible detail to a memory to make it seem more complete. This process takes place without the individual being aware of it.

MEMORY AND HEALTH

Much about our experience of health is dependent on memory. We have memories about our personal experiences of health and illness. We also have information from outside sources, such as what we have read, heard from others or seen for ourselves. This information influences our understanding of health, illness and disease, our reactions to those states, and the behaviours that we adopt in the differing roles.

DEMENTIA

Dementia is the loss of cognitive or intellectual functions. It is increasingly prevalent, related in part to the ageing population. Better health care can maintain life longer, but longer life can result in a longer time for deterioration in body structures. Alzheimer's disease probably receives most attention in the media, but there are seven types of dementia. They all involve damage to, or death of, nerve cells in the brain. The damage cannot be repaired, so the focus of treatment is to prevent more damage.

One of the first and most obvious functions to be affected is memory. Not surprisingly, the newest and least-established memories tend to be affected first, which explains why a childhood memory may remain although the sufferer forgets the name of their treating doctor. Even if biomedical sciences find a way to regenerate the damaged or dead nerve cells, this would only be able restore function: the memories stored in the original cells would still be gone.

There are over 100 known causes of dementia, including neurological disease (e.g. Alzheimer's and Parkinson's diseases), vascular disease (e.g. multi-infarct dementia, involving death of localised groups of cells due to loss of their blood supply) and infections (e.g. HIV). When the deterioration is progressive, other important mental functions—problem-solving, decision-making, judgment and understanding—are affected. This can result in the loss of a person's individual qualities. Such loss is accompanied by personality change.

Because of the loss of memory function, the sufferer becomes less able to care for themselves. This increases the burden of care on other people, which may in turn affect the carers' health.

6.4 CASE STUDY

JEMANA AND SAFE DRIVING

Jemana is a 17-year-old student who has just applied for her learner's permit, as she wants to be able to drive a car as soon as she turns 18. Since young people have faster reflexes than older people, she wonders why she needs to keep a record of her driving practice, and why she has to have so many hours of practice before she gets her licence. Her existing knowledge—gained from watching adults drive—suggests to Jemana that driving is easy. However, learning how to drive involves developing new manual skills such as steering, braking and watching out for other cars that she did not previously need. These new skills must be integrated with existing skills such as balance and visual scanning that she learnt from walking or riding a bicycle or skateboard. Gradually, Jemana realises that practice is vital in achieving these changes in behaviour. Adult drivers may have years of driving experience in a large variety of conditions. As a result, they have learnt not just basic skills but also a range of coping strategies for different conditions. For example, a driver may have developed coping strategies (e.g. driving more cautiously, slowing or stopping when in doubt) that result in them being in fewer situations that require fast decisions or speedy reaction time. Through practice, the coping strategies become so well learnt that they are automatic.

However, driving seems to come very easily to Jemana. After 10 hours of driving around an empty car park on Sunday afternoons, she feels that she is competent to drive anywhere and at any time. Jemana is a frequent user of her mobile phone, and can read and send messages quickly and confidently. She finds it difficult to ignore her phone, for fear of missing out on something. Having persuaded her mother to let her drive home after a practice session in the car park, Jemana becomes distracted when her phone rings. She drives into a parked car. Although the damage to both cars is minor, Jemana is very distressed and subsequently finds it hard to even think about driving without experiencing anxiety. Her parents think she is overreacting and being a bit phobic.

Finally, after getting used to riding with other people and after a great deal of persuasion by her family, Jemana gets back behind the wheel. She no longer objects to the long hours of practice, and gradually becomes confident enough to drive in different conditions: at night, during rainy weather, in heavy traffic and at higher speeds on country highways. She also completes a defensive driving course. She passes her driving test and receives her licence. However, she is disappointed to learn that because of her age and her accident she will have to pay much higher insurance premiums than her 25-year-old sister, and that most rental car companies won't even let her drive one of their cars.

1   How would an understanding of how people learn and remember skills help to understand Jemana's story?

2   How could one small accident result in a phobia about driving?

3   Might the accident and subsequent anxiety cause a permanent change in Jemana's driving behaviour?

4   What factors could influence her level of risk once she is a fully licensed driver?

Points to consider

Driving and texting both require attention, information-processing, decision-making and physical movement. As large areas of the brain and memory are involved, the same functions may be called upon by both activities. Anything that interferes with the behaviours involved in safe driving will increase the likelihood of accidents. It is estimated that the risk of using mobile phones while driving is similar to the risk of driving under the influence of alcohol or drugs. It slows reaction times, interferes with motor skills, distracts attention and prevents recall of important memories for coping with driving—just as alcohol and drugs do.

Insurance companies operate on the basis of probabilities, to reduce their risk of increased costs resulting from accidents. Statistically, slightly older drivers have learnt coping skills behind the wheel, and therefore have fewer and less serious accidents. Substance-abusing drivers are more likely to have accidents, and therefore may be refused insurance coverage or have to pay higher premiums.

CHAPTER SUMMARY

Learn more
Access additional resources to broaden your understanding of this chapter. See the Guided Tour for access details.

- In high-income countries, behaviour and lifestyle have replaced infections as the main sources of illness and death.

- Modification of behaviour can prevent much illness and help to promote health.

- Risky behaviours—including smoking, alcohol abuse, illegal or prescription drug abuse, obesity and dangerous activities—constitute areas in which behaviour change is particularly important.

- Health behaviours increase levels of health, while risk-reduction behaviours are aimed at reducing the health impacts of risky behaviours.

- The study of learning (i.e. a change in the organism as a result of experience with the environment) and memory (the processes by which experience is retained within the organism) provides a basis for understanding behaviour change.

- Simple models of learning, such as classical and operant conditioning, indicate that stimuli that lead to behaviour and the consequences that follow are critical to stability and change in behaviour.

- Memory processes provide the information that we use to understand health and illness. Dementia is a significant health problem in which memory is affected.

FURTHER READING

Denning P & Little J (2017) *Over the Influence: The Harm Reduction Guide to Controlling Your Drug and Alcohol Use* (2nd edn). Guilford Publications.

Doidge N (2008) *The Brain that Changes Itself: Stories of Personal Triumph from the Frontiers of Brain Science.* Scribe.

Doidge N (2016) *The Brain's Way of Healing: Remarkable Discoveries and Recoveries from the Frontiers of Neuroplasticity.* Penguin.

Hooker S, Punjabi A, Justesen K, Boyle L & Sherman M (2018) Encouraging health behavior change: Eight evidence-based strategies. *Family Practice Management* 25(2), 31–6.

7

Thinking about Health Behaviour: Cognition and Health

CHAPTER OBJECTIVES

By the end of this chapter, you should be able to:

» understand the common ways in which individuals make decisions and how this influences decisions about health and illness, and the clinical decision-making of health professionals

» describe and compare various models of health beliefs and action regarding health, including why this behaviour may not appear to be in the best interests of the individual

» understand the role of attitudes and expectations in regulating behaviour

» describe placebo effects and how they relate to expectations

» discuss the issues raised by the use of placebo effects in research and treatment of patients

KEYWORDS

» attitudes
» agent
» algorithm
» automatisation
» balance theory
» cognition

» compliance
» endorphins
» expectancy–value theory
» expectations
» heuristics
» nocebo effects

» perception explanation
» placebo effects
» stereotyping
» validation
» wonder drug effect

Introduction

In Chapter 4, we looked at the decisions that someone makes when they experience symptoms and about thoughts that people may have about their health. It is time to take a more detailed look at thinking and problem-solving in health and illness.

Cognition
A general concept embracing all types of knowing, judging, thinking, reasoning and so on.

Cognition is a useful psychological term that refers to all the mental processes that we use. In everyday language, this includes reasoning, judging, mulling, problem-solving, deciding, comparing and all the other ways we have of dealing with information. If we are to look at the ways in which people deal with health and illness, we need to look at the general processes underlying conscious (and possibly unconscious) thinking and decision-making.

One way of looking at these processes is to say that they involve the transformation of information that may come from memory, sensory input from the environment, or sensory input from within the body. This information is then dealt with in some fashion; for example, by deciding that it is unimportant and can be ignored, by relating it to other information, by comparing it to memories, or by deciding that it is worth holding onto against some future need. These transformations may take place in the forefront of our attention or they may just go on in the background without our paying too much attention to them. Some of the processing is relatively automatic, as when a smell produces a memory without our thinking about why it smells familiar. At other times the transformation requires a lot of effort, as when we are trying to learn a new set of concepts.

7.1 CASE STUDY

DAVID AND KNEE REPLACEMENT

This case study examines the ways in which decisions about health are made.

David, aged 60, has suffered from pain in his right knee for a number of years, but it is gradually getting worse. He was athletic as a young adult but has had to completely give up playing tennis, and is now struggling to play a round of golf before the pain makes him stop. He has been told by his doctor, Dr Teresa Ngou, that he has osteoarthritis and that the cartilage in his right knee is very badly worn. He has been taking painkillers recently, but the pain is not being controlled. Pain at night is starting to interfere with his sleep. Dr Ngou referred him to an orthopaedic surgeon for evaluation. The surgeon has told David that he believes there are only two options: to continue to try to control the pain with medication, or to have a total knee replacement. David and his wife Marta have been discussing these recommendations, and the factors involved.

1   What factors would affect David and Marta's decision about a total knee replacement?
2   How could they go about improving the quality of their decision?

Rational decision-making

Cognition often involves decision-making: choosing a preferred option or course of action from among several alternatives. We have to make many of these decisions every day, from major ones such as whether to get married or choose a particular career, to minor ones such as which brand of breakfast cereal to eat, or whether to take the first available parking spot or hope for another one closer to our destination. Decisions often have to be made on the basis of incomplete or uncertain information. How do we decide to take this parking space when we cannot know for sure whether there might be a closer one? Decisions often have to be made in the face of conflicting information; for example, your mother wants you to be a doctor, but your father wants you to be an athlete. Sometimes there is conflict regarding our own preferences; for example, whether to pursue a potentially huge but very uncertain income as a rock star, or gain the certainty of a more modest income as an accountant. The same issues arise with regard to health-related decisions.

It would be nice to believe that we are rational about our decisions, weighing up the costs and gains and picking the most sensible alternative every time. **Expectancy–value theory** is the name given to one approach to understanding decision-making. It suggests that it should be possible to predict our choices by mathematical modelling, based on our attitudes about alternative choices (Vroom, 1964).

Expectancy–value theory
A model that suggests that rational choices between alternatives are based on the perceived probability of occurrence of each option and its value to the individual.

PAUSE & REFLECT

Do you have a health behaviour that seems to be irrational? Do your friends?
Can you use expectancy–value theory to explain why that behaviour continues?

Expectancy–value theory assumes that behaviour results from conscious choices among alternatives whose purpose is to maximise gain and minimise loss. 'Expectancy' refers to the strength of the person's belief that an outcome is obtainable. This expectancy has probabilities ranging from 0 (it is impossible) to 1.0 (it is certain). The term 'value' describes the value of the outcome to that individual. To the extent that our decision-making is rational and based on the best evidence that we have available, we should be trying to select the alternative that produces the highest combination of expectancy and value. An individual who has low expectancy that smoking is harmful and values smoking highly, for example, may rationally decide to continue smoking. In their case, they gain more from smoking than the health cost they ascribe to it.

Expectancy–value theory can be written as a formula:

$$Behaviour = Expectancy \times Value$$

Expectancy–value theory helps to predict many decisions, but works best when the information we have is relatively complete. If we have to choose, say, between buying one car and another, we usually can find out exactly how obtainable each car is and the cost in dollars if the cars are similarly equipped. Similarly, gains in comfort and prestige will be fairly clear. But even in this case, we often waver and struggle to decide, and may be swayed by qualities that we would have trouble defining even to ourselves. It is difficult for expectancy–value theory to explain why people bet on lotteries, for example, since any analysis would show that each bet is likely to be a loss, and that over time the regular gambler is very unlikely to gain any benefit.

Analysis of why people get vaccinated against disease, or refuse vaccination, is an area that has been studied in some detail (Brewer et al., 2017), even before the COVID-19 pandemic. Although it would appear that avoiding any disease would have high value, and vaccination offers a high probability of preventing at least the most severe consequences of a disease, a proportion of the population still rejects vaccination. Health Direct, a site supported by all Australian government Health Departments, lists the seven most common reasons for avoiding vaccination. It shows that these are directly related to beliefs about probabilities and values on each side of the argument (Health Direct, 2021).

Algorithm
A mechanical routine or simple set of rules that can be used to solve all problems of a particular kind.

When we have complete information, we can use **algorithms** to reach decisions (Chabert, 2012). An algorithm is a mechanical routine or simple set of rules that can be used to solve all problems of a particular kind. Mathematical processes such as addition, subtraction, multiplication and division are algorithms. As long as you do not make a mistake while carrying them out, you will get the right answer. Many games—noughts and crosses and checkers, for instance—are simple enough that you can use algorithms and lose only if you make a mistake. The same is true of balancing your bank account.

If, as is often the case, we do not have enough information to enable us to use algorithms, then we run out of rules that can be guaranteed to provide a right answer. Chess, for example, has far too many possible moves for a player to be certain that they have considered them all. Daily choices tend to involve a lot of complex information that is relevant to the decision and a lot of extraneous noise that is not. The choice of what to eat for breakfast would take all day if we were to consider each possible ingredient in the light of rules about nutritional value, possible risk and taste preferences—our own and those of any other people who might be sharing breakfast with us. By the time we finally came to a decision, we would probably have starved to death. It is clear that much of our decision-making is less than completely rational.

Heuristics

Decision-making is often complex and is affected by many variables, including age, gender, experience, the influence of other people, and the beliefs that a person holds. Information about expectancy and value are often very incomplete and fuzzy, yet decisions still must be made—often urgently. The result is that individuals use other, less rigorously rational ways of making decisions. A large group of these are called **heuristics** (Myers, 2012), with simple ones often referred to as 'rules of thumb'. Examples include, "Keep your head down and your eye on the ball" in golf, or "Never talk to strangers". While these rules of thumb are often based on experience—our own or others'—and can be helpful, they can often lead to irrational decision-making.

Heuristics
Problem-solving strategies based on general rules that usually or often work.

One type of heuristic is means–end analysis. After deciding where you would like to end up, you choose actions that appear to get you closer to that end. If your end with regard to breakfast is to eat in time to get to work, you may select any combination of things that you encounter that can be eaten safely; all of them will get you fed. Imagine you are a novice chess player, and you have been told that chess players try to control the centre of the board because it greatly increases their chances of winning. If you were to play your first game of chess, you may well adopt this strategy in the absence of any other heuristics. However, while it might help you to lose more slowly, it would be unlikely to help you win against the expertise of seasoned players.

Another type of heuristic is reasoning by analogy. It is based on trying to use decision-making rules that have worked in similar situations. If you have tried standing between an opponent and their goal in one sport and it has worked, you might try this in another sport that has opponents and goals. This rule could be taken from basketball and successfully applied in football, but it is not advisable in golf.

A lot of problem-solving heuristics are aimed at simplifying the problem. The term 'simplification' is used in mathematics to describe a number of procedures that have been found to improve the ability to see a possible solution. Grouping similar terms is an example. Many non-mathematical problems can be broken down into smaller parts. In subgoal analysis, the aim is to break the final goal into a number of smaller problems with goals that get you part of the way to a solution, and then attempt to find solutions to each of the smaller problems.

PAUSE & REFLECT

What heuristics do you use when you are taking notes in class?

How do you simplify things so your notes are most useful for studying later?

We frequently use heuristics when making decisions about health. If you are suffering as a result of a cold virus, there is little you can do about the virus except let your immune system develop a defence. In the meantime, taking paracetamol for the fever and pain will get you closer to the goal of not suffering. This is known as a means–end decision.

Complying with the instructions of a health professional is often associated with getting better. By extension, it is probably going to be a good idea to comply with the instructions of the next health professional you consult. Health professionals often use subgoal analysis to decide how to treat the health problems of a particular patient.

Heuristics have two advantages over algorithms: they will work with incomplete information, and they are fast. They have the disadvantage that they can be (and frequently are) wrong. The heuristics related to COVID-19 vaccinations indicate the complexity of the issue, and problems with decisions based on flawed heuristics (Madison et al., 2021). The next section considers some heuristics relevant to health decisions and some of their shortcomings.

7.2 CASE STUDY

DAVID AND MARTA (CONT.)

David and Marta might try to make the most rational decision they could by using expectancy–value theory. This would involve establishing the degree and probability of risk of having surgery, and comparing that with continuing to manage the pain with increasingly strong medication. The first consideration is financial. They have top-level private health insurance through David's employer, and he has enough sick leave to cover the surgery and rehabilitation periods without loss of income. Marta might have to take some time off work to help David with his rehabilitation, and her employer doesn't have a generous carer provision. If she took time off, their income would decrease a little but they could easily cope. Then, they consider the possible risks of surgery.

There are several heuristics available to David and Marta. They could use the analogy mentioned above: that it is in general a good idea to do what the doctor says. People often reason by analogy with individual cases that they have known about. David and Marta talk to a neighbour, who tells them about a cousin of his who had a bad experience with hip replacement surgery, falling downstairs and becoming a wheelchair user. This information worries David and Marta, as it suggests that joint replacement surgery may bring permanent risks to David's health.

1 What problems are raised by making decisions based on stories you hear about a solitary case or anecdote?

2 What are some advantages and disadvantages of making health-related decisions by using heuristics such as analogy?

HEALTH HEURISTICS

Representativeness

People make decisions because they believe that a particular event is representative of a category of event. Consider a couple who had three sons. Although they had always wanted a daughter, they decided not to have any more children because they thought the next child was bound to be a boy. Was this a correct conclusion? Not really. In the absence of a reproductive problem, which had been eliminated in this case, each conception has approximately the same chance of producing a girl as a boy. The sequence of chances that had produced boys three times in a row for this couple was irrelevant to the sex of their next child. To take another example, consider a medical doctor who dismissed his mother's complaints of pain in her hip as not serious because she suffered from arthritis and frequently had pain in her hips. She was subsequently found to have broken her hip as a result of a fall. The doctor felt very guilty that he had biased his judgment of his mother's pain on this occasion by viewing it as representative of her typical kind of pain.

Availability

Because decisions are based on the information that we can call to mind or find in other ways, they will be influenced by the availability of the information—how easy it is to remember or to find. If our cultural background is Chinese or many of our friends are Chinese, we have a high likelihood of encountering individuals who have taken Chinese herbal medicines and become well. If few of our friends are Chinese, we may know very few people who have done so. Our judgment as to whether we should try Chinese herbal medicines will be affected by this information, but it should not be. Who we know does not influence the effectiveness of the medicines in any way. The sample we have knowledge of is a biased sample, in a statistical sense. If our cultural background is Chinese or we have many Chinese friends, we will find available examples easily. If we do not, examples will not be available.

Nisbett and Ross (1980) showed that vivid information is given more importance in our decision-making than less vivid information, apparently because it is more easily available.

Information is likely to attract and hold our attention to the extent that it is emotionally interesting, concrete, image-provoking and/or recent, nearby or involves someone we know. This can explain why media stories about miraculous new treatments attract so much attention and can lead to people trying something that does not have a good evidence base. Wonder drug stories are certainly vivid.

PAUSE & REFLECT

Think of a recent health-related story that has made a great impact on you.

What made the impact so strong?

Clinical decision-making

It may appear that the main difference between experts and others is that the expert has more knowledge. While the decision-making of health professionals about patients involves the same processes as those described above, expert health professionals' decision-making differs from that of less expert individuals in several ways.

Some algorithms are used. The process of making a differential diagnosis involves listing the diagnoses that a reasonable professional could make, based on the observed symptoms and signs. Results of the history obtained from the patient and tests that have been performed, along with any other data that can be found, are used to eliminate diagnoses from the list until the most probable one is identified. Other diagnoses of lower probability may not have been fully excluded; the competent professional keeps these in mind until they can be excluded.

Biomedical theories about how particular causes produce particular symptoms and signs lead to models of operation for health professionals. These theories may change as more knowledge is obtained but, to the extent that they represent how things really operate, they are algorithms. But they may well be incomplete or only partially accurate, in which case they resemble heuristics more than they do algorithms.

Health professionals use a variety of heuristics that may have been learnt from others or derived from the professionals' own experience (Fernández-Aguilar et al., 2021). These medical rules of thumb can be as simple as testing all adult patients for high blood pressure. Means–end analysis is frequently used to decide how to make a patient feel better as well as to treat the cause of their disease. In the absence of a specific diagnosis of a disease— which is very common in practice—subgoal analysis may focus on relieving symptoms, one at a time, until the problem goes away or the diagnosis becomes clearer. Simplification strategies could include identifying what the most important symptom is for the patient and concentrating on that first, or grouping problems that have similar treatments.

Pattern recognition is an important decision-making process. As a result of training or experience, health professionals develop an ability to recognise combinations of elements that may signal the presence of a meaningful pattern, which could include information from an observation of the patient's appearance and behaviour that leads to a feeling that the problem is likely to be a specific one. This can lead to the professional making correct choices about what questions to ask, how to ask them or how to respond to the patient— questions that speed up or smooth the process of diagnosis and treatment.

Automatisation
The carrying out of
patterns of behaviour or
thinking that are so well
learnt that they require
no apparent thought.

Automatisation refers to patterns of behaviour or thinking that are so well learnt that they require no apparent thought. Hand-washing becomes automatised for many health professionals, as does the care of equipment and touching of patients. Taking histories may also become automatic. A problem for students in the health professions is that their clinical teachers may forget that a decision-making process that is automatised for them will need careful step-by-step explanation for students. This is as true for diagnostic heuristics as it is for the proper way to give an injection. Automatisation is not restricted to the behaviour of health professionals, however. It is common through all aspects of our lives, from the way in which we hold our cutlery or chopsticks while we eat, to the way we type when we are writing an essay.

Health beliefs

Attitudes
An individual's
thoughts, feelings and
readiness to act in
relation to any object,
person or event.

The cognitions that an individual has regarding health are a major influence on health behaviour. An important part of these cognitions is **attitudes**. Attitudes consist of the thoughts, feelings and readiness to act that we have about any object, person or event. Our attitude to peanut butter, for example, may include knowledge about its nutritional value, feelings about its taste and stickiness, and readiness to eat peanut butter if it is offered, or to go out and buy some if there is none available in the house.

The sick role is discussed in Chapter 4.

To take an example from a health-related area, attitudes to exercise would include not only knowledge of what it is and what effects it can have on cardiovascular fitness, but also how exercising makes the individual feel and whether that individual is prepared to go out and exercise in the face of competing time and energy demands. Health psychologists— along with advertisers, politicians and many others—have an interest in understanding how we make decisions about health. One primary focus in the study of health behaviour has been on the interaction between attitudes—our thoughts, feelings and behavioural intentions—and their relationship to actual behaviour.

The influences of culture, social class and family are discussed in Chapter 14.

By understanding people's attitudes, researchers can use them in promoting health. Using a vivid emotional story, for example, may be more helpful in persuading people to adopt certain health behaviours than using statistics to convey similar information. A very important influence on health decision-making is being part of a group. Groups share knowledge, attitudes and biases. They also confer the rights and obligations of the sick role.

Because of differences in health beliefs between cultures, it is important that health professionals have at least a general knowledge of what those health beliefs are. For example, Vicary and Westerman (2004) found that many First Peoples in Western Australia did not think of depression as a disease that could be treated. Similar issues arise with First Peoples in other countries, and with immigrants and refugees.

The general principles of decision-making discussed above are all relevant to health decision-making, but a number of theories have been proposed that are specifically aimed at predicting important choices about health. The persistence of unhealthy behaviour— which should be very unlikely if decision-making is rational—indicates the importance of understanding the process. There are quite a number of theories about health behaviour, which is in itself a problem (Noar & Zimmerman, 2005; Weinstein, 2007) because it can lead to confusion and even be misleading. This issue is discussed after a brief presentation of some sample theories.

THEORIES ABOUT HEALTH BELIEFS

Theories are useful for assisting health professionals to change clients' behaviours. Theories can also help change the behaviours of health professionals themselves (Turner et al., 2021).

The health belief model (HBM) depicted in Figure 7.1 was developed by people who were interested in patient compliance with recommended health behaviours (Rosenstock, 1974; Scherr et al., 2017). There is a degree of resemblance between the HBM and expectancy–value theory. The degree of perceived threat (value) to individuals is made up of their general views about the importance of health, their personal vulnerability to a particular threat, and the severity of that threat if it were to occur. The individual's perception of the benefits that would come from a particular health behaviour and the barriers to that health behaviour are important in determining whether they will believe that the health behaviour is possible and likely to be effective in averting the threat (expectancy).

This model predicts some behaviour quite well (Sulat et al., 2018), but does not seem to account for all the cognitive factors involved in health behaviour (Allen, 1998). Noar and Zimmerman (2005) suggest that the HBM might be most useful when the health threat presented by a particular behaviour is obvious to the individual. The HBM has been used widely in health communication and awareness campaigns. It is most effective when all the components of the models are addressed: severity, susceptibility, perceived benefits, and perceived barriers in either a media campaign or in personal interactions with clients. Identifying and addressing perceived barriers is very important, and sometimes forgotten by health professionals. Behaviour change becomes much easier once barriers (real or perceived) are identified and addressed.

FIGURE 7.1 Health belief model

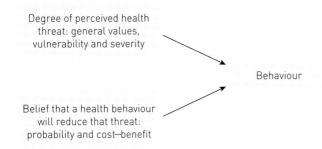

Rosenstock (1974)

PAUSE & REFLECT

Think about your attitude towards smoking.

Where did it come from? Have media campaigns played a significant part? Have your parents?

The HBM does not take into account the social influence of others (approval or disapproval of the behaviour) in the decision-making process (Fishbein & Ajzen, 1975). In many cases, people's decisions about health behaviour are influenced by what they hear from others, what is presented in the media, and what the general opinions of health professionals are. The theory of reasoned action (Fishbein & Ajzen, 1975; see Figure 7.2) tried to predict motivations for health behaviours, including social influence. Norms (a person's perception of what others believe should be done) and attitudes (a person's perception of the consequences of a behaviour) were seen to impact on that person's intentions to behave. This theory proposes that intentions would accurately predict actual behaviour.

FIGURE 7.2 The Theory of Reasoned Action

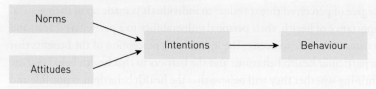

Fishbein & Ajzen (1975)

This model of decision-making about health has enabled people to predict health behaviours in a variety of settings, but it struggles when people either do not control the behaviour in question or at least believe that they do not control it (e.g. domestic violence or terminal disease diagnosis). This resulted in the theory of planned behaviour (Ajzen & Madden, 1986; see Figure 7.3) which includes the construct of perceived control (the belief that a person has or does not have control over a particular behaviour). This construct is closely related to the self-efficacy concept in social cognitive theory, which will be discussed later.

FIGURE 7.3 The Theory of Planned Behaviour

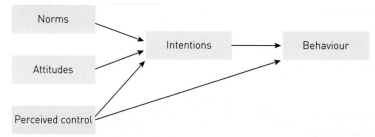

Ajzen & Madden (1986)

Neither of these models appears to take much account of the effect of the individual's past behaviour or habits on their present behaviour, unless we consider the impact of learning on norms, attitudes, perceived control and intentions. These two theories may be most useful when the connection between intention and behaviour is strong and clear to the individual. One way to use these theories is as a checklist when working with clients, either when interviewing them (e.g. "What do you intend to do over the next seven days?"), or when proposing strategies for behavioural change (working together with the client to change their social norms, attitudes, perceived control or intentions). A health professional can quickly assess a person's social norms, personal attitudes, control beliefs and intentions towards a behaviour of interest and make recommendations related to each of the constructs to ensure that behaviour change is likely. This is because a theory is most effective when all the components are addressed.

Clearly, the influence of our thought processes on our behaviour is complex. We cannot expect all health behaviour to be rational.

Too many theories?

There are thousands of studies that have looked at whether theories of health behaviour really explain health behaviour (Weinstein, 2007). The typical conclusion is that a particular set of cognitions occurs in those individuals whose behaviour changes, and does not occur in those whose behaviour does not change. This is usually demonstrated by correlations between cognitions and behaviours at the end of the process, which, unfortunately, doesn't enable us to be certain that it was the existence of the cognitions in the first place that led to the behaviour. There could have been common factors that produced both, or it could be the behaviour that led to the cognitions (Bandura, 1998).

Noar and Zimmerman (2005) suggest that this mass of research is not really advancing our knowledge about what regulates behaviour, and that we need a different approach if we are to move forward. They recommend comparing different theories within the same study to see if we can determine whether particular cognitions are more important than others. These studies would need to be carried out with many different behaviours, because any single theory may predict better in one situation than another. They would also need to begin before the behaviour change attempt started, so that the order of events could be studied all the way through the process. There is also a problem with the multiplication of concepts used in numerous studies. Weinstein (1984) suggested that we need to consider unrealistic optimism as a factor, and Rogers (1985) suggested including fear in the HBM. This increase in the number of concepts can result in confusion and a lack of comparability between studies. Ogden (2007) described the addition of ethical/moral norms, anticipated regret, self-identity, ambivalence, emotion, personality and self-prediction to various models, thus adding further to these conceptual issues.

Another problem with the large number of theories is that even though they use different terms, they don't necessarily differ from one another (Weinstein, 2007). A lot of the concepts are very similar. The most obvious case is the theory of planned behaviour, which was developed out of the theory of reasoned action by adding the concept of perceived control. How different is that from the importance of cognitions in the HBM regarding whether a healthy behaviour is possible and likely to be effective in averting a threat to health? Ogden (2003) advanced the view that while each of these theories may help predict some behaviours some of the time, they may lead to circular reasoning; that is, the conclusions drawn from them may be "true by definition rather than by observation" (p. 424). There are common elements in these theories that are almost certainly of importance. One of these is knowledge about a link between a particular behaviour and some aspect of health. If the person is not aware that a behaviour is unhealthy, they will not be motivated to change that behaviour. A second common element is the perceptions that a person has about their control over the behaviour. The person who doesn't believe that the behaviour is controllable, or who believes that they can't control it for some reason, is unlikely to make the effort. These beliefs about control may relate to barriers (e.g. they may not be able to afford professional help) or personal capabilities (they may have an external locus of control and believe that powerful others control their outcomes).

One way of simplifying these models is to look at how a variety of factors may act through a more general factor. The integrative model (IM) of behavioural prediction (Fishbein, 2008) focuses on how a number of the factors described above impact on motivation. In the integrative model, intention to behave in a particular way, along with relevant behavioural skills and environmental factors that allow or constrain the behaviour, are seen as exerting direct influence on behaviour. Understanding these three elements can lead to predictions about both individual behaviour change and the effectiveness of broader inventions aimed at groups or populations (Dai et al., 2017).

Most of the factors discussed in the previous paragraphs exert influence by changing the individual's intention to behave. For example, beliefs that a behaviour will affect health, or emotions such as fear, both act on our intentions to behave. If we have the necessary skills to carry out the behaviour, and nothing in the environment prevents it (or if something promotes it), we will have a higher likelihood of carrying out the behaviour. While is it more general than most models, the IM still does not necessarily answer all the objections given above. One general theory of behaviour (not just health behaviour) that takes these aspects into account is social cognitive theory (Bandura, 1986).

Social cognitive theory

See Chapter 16 for more about health promotion.

As applied to health behaviour, the emphasis of social cognitive theory is on the individual as the **agent** of change. The idea of the individual as agent of change is also central to the practice of health promotion (Chapter 16) and to self-managed models of care (Chapter 4). The links between the person and the outcome are efficacy beliefs and outcome expectations (Bandura, 1998). Efficacy beliefs can come about through four main influences. The most effective of these are mastery experiences. When the individual attempts to exert control and is successful, these mastery experiences increase their sense of self-efficacy; conversely, failure undermines self-efficacy. The second influence comes from vicarious experiences, in which the individual observes what happens to others (role models) when they exert control and succeed or fail. The third influence is social persuasion, which involves direct or indirect attempts to convey to individuals that they can influence their outcomes through their own efforts and that change is possible. In all of these situations, it is important not to overlook the fourth influence—the somatic (energy level) and emotional states of the individual at a particular moment in time. Tiredness can lead to a lowered sense of control, for example, even if it has resulted from illness rather than from efforts to exert control. Depression arises in biochemical processes within the brain, but has profound effects on cognitions. The depressed individual feels helpless to influence events or their own feelings, and the hopelessness that accompanies depression saps motivation to behave at all.

Agent
The person who has control over the stimuli and/or reinforcements for change.

Outcome expectations are cognitions that the individual has about what will follow a particular behaviour. This is related to expectancy in expectancy–value theory and elements of most HBMs. Bandura (1998) states that these expectations include beliefs about how the behaviour will make the individual feel (physical), what kinds of reactions the behaviour will produce in other people who observe it (social) and how the individual will view themselves following the behaviour (self-evaluative). This last aspect is, in Bandura's view, often overlooked in other theories about health behaviour.

The relationship between self-efficacy and reinforcement is discussed in Chapter 5.

PAUSE & REFLECT

Write a list of your outcome expectations regarding exercise.

How many are physical, social and self-evaluative?

One of the differences between social cognitive theory and many of the others described above is that it is more general; that is, it is intended to describe a broader range of behaviour than just health behaviour. As a result, it can be helpful in integrating theories of health behaviour and in designing ways to compare them. There are other theories of this more general sort, such as self-determination theory (Ryan & Deci, 2000). Attempts to compare theories are not common, however, and there appears to be a great deal of overlap between them. Cognitive theories are useful in explaining a variety of behaviours that are important to health. Compliance with healthy behaviour or treatment is one of the most important of these.

The steps to health behaviour change

Prochaska and DiClemente (1984) looked at the steps that people tend to go through when moving towards a change in health-related behaviour. Their transtheoretical model enables other theories to be brought together to map the process of change. Central to this theory is the idea that behaviour change is a process that can take a short (e.g. immediate smoking cessation following lung cancer diagnosis) or a long period of time (e.g.regular smoking cessation process when there is no immediate perceived threat to health). The theory can be used to guide thinking about what kinds of intervention are most likely to help people to move in a healthy direction of change. It also serves as a useful model of decision-making for health professionals. It is often described as a spiral model, because individuals frequently drop back from a higher stage to a lower one as motivation wavers, as accidents interfere with change or if relapses occur.

Illness behaviour as a process is discussed in Chapter 4.

1   *Precontemplation stage.* This refers to the time before behaviour change is considered. The individual either does not realise they have a problem or has no thoughts that the problem can be changed. Interventions at this stage need to be aimed at bringing about awareness of the problem.

PAUSE & REFLECT

What strategy might you use to encourage change in a patient who has no intention of altering their risky behaviour?

How could you introduce the idea of change (without confrontation) with, for example, a cyclist who won't wear a helmet?

2   *Contemplation stage.* This begins when the individual recognises that something is wrong and needs to be changed. This does not mean that a decision has been made to do something or that they have a plan for doing something. Interventions at this stage should focus on the probability that change is possible and that it would have a significant effect on the individual's risk of ill health.

3   *Preparation stage.* This refers to the time during which the individual is thinking of how to change a behaviour. They may be evaluating strategies they have heard about, talking to others who have made the change, and developing the commitment to try. Interventions at this stage aim at motivating and educating about change rather than just about the problem itself.

4   *Action stage.* This is when the individual has begun to modify the behaviour. It does not mean that the change has taken place or that it is certain to occur, only that the change attempt has begun. At this stage, it is best if interventions focus on encouragement and motivation.

5   *Maintenance stage.* Once the behaviour is changed for a while, the individual is in the maintenance stage. The importance of this stage is often overlooked in the enthusiasm over the fact that a change has occurred. Maintenance is critical: many well-planned change programs fall apart because the individual has no strategies for keeping the change going and dealing with relapses. Interventions here can look at the benefits gained from the change and what would be lost if the individual returned to the earlier behaviour. Specific relapse management strategies (see Chapter 8) and coping strategies to deal with temptation may be helpful.

Not all experts find this model useful. Bandura (1998) suggested that the boundaries between the stages of the transtheoretical model are fuzzy; they are matters of degree rather than true boundaries. How long, for example, does a person stay in the action stage before they are in the maintenance stage? One month? Six? Another criticism of the stages of change is that the most effective intervention for a particular individual may include several elements that are linked to different stages. In fact, a general criticism of all stage theories is that they don't allow for individual variation.

7.3 CASE STUDY

DAVID AND MARTA (CONT.)

Dr Ngou maintains that it would be a good idea for David to have the knee replacement, as she is concerned about the risks of increasing use of powerful painkillers. David and Marta decide to accept whatever she recommends, because they see her as the expert where matters pertaining to health are concerned (a heuristic).

Dr Ngou knows that much of the success of knee replacement will rest on David's compliance with his rehabilitation program—physiotherapy, special exercise programs, and giving himself time to fully recover. She also knows that David will have to modify some of his activities following the replacement, as there will be some limitations.

Dr Ngou decides that, as far as surgery is concerned, David and Marta are in the contemplation stage because they are thinking about it. She knows that she should try to increase their knowledge about the effectiveness of a knee replacement in greatly reducing or eliminating David's pain, and the importance of that for David's quality of life. By talking to David and Marta about surgery in general, Dr Ngou is providing them with norms, with the aim of modifying their intentions. This will encourage them to behave in a way that Dr Ngou believes is in David's best interests.

David has his knee replacement. Talking to health professionals and other patients during his post-surgery exercise and physiotherapy sessions, he finds that most expect positive outcomes. A few focus on the immediate post-surgical pain and limitations and grumble about the rehabilitation, but most are keen to participate. David begins to think that he is likely to have good outcome, and begins to feel better quite quickly (this is a variety of placebo effect).

1 How would David's experience affect his thinking about future treatment if his other joints were to become painful due to osteoarthritis?

2 Could David's expectations about rehabilitation make it more likely that he will feel better, and that he will comply with the exercise program?

3 Could surgery produce placebo effects?

Compliance

Given that we like to think of ourselves as rational beings, it is instructive to note that non-compliance with advice and instructions from health professionals is a serious and common problem. A majority of patients do not, for example, take medication in the doses or time patterns that doctors recommend. Sometimes this is because the patient did not understand the instructions, but usually it is because the patient was not motivated to follow instructions that they did understand. Shelton (1994) lists the following as factors that reduce **compliance**: low levels of experienced distress, denial of the illness, poor communications, complexity of the treatment program, embarrassment about the treatment, side effects, and gains from remaining ill. Factors that encourage compliance include effective communication, simple programs, clear instructions, positive reinforcement of compliance and, of course, any decrease in distress that comes with following the treatment program (Krot & Sousa, 2017).

> **Compliance**
> Obeying another person's instruction, or acting as they would like. It does not necessarily mean agreeing with the reasons behind the instructions.

It is clear from this that compliance will be particularly low when the individual's diagnosis is not accompanied by a sense of being ill, such as treatment for high blood pressure, treatment for asthma aimed at preventing rather than relieving attacks, or antibiotic treatment where the individual should take the entire course of tablets regardless of whether the symptoms have gone. Compliance will also be low if the side effects of treatment are unpleasant or embarrassing, such as when drugs cause stomach upset, headache or drowsiness.

There is much that can be done by both the health professional and health education to improve compliance. It is perhaps surprising that little is being done when the problem is so significant. The reason may lie in the assumption that we are all more rational in our thinking and decision-making about health than in other areas of life—because of the benefits to be gained and risks of not complying—but the study of health beliefs tends to indicate that this is not necessarily the case.

Expectations and healing

As these health beliefs models indicate, a wide variety of expectations may influence our behaviour: the beliefs of important others, our past experiences and our expectations about how the world works. These expectations play a very large role in regulating our thoughts, emotions and behaviours.

EXPECTATIONS

Expectations
The cognitions held by an individual about what is likely to happen in a given situation.

Expectations are the cognitions that individuals have about what is likely to happen in a given situation. When we flip a light switch, we expect to get light, not water. When we say to someone, "How are you?" we expect to get a ritual response such as "I'm fine", not details of digestion and respiration. Expectations allow us to simplify our interactions with the world so that they are predictable. Remember that beliefs are expectations about the workings of the world, while health beliefs are expectations about the workings of health.

Not surprisingly, we like to have our expectations confirmed. When we expect to do well in an examination, and we do well, we are pleased. If we do not do well, we are disappointed. When we do not expect to do well and do not, it gives us some satisfaction to prove ourselves right. Punishment can be satisfying if it confirms our expectations. It means that the world is a predictable place and that we can organise ourselves to meet it. A stable life is predictable. Research on life stress—the effect on someone's health of the events that occur to them—has shown that change is always stressful, whether it is positive change such as a promotion, or negative change such as loss of a job. In either case, change decreases our certainty about how to behave and what to expect.

Life events and stress are discussed in Chapter 12.

Balance theory (Heider, 1967) suggests that consistency is the organising principle of our cognitions. Thus, if our cognitions are consistent with one another, we are in a state of balance—a satisfactory state. For example, you might want all of your friends to like one another. If your two best friends hate one another, it creates a state of imbalance within you, and you will work to produce a more balanced state. You might drop one friend, deciding that the other friend is right and the dropped one is really not so nice after all. You might work to change both your friends' minds by getting them to like one another. If all else fails, you may deny the imbalance by convincing yourself (inaccurately) that they really do like one another but just can't be in the same place at the same time because of chance factors. Consistency is important to the way in which we form expectations about people.

Balance theory
An approach that suggests consistency is the organising principle of an individual's cognitions.

PAUSE & REFLECT

Think of a time when your cognitions were unbalanced or you felt stressed because things didn't seem to make sense.

What were your coping strategies?

Did you choose to change some of your thinking to make yourself more comfortable?

The importance of the individual's expectations of a medical treatment to its outcome was demonstrated in a study done by Dix (1985), who looked at the expectations of patients with long-term pain resulting from osteoarthritis of the knee. All patients took part in three treatment conditions over a three-month period. At the end of this period, the subjects who reported the most improvement were those who had moderate expectations at the beginning. By comparison, those who had either low or high expectations showed little improvement. Those with low expectations got what they expected—not much. Those whose expectations were too high could not have been satisfied by any treatment and were disappointed. Moderate and realistic expectations seem to be crucial to the achievement of improvement, whatever the treatment.

PLACEBO EFFECTS

Historically, a placebo (from the Latin for "I will please") was thought of as a sugar pill: a substance of no worth given to humour a difficult patient. A clear distinction has existed in people's minds between treatments (which work) and placebos (which do not). Every health professional will encounter patients who have been cured by a faith healer, a magic device or a sugar pill. The patient will not be lying or crazy. The health professional will find that clear clinical signs of an infection, an emotional symptom or even a tumour have disappeared. Such incidents cannot be dismissed as simple coincidences. They demonstrate the strength of **placebo effects** (Colloca, 2018a).

Placebo effects
The non-specific effects that any treatment produces.

The very best treatments do not always work, and so-called placebos often do (Colloca, 2018b). Recognition of this fact has led to a change in the way treatments are understood, especially in the way in which treatments are evaluated. Any treatment has specific effects; for example, diuretics are drugs that cause cells to lose water, morphine is a drug that binds to receptors on cells that respond to pain. Every treatment will also produce some non-specific effects; that is, ones for which no direct consequence of the treatment seems responsible. Placebo effects refer to these non-specific (or non-pharmacological or non-surgical) effects that a treatment produces.

A placebo effect is generally defined by the proportion of subjects who respond to a (supposedly) inert treatment in a randomised control trial, preferably double-blind; that is, a trial in which neither the researcher nor the recipient knows whether a real treatment or a placebo is being administered. A randomised control trial is one in which patients are assigned at random to receive either the experimental treatment or a placebo. Beecher (reported in Balis, 1978) studied the effects of morphine on post-surgical pain. Patients who had undergone abdominal surgery, which is extremely painful, were given injections of either morphine or sterile saline. Saline is considered a placebo in this case because there is no particular reason for assuming that it will have any effect on pain. It was estimated that about half of the effect of morphine could be attributed to its placebo effects. It is worth remembering that the patients given morphine knew that there was a 50:50 chance that they were getting saline. As a result, they may have been experiencing a nocebo effect (discussed later in this chapter).

PAUSE & REFLECT

One major difference between treatments prescribed by health professionals and complementary treatments such as herbal remedies is that the former have been tested in randomised control trials and most of the latter have not.

What health risks might result from the lack of scientific testing?

Because of the strength of placebo effects, most new treatments undergo rigorous testing involving double-blind, placebo-controlled trials, which has provided a considerable amount of information about the scope of placebo effects. When tested without a placebo control condition, treatments are very much more likely to be judged to be effective. Unfortunately, many alternative or natural treatments have never been tested against placebos. This means that they may seem at first glance to be more effective and less prone to side effects than scientifically validated medical treatments. When rigorously tested, many of the untested alternative treatments turn out to be ineffective, to interfere with other treatments or even to have dangerous side effects. Without such testing, any effects that these treatments may appear to have may simply be placebo effects.

Placebo effects are reported by 30–50% of subjects in all treatments when controlled studies are done, although some authors report the range to be 0–100%, depending on the conditions (Shapiro & Morris, 1978). The proportion of placebo responders tends to vary depending on the treatment, with higher proportions of patients responding to placebos in trials of mood-altering treatments, for example, and lower proportions in trials of pain relievers.

Results produced by placebos can include every effect produced by any treatment (Balis, 1978). They have been shown to affect not just symptoms such as pain, headache, coughing, nausea and depression, but also underlying bodily states. They have been reported to be able to produce dilation of airways, reduce blood sugar in people with diabetes, reduce swelling following injury, improve (or impair) immune function, and even slow or reverse tumour growth. Spiro (1986) examined a large number of reports and concluded that there is better evidence that placebos affect illness than that they affect disease.

This finding includes surgical procedures. In the 1950s, one treatment for angina pectoris (chest pain resulting from coronary artery disease) was internal mammary artery ligation, a procedure that involved operating to tie off the internal mammary artery. Many patients reported considerable, although usually temporary, pain relief after the operation. Dimond et al. (1960) reported the results of a placebo-controlled trial using sham surgery, in which some patients (double-blind) received an anaesthetic, had their chests opened and then immediately sewn back up. The results were quite clear: the same proportion of sham-operated patients reported pain relief as for the ligation patients, and some reported greater pain relief than most of the ligation patients. The authors summed up their discussion by referring to the powerful psychological effects of surgery. Needless to say, internal mammary artery ligation is no longer performed. Ethical restrictions were less strict at the time of this research, and because the experiment involved deception and unnecessary anaesthesia it would be considered unethical by current standards.

Placebos also produce side effects. If the common side effects of a real treatment are well known, a placebo will often produce them (e.g. gastric symptoms with placebo antibiotics). Logically enough, the more medicinal a placebo, the more effective it is likely to be. A big pill would work better than a small one, a capsule better than a pill, an injection even better, and a painful injection best of all. Side effects resulting from placebos are so consistent that it is hard to remember that we are discussing the effects of inert substances.

Factors affecting occurrence of placebo effects

It has often been assumed that placebo responders are a particular group—neurotic perhaps, or unintelligent. However, there is little evidence to suggest that they can be identified as a particular group. Whether an individual responds to a treatment seems more related to their outcome expectations for that treatment at that time, than to any enduring characteristic of the patient (Shapiro & Morris, 1978). Scientifically oriented people may be less likely to respond to a spiritually based treatment, but may in turn be more likely to respond to a plausible scientific placebo than might a religious person. In fact, placebo effects vary within a given individual over time, across bodily systems, between types of treatments and from one treating health professional to another. If there are any characteristics that comprise a placebo personality, they include a lack of confidence about knowledge in a particular area, and persuasibility. Even these characteristics can, in a particular case, be overwhelmed by situational factors.

Different health professionals get differing levels of response from their patients to almost any treatment. Placebo treatments are just another case. The enthusiasm of the health professional for the treatment is important, and one of the major factors behind the **wonder drug effect**, which is the observed tendency for a new treatment to appear to work better than existing ones only while it is new to the market (Wieseler et al., 2019). A better relationship with patients produces bigger placebo responses. It is likely that these things lead to greater trust by patients of the health professional and, as a result, better expectations for outcome.

Wonder drug effect
The observed tendency for a new treatment to work better while it is new to the market.

The situation in which treatment takes place has all the elements of **stereotyping**. Health professionals often wear uniforms and have professional manners. Walls and desks are covered with the symbols and tools of the trade, and interaction tends to proceed in a stereotypical way. The setting and interaction themselves can have healing effects, some of which may result from conditioning. As a person gains experience with attending health professionals, they experience repetition of the pattern: "See a health professional—get better." Since the natural history of most disorders is to get better, this repetition of stimulus and response will tend to occur whatever the health professional does. The person may become conditioned to get better. Certainly, patients' anxiety levels drop considerably when they have seen a health professional (in most cases) because they have a clearer idea of what to expect, including that they will get better.

Stereotyping
Assuming that a member of a category of people will share all of the characteristics attributed to that category.

Stereotypes are biases in person perception, as discussed in Chapter 4.

One important element of the doctor stereotype is that the consultation usually ends with a prescription. If the patient does not get the prescription—whether or not they need one—they may be unhappy. This puts pressure on the doctor to give something, even where nothing is likely to help the patient, just to humour them and take advantage of any placebo effects. This shot-in-the-dark approach is often justified on the basis that it does little harm. Unfortunately, many of the substances given in this way, such as antibiotics, do have considerable potential to do harm. In addition, going along with the situation stereotype tends to lead patients to trust medication rather than their own resources. More and more doctors are recognising that patients can accept reassurance and behavioural interventions, and will show the same kind of conditioned healing with many fewer side effects. The Australian government encourages doctors to give behavioural prescriptions, written on a standard prescription form, to take advantage of this stereotype.

PAUSE & REFLECT

Imagine that you are being treated by a health professional for some health problem.

What stereotypes are present in your image?

Psychological explanations of placebo effects

A number of psychological explanations have been offered for placebo responses. Most of these have been mentioned already in relation to expectations, but a review may help to organise them. All are true in some degree, which is why they have continually been referred to in the plural—placebo effects. There are as many placebo effects as there are explanations, conditions, treatments and patients.

Conditioning was discussed above. Prior experience with treatments in general leads to conditioned healing. It does not give a precise explanation for the mechanism by which change takes place. The other explanations given below may provide that mechanism.

Perception explanations suggest that placebos actually affect the perception of the symptom rather than the symptom itself. If a person has pain and takes a sugar pill, the pain is still the same as it was, but it seems to be less severe. There is a large body of work that supports this explanation, and it is undeniable that placebos have a major influence on our perceptions. It is not the whole explanation, however, since placebos have been shown to affect underlying conditions as well. It is difficult to see how altered perception could lower blood pressure, for example, or increase someone's resistance to infection.

Perception explanation
The idea that placebos affect the perception of the symptom rather than the symptom itself.

Validation is based on the idea that patients will assume that a health professional will not give them a diagnosis or a treatment unless they have valid reasons for seeking them. When a health professional gives a patient any treatment, they have done several other things: they have validated the illness by saying, "Yes, you really are ill", and indicated that the illness is significant enough to merit treatment and that the effort of providing that treatment is worthwhile—all this can give the individual hope that improvement in their condition is achievable. As well as improving their mood, this validation can mobilise the patient's resources to their own benefit (Frank, 1973) and also mobilise others to help them. Subsequent effects might be produced by the hope and the mobilisation of resources. The role of validation in placebo effects should not be overlooked.

Validation
The idea that patients assume that a health professional will not give them a diagnosis or treatment unless they have valid reasons for seeking a diagnosis or treatment.

Theories of placebo effects are often based on suggestion, by either the health professional or the patient, which leads to the individual being persuaded that they are getting better. This leads to actual improvement. Suggestion may arise from direct attempts to influence the patient, the nature of the treatment relationship (sometimes called transference), role demands (Shapiro & Morris, 1978) or possibly even hypnotism. Persuasion certainly occurs in healing, but the question remains: If we have that much control over our bodily processes, why are we unable to learn to use it without the intervention of some inert treatment?

People try to get their responses to treatments to add up and make sense. This leads them to expect change, then to evaluate the results that appear to come from the treatment, and then to re-evaluate their thinking about their illness and the treatment. This can lead to placebo effects but can also lead to the opposite, known as **nocebo effects.** These can include the patient feeling worse or having side effects or adverse experiences from a placebo, but also from a genuine treatment (Howick et al., 2018). The study by Dix (1985) cited earlier would indicate that such mental arithmetic occurs in patients who expect too little or too much from their treatment.

Nocebo effects
Negative experiences which follow a treatment, such as side effects or failure to work, that result from patient expectations and not from the treatment itself.

Storms and Nisbett (1970) suggested that some people get little benefit from sleeping pills due to a nocebo effect based on mental arithmetic. These individuals take a pill, go to bed and begin to think: "I have taken the pill, so I should sleep. But I am not sleeping, therefore I must be worse than I thought." Then they lie there and worry about the significance of the sleeping pill not working. The researchers suggested that, if this occurs, giving people an arousal placebo might work better than a relaxation placebo. Subjects could then attribute feeling awake to the effects of the pill, which would lead them to stop worrying about their state of alertness and go to sleep. Subjects who received the arousal pill went to sleep sooner and reported better sleep than the subjects given the relaxation pill. While mental arithmetic probably serves to modify increasing or decreasing placebo effects, and may be particularly useful in explaining side effects of placebos, it is too narrow an explanation to cover very much.

All of the above explanations, and others, ultimately result in a reduction in a patient's uncertainty about the future. This can decrease anxiety, improve compliance and alter risky behaviours.

Physiological explanations

In addition to—or resulting from—these psychological factors, placebos produce biochemical and physiological changes that can help explain the observed phenomena (Colloca, 2018a). A few of these explanations are given here.

The body produces a number of substances that can change physical states or affect ongoing physical processes. Examples include **endorphins**, which are considered to be the body's own pain relievers and bind to the same sites as morphine. Circulating levels of endorphins are known to increase during exercise, (sometimes) in yoga, and in chronic pain. Levine et al. (1978) suggested that endorphins may help to account for placebo pain relief (analgesia). They analysed blood from pain sufferers who had been given a placebo treatment for pain following the extraction of wisdom teeth and found higher levels of circulating endorphins in placebo responders than in non-responders. When subjects were given a blocking dose of a drug (an endorphin antagonist called Naloxone), placebo effects were significantly reduced. Although other researchers have failed to replicate the results quite as clearly, this research suggests an interesting model for the physiological process underlying placebo pain relief. However, it relates only to pain relief, and while it explains the 'how' it does not offer much help on the 'why' of placebo responding in that area.

> **Endorphins**
> Endogenous substances that are considered to be the body's own pain relievers, binding to the same receptor sites on neurons as morphine.

It has been noted that immune function can be affected by a variety of events at the cognitive level. Stress, anxiety and depression have all been linked to poorer immune function. Treatments aimed at reducing stress (e.g. relaxation, hypnosis, meditation and mental imaging) have all been linked to improved immune function. It is not surprising, therefore, to find that placebos may have a considerable effect on immune functioning, which may help to explain how things as varied as AIDS, colds and cancer may be affected by placebos. This is closely related to the next explanation.

> *Psychoneuroim-munology is discussed in Chapter 10.*

Placebos may cause a reduction in damping effects caused by stress. Stress has a mobilising effect on the organism. Partly as a result, some bodily systems are put into an emergency mode, which may be detrimental to the body over the long term. The immune system seems to be changed considerably by stress. The body begins to patrol aggressively for intruders. The cardiovascular system also responds by raising the output of the heart and, coincidentally, blood pressure. On the recuperative side (i.e. healing functions and the replacement of resources) things seem to be damped down or put aside until the organism has leisure to spare from the emergency. If the organism is continually stressed, this damping down may interfere with long-term healing. Placebo effects may decrease this damping down by redefining the situation as no longer an emergency.

Therapeutic uses of placebo effects

It is possible to use placebos and placebo effects in clinical practice (Evers et al., 2018.; Klinger et al., 2018).

The health professional also functions as a placebo. The non-specific effects of the professional's behaviour on the patient's health result from the same causes as the non-specific effects of drugs. The professional's value—validating the patient's illness, providing stimuli that have been conditioned to healing, and just being present—can add to the real effect of every treatment that they provide. This additional effect can be encouraged by the professional by providing patients with positive, but also moderate and realistic, expectations for the outcome of the treatment, by validating the patient's sense that something is wrong and needs attention, and by mobilising the patient's own resources, including physiological ones, in healing (Howe et al., 2017).

Significant ethical issues are raised when using inert substances in an attempt to humour the patient, particularly if the patient is considered by the professional to be a hypochondriac or neurotic. It is under these conditions that placebos are most likely to do harm, first through mental arithmetic leading the patient to believe that they are sicker than they previously thought, and second by encouraging a dependence on pills for what are really problems of communication between doctor and patient.

7.4 CASE STUDY

MALIK AND FLOSSING

Malik is a 30-year-old accountant. He is married and has children aged four and two. During a routine dental check-up, he is told that he has a lot of plaque in between his teeth and needs to use dental floss after every meal, or at least before going to bed every night, if he is to avoid increasing problems with decay. Malik has never used floss. Flossing is a risk-reduction behaviour that he hasn't given any particular thought to, but now his dentist has indicated that it is important. This makes Malik think about flossing for the first time. No one in his family uses dental floss, so there is none in the house. However, he doesn't want to have decay or gum disease.

Up to now, he has gained most of his ideas about flossing from second-hand sources. For example, one of his friends said that they tried flossing and it caused a lot of bleeding from the gums. Malik feels very queasy when he sees blood, so this makes him anxious about having 'a lot' of blood in his mouth. However, he has to integrate new information, from a health professional who he trusts, into his existing beliefs. Malik already has a number of good health habits, such as doing regular exercise, and believes that healthy behaviour is important. He also has a strong belief that he can do new things if he wants to. He asks another friend who flosses regularly about the bleeding problem and is told that the bleeding stops quickly once regular flossing is established. While in the supermarket, Malik sees floss on special, so buys some to try out.

After using dental floss for the first time, he discovers that it is mint-flavoured. He likes the taste and his mouth feels fresher. A colleague tells Malik that she used to avoid him because of his bad breath, but has noticed that this is now gone. He also finds that the bleeding is slight, and quickly decreases as he flosses regularly. He finds flossing easy and quick.

After a few weeks, flossing has become part of Malik's regular teeth-cleaning routine, so that he no longer has to even think about doing it. If he forgets, he finds that he becomes aware of an unpleasant taste in his mouth, and this reminds him about flossing. He even suggests to other family members that they should start flossing. His parents have had a lot of trouble with dental disease, both tooth decay and gum problems, and Malik doesn't want his own children to face these problems in the future.

1   How much influence do simple environmental effects (e.g. the lack of dental floss in the house) have on your own health behaviour?

2   What could Malik's dentist have done to improve the likelihood that Malik would begin to floss? How could the knowledge of Malik's stage of change have guided the dentist's behaviour?

3   Flossing is a fairly simple health behaviour with hardly any side effects. How does modifying it differ from modifying a major health behaviour such as compliance with medication for lowering blood pressure?

4   Over time, are any other changes in behaviour likely to be observed as Malik continues to use dental floss?

Points to consider

A number of theories of health behaviour can be seen in this case study. Malik has progressed through the stages of change from pre-contemplation (when he hadn't given much thought to using dental floss as a health behaviour), through contemplation to action and maintenance. He has experienced changes to his cognitions about dental health. Some of these relate to the link between the behaviour of flossing and the outcome of dental health, and some are about the likelihood that flossing will produce the desired change in his risk. He has encountered barriers to the behaviour: unavailability of floss, and negative feelings about bleeding. He has sought information about possible effects of the behaviour, and found some good and bad sources of information. Self-efficacy has played a significant role in his behaviour change and, in return, the behaviour change has probably increased his sense of self-efficacy.

CHAPTER SUMMARY

Learn more
Access additional resources to broaden your understanding of this chapter. See the Guided Tour for access details.

- Cognition refers to the variety of thinking processes that people use. We would like to believe that our thinking and decision-making are rational, but we often ignore objective information and instead make subjective evaluations of the likelihood and value of particular outcomes.

- Instead of using algorithms (mechanical routines that guarantee a correct solution but are slow) we frequently use heuristics (rules of thumb that are fast and can work with incomplete information but may lead to incorrect decisions).

- Health professionals may use heuristics of various kinds to assist clinical decision-making; the same issues arise from this use.

- A number of models have been developed to try to explain our thinking and decision-making about health. Most of them are only partially effective in explaining behaviour, but can give some assistance in explaining why that behaviour is often not very rational.

- Compliance with the recommendations of health professionals is often poor. Many of the reasons for this are related to health beliefs.

- An understanding of how expectations affect behaviour can be useful in the study of health and illness.

- Placebo effects provide a good example of the ways in which expectations can produce outcomes that differ from those that an objective observer might expect. Placebo effects may arise from a variety of psychological processes and the ways in which these processes influence the physiology of the body.

- It is important for health professionals to recognise the power of placebo effects and to use them ethically in the treatment of patients.

FURTHER READING

Fishbein M (2008) A reasoned action approach to health promotion. *Medical Decision-making* 28, 834–44.

Higgs J, Jones MA, Loftus F & Christensen N (2008) *Clinical Reasoning in the Health Professions* (3rd edn). Elsevier.

Maher P (1999) A review of 'traditional' Aboriginal health beliefs. *Australian Journal of Rural Health* 7(4), 229–36.

Noar SM & Zimmerman RS (2005) Health behavior theory and cumulative knowledge regarding health behaviors: Are we moving in the right direction? *Health Education Research* 20, 275–90.

Turner K, Weinberger M, Renfro C, Powell BJ, Ferreri S, Trodgon JG et al. (2021) Stages of change: Moving community pharmacies from a drug dispensing to population health management model. *Medical Care Research and Review* 78(1), 57–67.

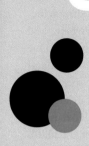

8

How to Change Health Behaviour

Introduction

Changing health-related behaviours was brought into sharp focus during 2020 and 2021. Public health messages relating to hand-washing, mask-wearing, social distancing, self-isolation and vaccination to reduce the risk from COVID-19 were everywhere, and discussion of how to change these behaviours was a daily occurrence in the media. Due to the time it takes to design and complete scientific research, have it peer-reviewed and then published in a journal, there is actually not much completed research specifically about COVID-19 in the literature. However, this research is being done, and evidence is gradually building (Ashchwanden, 2021). None of the issues on changing health behaviour are completely new, however, and research in this area has a long history (Bavel et al., 2020). This chapter looks at what is known about factors affecting all health behaviours.

Motivation for change

"How many psychologists does it take to change a light bulb?" Answer: "Only one, but the light bulb really has to want to change." As this joke indicates, the most important factor in determining whether an individual will modify behaviour is how motivated they are to change. Before considering strategies for change, it is necessary to consider the general issue of motivation.

When we are hungry, we eat: this is a simple case of motivated behaviour that we can easily understand. However, many people in the world would, and do, starve to death rather than eat readily available and perfectly nutritious food. Think about the following examples. Nearly 195 million people in India are undernourished and yet sacred cows wander freely and are never slaughtered. How easy would you find it to eat insects? Many people around the world eat them. It might depend on whether you knew you were doing so (crayfish and crabs, for example, are *Arthropodae*—related to spiders). It might also depend on whether eating insects was your only way of staying alive. People suffering from anorexia nervosa starve themselves in the midst of plenty in order to attain their ideal of body shape. The further we get from the simple case that we started with, the harder we tend to find it is to understand what motivates the behaviour.

Motivation
Factors that arouse, sustain and direct behaviour.

Most people think about **motivation** in terms of needs that must be met to achieve a state of comfort. When behaviour occurs, we assume that it has been done to achieve some goal. If the behaviour succeeds, the result is satisfaction; if not, frustration. The study of motivation, therefore, is concerned with those factors that arouse, sustain and direct behaviour.

One useful analysis of human motivation (Maslow, 1970) suggests that we have a hierarchy of needs that we will be concerned with satisfying. Our most basic needs come first, after that we are able to direct energy at higher-level needs (see Figure 8.1). The most basic needs are the fundamental physiological ones: hunger, thirst and avoidance of pain. Only when these are satisfied are we able to worry about the next level, which Maslow described as safety needs: to feel secure and out of danger. The next level of needs is seen to be social: the need to belong to a group, to be loved and wanted. Esteem needs come next: the need to feel competent, to achieve something, to gain the approval of our peers. Maslow completes his pyramid of needs with the need for self-actualisation: to be the best that we possibly can be, to fulfil our own unique potential.

FIGURE 8.1 Maslow's hierarchy of needs

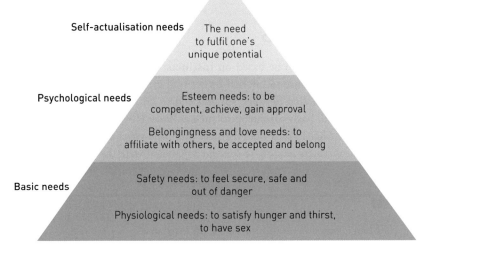

Maslow (1943)

8.1 CASE STUDY

DANIELLE AND SLEEP

Danielle is a 19-year-old university student enrolled in a Bachelor of Nursing degree, and she hopes to eventually work in intensive care. She has read in textbooks and on social media that older teenagers—like her—and young adults need seven to nine hours of sleep each night in order to perform at their best. She has been getting only about five hours or less on weekdays, because of classes, a busy social life, part-time work, and studying. Until recently she had thought she was coping, as long as she slept in for a few hours on Sunday mornings to catch up. Lately, she has noticed that she is finding it hard to stay awake during lectures, and frequently loses concentration while studying. However, a lot of her fellow students follow the same sort of low-sleep lifestyle and seem to be coping. She also knows an ICU nurse who claims that she can cope perfectly well on four hours sleep a night. At this point, Danielle's behaviour is unlikely to change unless there is a change in her motivation.

1   What might stimulate such a change for her?

2   Who should be responsible for making sure that students training for high-pressure health professions get enough sleep?

While Maslow's theory makes good intuitive sense, a number of objections have been made to it. All of us can think of times when we ignored a basic need to look after a higher one, and examples of people who have sacrificed their own security for the benefit of others are too common to ignore. Clearly, circumstances can lead to a reordering of the hierarchy. Maslow's theory does not really give a detailed picture about how 'needs' work: where they originate, how they push or pull behaviour, and why humans do things that are quite clearly not in their own interests. To begin to understand, we need to examine genetic, biological and higher mental (cognitive) factors that influence motivation.

Genetic factors

Instincts
Patterns of behaviour that are genetically programmed to occur in response to internal or external events.

Much of animal behaviour seems to be based on **instincts**: patterns that are hard-wired or programmed to occur in response to internal or external events, including events such as the migration of birds, aggression between species, and so on. What holds for animals might hold for humans as well. Early psychologists such as James (1890) believed that social behaviour showed patterns that looked like instinct, while the psychoanalyst Freud (e.g. Hall, 1979) believed that instincts relating to sex and aggression were the basis of much of human behaviour.

PAUSE & REFLECT

How much of your behaviour do you think is based on instincts?
Can you give any additional examples to those in the text?

Some patterns of human behaviour appear to be so universal that an instinctual basis seems likely. One example is the protectiveness that almost all adult humans feel for babies. The head size and the shape of a baby's facial features seem to produce in adults an internal state and a readiness to respond protectively. Stimuli that perform this kind of preparatory function are called 'releasing stimuli'. Releasing stimuli in lower animals may produce mating behaviour (e.g. the mating dances that many birds perform) or aggression (e.g. attacking any bird that approaches too closely to the nest). Some authors have considered which human behaviours appear to be most instinctive. Attention has generally focused on behaviours that ensure the transmission of genes to the next generation. Attachment in mothers and babies helps to ensure the survival of those who share genetic endowment; some authors have suggested that territoriality and dominance in males serve the same purpose. In humans, most behaviours are too variable to have been caused by instinct. There is quite clearly a heavy overlay of learnt behaviour.

Attachment is considered in more detail in Chapter 2.

Biological factors

Primary drive
An unlearnt drive, for which there is an organic or physiological basis.

Some drives quite clearly ensure the survival of the individual and are so based in bodily states that they must have a key biological focus. Physiological needs, in Maslow's terms, give rise to internal states focused on satisfying those needs. These states are commonly referred to as **primary drives** (Hull, 1943). In a primary drive, either deprivation (e.g. of food or water) or stimulation (e.g. pain or sexual arousal) produces a need state in the organism, which in turn gives rise to a drive to satisfy that need. This drive is not just a general state; it also has a direction. In the case of hunger, this direction is to find food; in the case of pain, it is to move away from the source. Thus, a drive not only produces behaviour, it also produces certain specific behaviours related to the desired goal. The behaviours may succeed in reaching the goal, in which case the need is reduced. If not, the drive state continues to produce behaviour aimed at the goal until either the need is reduced or the organism is exhausted (see Figure 8.2).

FIGURE 8.2 Drive cycle

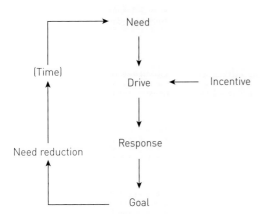

Sometimes, even after we have eaten until we are full, an especially desirable food can tempt us to eat again. This ability of an object to draw out behaviour is called **incentive**. Pain avoidance and sex are essentially incentive-based drives. No one ever died from a lack of pain or a lack of sex, which are needs based on the presence of environmental (or, less commonly, internal) stimuli.

Not all of our behaviour is related to the reduction of a handful of biological needs. Why, for example, are we willing to work hard just to receive a few words of praise or a mark on a piece of paper? Most theories that consider drives to be the basis of behaviour have argued that such behaviour is based on learnt drives (acquired drives) gained through association with primary drives. Because our experiences of the satisfaction of hunger and thirst during the dependency of infancy are closely tied up with the social relationship between infant and caregiver, we learn to have a need for social contact. This learnt state of need gradually becomes more or less independent of the physiological need that gave rise to it. The occurrence of a state of need leads to a secondary (learnt) drive, aimed at reducing the internal need state. All sorts of learnt drives have been proposed (Murray, 1938; McClelland, 1961)—for affiliation, approval, nurture, succour, achievement and dominance, among others. Although few of the proposed lists have satisfied everyone, there seems to be general agreement that learnt drives act very much like physiological drives with both deprivation and incentive effects.

As Figure 8.2 indicates, need reduction theories describe a feedback system, with the arousal of a need producing a change in the system. This change results in a drive to attain a goal in order to return to a state where the need has been reduced. The concept of **homeostasis** (Kimble, 1992) describes the nature of this process. Like the thermostat on a heater or air-conditioner, there is a regulatory mechanism that responds to deviations from some desired level by producing system activity. Once the desired level is achieved, activity is turned off. In terms of our biological homeostasis, much of this regulation appears to take place in the **hypothalamus**, a small structure in the midbrain involved in temperature control, pain and pleasure, and emotional regulation. Electrical stimulation of parts of the hypothalamus produces effects on regulation of behaviour: stimulation of some spots can, for example, produce gorging of food or water in already full animals; others can produce a refusal to eat or drink.

Incentive
An external object or stimulus that draws out behaviour or creates motivation in the absence of a need.

Homeostasis
The tendency of the body to maintain internal constancy, and to try to restore equilibrium when that constancy is disturbed.

Hypothalamus
A small structure in the midbrain that regulates behaviour to maintain homeostasis.

Cognitive factors

The fact that motivated behaviour has direction (e.g. we tend to refrain from eating until we can eat preferred foods) clearly indicates the role of cognition (thought processes) in motivation. As already mentioned, motivation can be modified by learning, which means that higher mental processes can play a significant role in our understanding of motivation and our responses to it. Much (if not most) of the time, our behaviour appears to be mindful; that is, rational and sensible. We do not usually grab and eat other people's lunches just because we are hungry. There is a considerable degree of cognitive regulation at work. We balance the costs and returns of our behaviour to produce the maximal overall outcome (dependent on the probability and desirability of each outcome). If we behave in ways that are asocial or antisocial, other people will regulate our behaviour for us in undesirable ways (e.g. imprisonment, rejection or physical threats).

Cognitive factors are discussed in more detail in Chapter 7.

In some cases, cognitive appraisals—judgments that people make about the situations they are in—lead individuals to make regulatory decisions that look pretty irrational in terms of their biological needs. Some people have chosen to be arrested, tortured and even executed rather than fight in a war, while others may be willing to fight to the death over a minor insult. Although we may need to be recognised, most of us would stop a long way short of self-mutilation to get that recognition. Another way we regulate behaviour is by the postponement of gratification; we are far better at this than are most other organisms. Graduation, for example, is hard to predict on the basis of biological needs, yet many people work hard over a number of years to become university graduates.

As discussed in Chapter 7, cognitions about health are critical to our motivation towards behaviour change. The integrative model of behavioural prediction (Fishbein, 2008), like other cognitive theories about health, focuses not just on our cognitions about disease and health and what causes them, but also on our beliefs about our own capacities and limitations (behavioural skills), whether or not the costs and gains of a behaviour change come out in favour of going through with it (intentions), and whether or not we believe that factors which we can't control (environmental factors) will be likely to assist or block us in trying to change.

MOTIVATIONAL INTERVIEWING

One approach to changing behaviour specifically by targeting motivation is motivational interviewing (MI) (Miller & Rollnick, 2012). The basis of this approach is that people are often ambivalent about changing health-related behaviours; that is, they have positive and negative motivations. For example, most people who smoke or are very overweight know that they should change their behaviour in order to improve their health (positive motivation towards change). However, they don't want to give up their established behaviours, or the comfort that they may get from them, or are concerned about the unpleasant feelings that may arise from trying to change (negative motivation towards change). MI involves counselling people to explore their feelings about behaviour change, with the aim of helping them to resolve the ambivalence and find strong enough motivation to bring about action. There is a substantial literature that shows that motivational interviewing —whether carried out by psychologists, mental health nurses, social workers or other health professionals— can be quite effective in changing behaviour.

As with all approaches to behaviour change, MI is likely to work best when seen as just one element of the behaviour change process. Motivation is critical to bringing about change, but is usually insufficient on its own. This is often because the individual simply doesn't know how to go about it even if they are highly motivated to change. They need to have strategies as well. We focus on how strategies are developed and carried out later in this chapter.

PAUSE & REFLECT

What is it that motivates you to do well at university?
Where do think your motivation comes from?

In summary, motivation is an interaction of influences that come from the genetic, biological, cognitive and social levels.

MOTIVATION WITHOUT NEEDS OR DRIVES

What happens when all drives are satisfied? The organism does not just sit there waiting for a need to develop. A lack of stimulation is perceived as unpleasant and, if deprived of it, we will seek it out. **Optimal level theory** suggests that we have a preferred range of environmental stimulation. If there is too little stimulation, we seek more; if there is too much, we seek to reduce it. This relates fairly clearly to homeostasis and the idea that we have certain set points for internal regulation.

Even when we obtain the right amount of stimulation, we tend not to be satisfied for long. As we become accustomed to a given stimulus—a process called **habituation**—it becomes less pleasant to us. It has been shown, for example, that once we have become habituated to a particular stimulus, our preferred level of stimulus is one just slightly different from it. Imagine that you place your hand in a pan of cold water. At first it may be uncomfortable, but after you habituate you will find that water is more pleasant when it is just a little warmer or colder. Water that would have been pleasantly warm at first may now be too warm. Figure 8.3 represents this in graphic form. Experimenters have shown that animals placed in a boring environment will actually work fairly hard to earn a little stimulation, such as the opportunity to watch the outside world or watch a toy train going around in circles.

Optimal level theory
The idea that organisms have a preferred range of environmental stimulation, and that they will work to maintain themselves in that range.

Habituation
Adaptation to a stimulus so that it no longer arouses the level of response that it originally aroused.

FIGURE 8.3 The pleasantness of an unfamiliar temperature

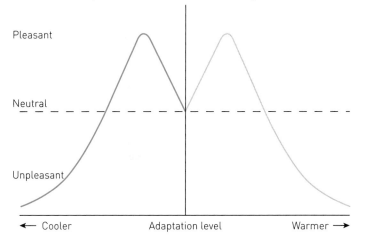

Opponent–process theory
The idea that there are always two processes in motivation: the primary motivation or process, and a secondary and opposite process set up within the nervous system.

One way of accounting for this kind of phenomenon, and others such as drug addiction, is **opponent–process theory** (Solomon, 1980). This proposes that there are always two processes in motivation—the primary process and a secondary and opposite one, set up within the nervous system. This secondary process comes on more slowly than the primary, but also fades more slowly. Its purpose is to protect the system from intense stimulation. Thus, in the cold water example, the primary process of discomfort with the cold water is opposed by a secondary process that decreases the discomfort. At this level of adaptation, a new opposing process diminishes our pleasure in this comfort to the extent that we prefer a change.

In the case of heroin addiction, the novice drug user experiences a strong primary rush, which, because of a secondary opponent process, reduces to a pleasurable state. When this pleasurable state fades with the drug, the secondary process (fading more slowly) is experienced as unpleasant. With continued use, the secondary process becomes better and better at reducing the rush to protect the nervous system from overload. The user has to take more drugs to continue to achieve a pleasurable state, and withdrawal produces a more unpleasant set of sensations.

Strategies for behaviour change

It is possible to modify behaviour by using the same principles of perception, learning and memory, and motivation that produced those behaviours in the first place. There are some basic assumptions implied by that statement, and it is important to make those assumptions clear in order to understand the ways in which behaviour can be changed (Berkman, 2018).

The first assumption is that we need to be able to see what it is we want to change; that is, we can only work with observable behaviour. We also need to have clear goals for how we wish the behaviour to change: in what ways, how much and within what time frame. Then we need to assume that maladaptive behaviours are learnt, and therefore can be unlearnt or replaced by adaptive behaviours. It is not particularly important in most cases to know just how a behaviour was learnt in the first place. It is not possible to go back and change events that produced that learning. Change has to take place in the present. This does not mean that we can't benefit from looking at past experience. Doing so can help us to pick methods that are appropriate to the behaviour we wish to change. Finally, it is much easier to change a behaviour if we have evidence that the behaviour is actually changing.

Some basic principles should be kept in mind in planning how to modify behaviour (Bailey, 2017).

PICK APPROPRIATE BEHAVIOURS

Extinction
The gradual lessening of a conditioned response when reinforcement is removed.

The techniques described in this chapter, based on simple psychological principles, are mainly aimed at producing small and gradual changes in behaviour. The importance of this kind of small and gradual change should never be underestimated. Behaviour change has several advantages: it is realistic, it is cheap, once change has occurred it tends to be resistant to **extinction** and, unlike many medical interventions, it doesn't have side effects.

It should be noted that behaviour change will never entirely replace medication, whether that medication is for the treatment of infectious diseases or major depression. Nor will it replace more intensive psychological treatments. People who have major psychological or physical health problems should always work with a qualified health professional to manage their conditions; however, behaviour change is often useful or necessary in combination with medical or surgical treatments. Evidence indicates that different approaches can help to change health behaviours linked to medical conditions such as type 2 diabetes (Galaviz et al., 2015) and cardiovascular disease. For example, total lifestyle programs such as the Ornish program (Ornish & Ornish, 2019), which involve medication, diet, exercise, coping skills and relaxation, can greatly decrease the incidence of heart attacks and strokes in those at risk. However, behaviour change cannot, and should not, entirely replace other medical treatments in serious conditions.

Individuals can improve their chances of a successful behaviour change by selecting appropriate behaviours. We can use a mnemonic (memory jogging) strategy to help choose behaviours that are appropriate for change. A common one is SMART (Ogbeiwi, 2017). Goals should be *Specific* (say exactly what you want to achieve), *Measurable* (have a clear way of determining what you have achieved), *Actionable* (define what action is needed to meet the goal), *Realistic* (neither too easy or too hard to achieve) and *Time-bound* (define when the goal should be met).

PAUSE & REFLECT

What health-related behaviours do you think you need to change?

Are there others that you would like to change?

Are there others that you think you will need to change at some time in the future?

PICK APPROPRIATE METHODS

Some methods of behaviour change are appropriate for some behaviours or for some people, but not for others. It is important to understand the nature of the behaviour targeted for change before selecting methods. Like the selection of appropriate behaviours, this is related to the 'specific' part of the SMART model. Some problems will be best handled with the behaviour change approaches discussed in this chapter; others will require stress management approaches.

Just as losing weight is best handled by increased exercise combined with changes in the food eaten (not necessarily dieting), some health behaviours need more than one technique. Given the demonstrated benefits of relaxation and stress management, there is probably no one who would not gain from improved technique and practice, but even these will not help with all healthy or risky behaviours. Some guidelines for selecting methods are included in later sections of this chapter and in Chapter 13.

Stress management is discussed in detail in Chapter 13.

DO NOT EXPECT TOO MUCH

The most common reason for failure of any treatment procedure is unrealistic expectations: the 'realistic' part. Around 70% of smokers trying to quit will fail at first, no matter what method they use. Eventually, though, more than 70% will succeed in quitting. It is more realistic to aim for a partial change (e.g. cutting down) and once that change is achieved to change the target. Success in meeting interim targets will add to feelings of confidence that the ultimate target can be reached as well, which is one of the reasons why it is so important that behaviours be 'measurable'.

GIVE METHODS A CHANCE TO WORK

Closely related to expecting too much, methods frequently fail because the individual gives up too soon or fails to stick to the rules. Behaviour change programs need to deal with slow progress, temporary setbacks and small (and even big) lapses without the individual giving up. But they also can't be open-ended, which is why 'time-bound' is essential. To maintain a behaviour change, some basic characteristics underlying the behaviour need to change and stay changed. In some cases, this will be for a fixed period of time; in others, forever. Patience is needed, and enough time for success to be achieved. To take the weight-loss example, crash dieting simply does not work.

PEOPLE ARE NOT FAILURES, ALTHOUGH METHODS MAY BE

If behaviour does not change dramatically in a short period of time, it does not mean that the person who tried it is weak or flawed. Most habitual behaviours are hard to change. If they were not, unhealthy habits would not exist. Low self-esteem can be a cause of risky behaviours; if behaviour does not change, self-esteem can be lowered as a result, thereby creating a vicious cycle. There are many ways to prevent this, the most important of which is for each individual to select the right behaviour and method for themselves.

8.2 CASE STUDY

DANIELLE (CONT.)

After reading articles about exhaustion and burnout being common problems for ICU nurses, Danielle realises that she may need to develop better sleeping patterns, and set aside more time for sleep. Having found motivation for this change, she begins to look at what affects when and how much she sleeps. She notes that she sleeps less well when she has been studying late at night, or when she has been up late messaging friends on social media. She has an old pillow that frequently needs to be adjusted to make it comfortable. She sleeps better on days when she has exercised or done relaxing things like talking to friends during breaks. She tends to go to sleep at odd hours and get up at odd times because of classes or work shifts.

She starts by buying a new pillow and making sure that her bedroom is dark and quiet during sleep time. She changes the settings on her phone and computer to sleep mode so notifications don't wake her except for urgent messages. Changing triggers like this is stimulus control.

Next, she reads materials about sleep hygiene. The recommendations are fairly basic, and include the things she has already done. Also, she should go to bed and wake up at the same time each day, try to avoid napping during the day, use the bed only for sleep (and, maybe, sex) and learn how to use some relaxation methods such as muscle relaxation or meditation.

1 What kind of behaviour change process has Danielle gone through with this analysis?

2 What changes could Danielle make in her health cognitions that would increase her motivation to get seven to nine hours' sleep each night?

PAUSE & REFLECT

Think of someone you know who has tried and failed to change a behaviour.

How did it make them feel?

What effect do you think it had on their future behaviour?

Changing behaviour by changing stimuli

In order to change a behaviour, we need to know two things about it. The first of these involves **antecedents**: the stimuli that precede its occurrence and lead to the behaviour. The second involves reinforcements: the consequences associated with the behaviour that keep it occurring.

Antecedents
Stimuli that precede and lead to the occurrence of a behaviour.

ANTECEDENTS

There are many things that trigger behaviour. Some of these are obvious, such as looking at the clock, seeing that it is time to go to work, and going. Some are a lot less obvious, such as why we looked at the clock in the first place. Sometimes, the best way to explain a behaviour is habit: we do something because we have learnt through experience to do it. We do not give much thought to tying shoelaces, for instance, but when we put on shoes with laces, habit takes over and we tie them. If we had to describe how we tie shoelaces to someone else, it is likely that we would have a lot of trouble. If we wanted to change our method of tying shoelaces, our habits would interfere. We might have to do some unlearning before we could learn a new approach. Many of our habits are so well learnt that we are not especially aware of the behaviour, much less what triggers it, which frequently produces problems when we want to change a behaviour. So, step one is to identify the antecedents. This self-monitoring is an important component of successful health behaviour change (van Achterberg et al., 2011). There are several useful tools for doing this.

Think back to past behaviours

If an individual would like to eat more fruit, they need to think about times in the past when they have eaten fruit with pleasure and try to decide what preceded eating. Was the fruit given to them? Was it new and interesting? Was it simply handy at the time they were eating something else? Did it look particularly good? Were they especially hungry? These kinds of clues to antecedents for fruit-eating will provide hints as to how to increase it.

Observe present behaviours

When does the individual eat fruit? How do they feel before they eat it? When do they think about eating fruit? When do they think about eating fruit without actually eating any, and what stops them at that particular time? There is considerable research which shows that present behaviour is the best predictor of future behaviour.

Keep a formal record

This goes together with points one and two. When eating fruit, or thinking about eating fruit, it is useful to keep a record that can be analysed for clues about antecedents. Diaries are often used in behaviour change programs, because time can be an important trigger for many behaviours. If we regularly eat fruit at breakfast but never at other times, then the time of day may be an antecedent to fruit-eating that the individual can work with.

This kind of monitoring of our own behaviour can be enough to change the behaviour. Thinking about why we do something alters the way we think about that behaviour, and this in itself changes the antecedents. People may say that they quit smoking by sheer willpower and without a plan, but by willpower they really mean that they thought about the stimuli for doing it and for not doing it, and this changed the antecedents of the behaviour. It is often the case that their willpower was boosted by thinking about the damage a cigarette would do or by keeping the mouth busy with something else, such as chewing gum or sucking on a blade of grass or a toothpick instead of smoking. This is the other side of behaviour change—motivation—and methods for changing this are discussed later in the chapter.

STIMULUS CONTROL

Stimulus control
Changing a behaviour by changing its antecedents.

The basis of changing behaviour by changing its antecedents is called **stimulus control**. Sometimes this involves eliminating a stimulus that produces the wrong kind of behaviour. If an individual scrolls through social media on their iPhone in bed they may find it harder to fall asleep, as they have become conditioned to associate bed with interesting and exciting events rather than with sleep. They can control the stimulus by using the bed only for sleeping. This means that the stimuli associated with the bed are all clearly and solely connected with sleeping.

Sometimes a stimulus that leads to a behaviour is not eliminated but modified, perhaps by changing its meaning or making it a stimulus for a different and competing behaviour. Instead of sitting in front of Netflix on arriving home, an individual might go for a run and listen to a podcast instead. The same stimulus—coming home—becomes the antecedent for a different behaviour.

Other people can serve as stimuli to trigger behaviours. Problem drinkers often find that the hardest thing to control is their friends. If the individual's social life revolves around the pub or friends who drink quite a lot, then it may be necessary to change those elements to reduce drinking. Sometimes others can be motivated to change, as when a parent changes the family's food-buying habits and menus to improve their child's diet. At other times, certain people or places may need to be avoided. Smokers often go to specific places—

special rooms in the house or outdoors—to smoke. Someone who is quitting is well advised to avoid those places because they will be full of smoking cues: smells, sights, cigarette butts and ashtrays, smokers and their positive comments.

Table 8.1 gives a summary of some antecedents for health behaviours, and some techniques that can be used to control them.

TABLE 8.1   Summary of stimulus control

ANTECEDENT	STIMULUS CONTROL METHOD
I forget to (exercise, eat fruit etc.)	Provide reminders for the behaviour.
I don't have the time to …	Schedule a regular time; reorganise program to make time; eliminate wasted time.
I never seem to have the right (food, equipment, material etc.)	Put the equipment in a convenient place; get it ready ahead of time.
(A healthy meal, gym time) is too expensive or too hard to find.	Take your meal with you from home; buy tickets in bulk; join a club.
I'm not aware that I'm …	Create a signal so that you can't do the behaviour without being aware of it; organise surveillance; ask others to tell you when you are doing it.

PAUSE & REFLECT

Think about where, when and how you study.

How could you use stimulus control methods to improve your study behaviour?

Increasing and decreasing behaviours

Behaviour change can be categorised into three groups: behaviours we want to increase (health behaviours), those we want to decrease (risky behaviours) and behaviours that we are not particularly aware of doing (**low-awareness habits**) that we want to increase or decrease. Slightly different techniques are useful with these three types of behaviour change, although there is considerable overlap.

If the goal is to increase a behaviour, such as exercise, the problem is often that there are not enough relevant stimuli for exercise in the ordinary environment. An important step in changing the behaviour is to change the environment so that those stimuli are present. The hopeful exerciser could, for instance, put up posters featuring exercise, set reminders on their phone, and keep exercise equipment in an obvious and easily accessible place. Someone who wanted to eat more fibre might keep high-fibre recipes on the fridge, or a list of the fibre content of snack food on the pantry door.

Decreasing behaviours involves reducing either the occurrence of stimuli related to those behaviours or changing the meaning of those stimuli. If an individual stops at a vending machine to buy chocolate every time they go down a particular staircase, simply finding a different path may be enough to stop the behaviour (Samdal et al., 2017).

Low-awareness habits
Habitual behaviours that the individual carries out without being particularly aware that they are doing so (e.g. nail-biting).

Eating and sleeping are heavily habit-dependent, a fact that often surprises people as we tend to think of them as bodily processes that are not consciously controlled. A common trigger for eating is the presence of food. Eating and sleeping often respond very well to stimulus control. For this reason, weight-management programs often ask people to develop different eating routines that might include rules such as never eat standing up; eat only in the dining room with the table set, others present and no television or other distractions; always wash dishes and utensils as soon as eating is finished and put them away out of sight; keep all food in difficult-to-access cupboards so that it is harder to get to; and never have food lying around unless it is part of the diet plan.

LOW-AWARENESS HABITS: A SPECIAL CASE

Low-awareness habits include chewing fingernails, lips or objects such as pencils; picking or pulling at skin or hair; slouching, fidgeting or grimacing; making noises such as grunts; and knuckle-cracking. Some of these habits have health consequences that are obvious. Nail-biting can lead to deformed nails, infections and the spread of disease. If other people in the vicinity find these habits odd, funny or unpleasant, they can lead to lowered self-esteem and associated problems with emotions. Almost always, the trick is to make the individual aware of the habit while it is occurring. Usually, once the person becomes aware, they are motivated enough to quit. There are several ways to make people more aware of these habits; for example, painting fingernails with a foul or bitter substance to keep children from biting them. This combines stimulus control (the bitter taste signals that the low-awareness habit is occurring) with reinforcement (the taste is unpleasant). This technique does not always work. Perhaps the habit has too many positive reinforcements associated with it, the habit is too strongly established, or the taste is not regarded as too unpleasant. Also, as this approach is based in part on punishment, it shares all the problems of punishment.

Other signalling methods can be used with low-awareness habits. Scheduling a mobile phone notification of something is a type of stimulus control, but anything that interferes with carrying out a behaviour could be used. A nail-biter will not be able to perform their habit if each fingernail is covered with a bandage; however, they may have to explain the reason to others. Most people are not aware when they are slouching, which can cause muscular pains or aggravate stomach or bowel problems. Techniques to raise awareness of slouching include wearing wide belts inside or outside of clothing that dig into the individual when they slouch, but are comfortable when they are sitting up straight (again, this includes punishment). A computerised strain gauge worn vertically around the body has been used to prevent the worsening of, or to improve, scoliosis (curvature of the spine) in young people. This gauge uses sound or vibration signals to tell the individual when their spine is not being held straight; the signals can be graded to be more obvious if the spine is not straightened within a pre-specified time.

The role of others in providing surveillance for low-awareness habits raises a number of issues. Although friends and family may be concerned about the habit and be willing to let the person know when it occurs, they may be reluctant to do so under some conditions. Suppose a person who picks at their earrings and causes irritation and infection asks friends to tell them when the behaviour occurs. If the behaviour and reminder happen in a public place, it may cause embarrassment for one or both parties. But the main problem with surveillance is that the person being watched may come to resent it. Even long-time friends or partners may find their relationship is strained by an action that can come to be seen as irritating. Still, surveillance can be used to good effect in many instances.

Earlier in this chapter, you were asked to think about health behaviours you would like to change. Pick one of them.

Which stimulus control methods might be appropriate to changing that behaviour?

Changing behaviour by changing reinforcements

This section deals with changing motivation related to problem behaviours, and this involves changing reinforcements. Reinforcements follow a behaviour to make it more or less likely to happen again. We eat because the tastes during the meal are pleasurable or to feel more satisfied afterwards—these are reinforcements. Another way of thinking about reinforcements is in terms of gains and costs. Talking to people about why they do not exercise as much as they should, they will often list the gains ("It makes me feel good and I sleep better") followed by the costs ("It takes too much time, and I feel tired afterwards"). In any attempt to change behaviour, it is useful to look at the reinforcements and whether they can be changed. Nicotine patches or chewing gum are two of several ways that the reinforcements of smoking can be changed by reducing the costs of not smoking related to nicotine withdrawal.

Reinforcements are discussed in detail in Chapter 6.

The longer it has been since we ate or drank, the more likely it is that we will feel hungry or thirsty. When we eat or drink, the reduction in tension is reinforcing (negative reinforcement). Whether or not we wish to lose weight, we do not want to eliminate eating entirely. Modifying eating means changing the way we eat, not the fact that we eat. The addictive nature of nicotine, as with other drugs, produces an increasing need as time passes. Satisfying this need is not essential for survival, so we can eliminate it without risk.

The general principle of reinforcement is to reduce the costs and increase the gains of desired behaviour. This may also involve increasing the costs and reducing the gains of undesired behaviour. A person who wishes to include more fibre in their diet may find that the foods they like do not contain a lot of fibre, and the ones that do contain fibre do not appeal to them. They could increase the gains of eating fibre by finding attractive foods that are higher in fibre (increasing the gains of the desired behaviour) or in some way adding fibre to the foods they like (decreasing the costs). Alternatively, they could use punishment: not eating desirable but low-fibre foods (reducing the gains of avoidance) or putting money into a charity jar when they do not eat fibre (increasing the costs of avoidance).

Positive reinforcement approaches

In general, any behaviour that is followed by positive consequences will increase in frequency. Training a child to use a toilet involves making the consequences positive ones. We try to make the process pleasant by having a comfortable seat for the child to sit on, and by giving praise and cuddles when the child uses the toilet. All of these are intended to increase the behaviour of using the toilet, and are usually successful.

The giving of positive reinforcement is one of the essential methods of behaviour change. If a person wished to do more exercise, they could arrange for a direct payoff by having a nice snack or coffee with friends immediately afterwards, have someone praise them for exercising, or have someone give them money.

Part of the problem with exercise—and this is true of many health behaviours—is that the direct benefits are long-term while the costs are short-term. Once people have exercised for a period of time, they are fitter, probably look better, almost certainly feel and sleep better, and have better general health. For most people, these gains tend to be a bit abstract compared with the short-term costs of effort, getting sweaty, missing out on socialising, and paying for equipment or facilities. This means that ways need to be found to make the rewards more immediate, or to reduce the costs.

One very useful technique involves making the payoffs part of the behaviour itself. Instead of sacrificing time with friends for exercise, they could exercise with their friends. Most people who exercise regularly report that part of the reason is social. They spend time with others, make friends, gain public respect for their skills or effort, and have a network of people who share their interests and values. Solitary exercise purely for the sake of fitness does rather poorly by comparison. The greater success of weight-loss groups over solitary weight-loss programs is primarily related to the social gains involved in having others who not only know and value what the individual is trying to do, but who also understand the difficulty involved in the process because they share it.

PAUSE & REFLECT

Think about exactly what motivates you to study in the first place.

How would you go about changing the costs and gains of studying?

Schedule of reinforcement
The pattern on which reinforcement is given. It may be continuous (every behaviour) or intermittent (less than every behaviour).

The **schedule of reinforcement**—when and how you get reinforcement—is also important. When beginning to reinforce a behaviour (when the behaviour is new and relatively unlikely to occur), it is important to do so frequently. If you wanted a child to smile more, you could give them a sweet every time they smiled. Once smiling became common, the sweets might be coming so fast that they lose their appeal, or even became a punishment by making the child feel sick from overeating. As time passes, the schedule of reinforcement needs to change to a less frequent one.

Occasional reinforcement makes a behaviour harder to get rid of than does constant reinforcement, largely because the lack of reinforcement is not so obvious. Problem gamblers find this a particular difficulty. They win just often enough to keep them gambling, although overall they lose a great deal more than they win. They keep thinking that the next win must eventually happen and that it could be big enough to make up for all the losses. The immediate gains of a big win are enough of a lure that they lose sight of the cost of a large number of small losses. Dealing with this kind of problem involves making the gambler more aware of the overall costs: not just the loss of money, but also of the things that the money could have bought, the loss of others' respect, family problems and so on.

On the other hand, knowledge about schedules of reinforcement can be used to produce positive changes by starting out with frequent rewards and gradually expecting more before a reward is given. Imagine, for example, that an individual wants to exercise three times a week and decides to use money as a reinforcement. At the beginning, they might put aside money to buy a small item of clothing each time they exercised. Once they have begun to develop the habit of exercising, they might only provide money if they have reached a particular target, such as running a certain distance within a set time. Ultimately, the goal is to have the reinforcements that arise from the behaviour itself replace outside rewards. People who continue to exercise report that the feeling of well-being is addictive, and that they miss that feeling badly when they do not exercise.

There are many reinforcements that can be used in behaviour change; for example, money, punishment, food, praise, time off work, fun and other people. Most of the techniques discussed are simply well-established ways of using those common reinforcements. One of the most important is self-reinforcement.

SELF-REINFORCEMENT

Everyone wants to have a good opinion of themselves: to feel that they are good, strong, worthy, interesting and attractive. This makes self-esteem—how good a person feels about themselves—a powerful reinforcement. There are various ways in which this can be used to modify health behaviours. The simplest is for the individual to praise themselves when they perform the desired behaviour, which tends to happen anyway: we feel good when we have done something that we are proud of. A difficulty arises when we are doing things that are considered to be good for us. We are more likely to feel bad when we have not done them than we are to feel that we have done anything praiseworthy when we have done them. Most of us do not pat ourselves on the back when we remember to brush our teeth before going to bed—we think of it as just basic sanitation—but will feel bad if we forget. Often, the trick with self-reinforcement is to recognise that a worthy behaviour deserves reinforcement.

PAUSE & REFLECT

Think about when you most often use self-reinforcement.

Is it mostly when you have been successful in your work? Do you ever reinforce yourself when you have had a successful study period? When you eat food that is good for you?

Self-reinforcement does not simply involve a person feeling good about themselves. It can include reinforcement with other desirable elements such as money, time, fun and social activities. The control over these reinforcements is in the individual's own hands. They decide when and how much reinforcement, and do not rely on others. Achieving for yourself often means more than achieving for someone else, and the main area of gain is **self-efficacy**. Self-efficacy refers to the sense of capacity that enables a person to control

Self-efficacy
The perception held by an individual that they can influence and control their own outcomes.

Self-efficacy is
also discussed in
Chapter 7.

their actions and determine their own limits. Self-efficacy has long been recognised as a key component of successful change (Bandura, 1977a). As the person succeeds in producing a small change, they not only gain small rewards but also an increase in self-efficacy. This is a powerful reinforcement, in part because it motivates the individual to go on changing.

A person who has made a number of attempts to quit gambling without success will have a low sense of self-efficacy, at least in this respect. Suppose that a person with a gambling problem does not set the target of quitting and never gambling again, but aims to limit the amount of money gambled on a given day. Most people who gamble find a proportional change such as this fairly easy to achieve. It can be regarded as a success if the person chooses to praise or otherwise reward themselves for it, and self-efficacy is increased for their attempt to further reduce expenditure on gambling. The setting of progressively more difficult targets is very useful, because it allows regular reinforcement and increases self-efficacy regarding the target behaviour.

8.3 CASE STUDY

DANIELLE (CONT.)

The process Danielle has gone through is not unlike motivational interviewing, in that she has been trying to reduce her ambivalence about sleeping longer hours by clarifying her motivations. Next, she decides that for the change in her behaviour to succeed in the long term, she needs to look at the reinforcements of the behaviour. First, the intrinsic motivation is that she feels better. She also has to study for fewer hours because her concentration has improved. Praising herself for remembering to follow her sleep hygiene guidelines increases her sense of self-efficacy, and makes her more confident about her coping skills. If her example influences others to change, she will feel that she has made a broader contribution.

1   What policy changes can you think of that would be likely to improve sleep hygiene among students at university?

2   How effective would it be for a university to begin punishing students for poor health habits, such as not exercising, eating poorly or not sleeping enough?

PUNISHMENT

The drawbacks
of punishment
are discussed in
Chapter 6.

It is always important to remember that punishment has drawbacks: it does not give any information about desired behaviour, it tends to produce avoidance of the whole situation and negative reactions to whoever is doing the punishing, and it can generalise to desirable behaviour that is associated with the undesired behaviour. If we want someone to eat less because they are overweight, then reminding them that they are overweight will simply make them feel angry towards the person doing the reminding. It will also lower their self-esteem and reduce their sense of self-efficacy. The overweight person is highly likely to start avoiding the 'helpful' person. Whenever we use punishment in behaviour change, it should be combined with positive reinforcement.

GOOD BEHAVIOUR BONDS

One technique that is often used very successfully in behaviour change is the **good behaviour bond**. Usually, this is a sum of money that is set aside and returned only if the behaviour change program is successfully completed. On the surface, this may look like punishment since failure to change results in losing money, but these bonds are very useful in motivating people to stay in programs even if behaviour does not change very much or at all.

An example is provided by weight-loss programs. Some may require each participant to pay an up-front bond equal to, say, a week's salary. If the participant sticks with the program until its conclusion, they get their money back. If not—and this is vitally important—the bond is forfeited, but never to the person running the program because the person running the program must not be seen to have a vested interest in participants' failure. Some programs give the money to charity, others use it to fund future programs or give it to recipients chosen by the participant. Some behaviour change experts feel that the bond is most effective if the money goes to a cause that the participant hates; that way, the participant cannot take comfort in the fact that although they have lost their bond, at least it is doing some good.

Bonds are often most effective when used to enforce participation rather than achievement. If the participant attends all sessions, keeps all the appropriate records and still does not modify their weight, they nevertheless get their money back. In this way, they at least leave the program with knowledge of the methods and a sense of self-efficacy, both of which can be useful in future attempts to lose weight. It is probably more common to link bonds to performance goals. This can be progressive. Each time the individual loses a certain amount of weight, they recover a portion of the bond. This gives immediate reinforcement during the program and keeps the individual from feeling that it is an all-or-nothing outcome. Sometimes programs mix performance and participation rewards—so much for attending, so much for weight loss etc.

Bonds do not have to be money; they can also involve goods or services. An individual could buy themselves a desirable object, but put it in the hands of someone else to keep or give away if behaviour change goals are not reached. Where money is a problem, the bond could consist of time or work. The individual could agree to provide 20 hours of unpaid work for someone and recover the hours through participation or performance. Bonds can also be used in support of a variety of other approaches.

Good behaviour bond
A sum of money (or equivalent goods or services) that is set aside to be returned only if a behaviour change program is successfully completed.

SUMMARY OF REINFORCEMENT METHODS

- Specific and clear targets should be set, that need to be reached before reinforcement occurs.
- A number of smaller targets that can be reinforced progressively is usually better than one big, far-away target.
- Reinforcement must be reliable; that is, if the individual reaches the target, reinforcement must be given.
- Success builds self-efficacy, which in turn encourages further change.
- Punishment should only be used in support of positive reinforcement.
- Reinforcement should occur frequently at first, then less frequently as behaviour changes. Intermittent reinforcement is best for maintaining behaviour.

- Reinforcements that arise directly from the behaviour change are the best kind; for example, the good physical feeling that follows exercise, or social contact from programs with others or as part of a group.
- A reward that can only be used if change is successful (e.g. a dress that will only fit if a certain amount of weight is lost) can be useful, but can also cause problems if, for instance, the target is too hard to meet.

Managing lapses

Lapses are likely to occur with any behaviour change program, and often result in the attempt to change being abandoned (Marlatt & Gordon, 1985). It is always a good idea to have plans for managing lapses. The most important is to ensure that lapses are not seen as failure. If a person thinks smoking a cigarette during an attempt to quit means they are a hopeless case, have no willpower or are permanently addicted, they will find it hard to resume the behaviour change program. If they see it as a momentary lapse—that is, not desirable but predictable, and to that extent acceptable—they are more likely to stick to or return to the program.

There are many techniques for dealing with lapses, including procedures for preventing them, minimising the damage they cause, and relabelling them as part of the change process (Marlatt & Gordon, 1985; Klein, 2021). Weight-loss programs often use averaged changes, or trends in change, to avoid the perception of failure if there is a temporary lack of weight loss or a short-term weight gain.

In exercise programs, injury is a cause of relapse that must be foreseen and dealt with. If the person quits exercising completely while injured, the gains that they have made in general fitness, time management and other benefits can quickly be lost. It is a good idea to keep the individual involved in appropriate exercise that will not aggravate the injury until they are fit enough to return to the original program. Injury is usually not seen as a failure on the part of the individual, and so the consequences for self-efficacy will be less. If they continue to participate in a limited exercise program, injury may not be seen as a lapse at all.

As we age, we may have to change exercise to suit changes in the body. If these changes are accomplished gradually, they usually do not affect the individual's view of themselves as a fit person.

8.4 CASE STUDY

SAKNGEA AND GAMBLING MOTIVATION

Sakngea is a 32-year-old temporary migrant. He entered Australia as a trained machinist to work in the mining industry in Western Australia. His main reason for coming was to allow him to support his extended family in Cambodia. At first, he felt very isolated as the only Cambodian working on a rural mine site, but gradually he became more comfortable as his English improved and as he took a greater part in social activities. These mostly involved gambling, particularly at mealtimes. He found playing cards with his workmates exciting, and his wins and losses were generally small.

Problems arose, however, when the company transferred him to Perth, where he didn't know anyone and felt very isolated again. While wandering around the city, Sakngea went to the casino and discovered that the excitement of gambling on cards made life more enjoyable and filled his empty weekends. Gradually, he discovered that he was spending most of his weekends in the casino, and didn't feel nearly as isolated or bored. However, he was losing far more money than he had realised at the time. Once, when he didn't have enough to make the usual transfer to his family, he borrowed the money from a workmate. Luckily, he managed to win enough the next weekend to pay this back, but he eventually fell so far behind that he took out a bank loan to cover his debts. Although his financial problems were getting out of hand, he was unable to resist the excitement of gambling. He believed that he would eventually have a big win that would pay off everything and get him back on track.

When Sakngea discovered that he couldn't afford to both make the repayments on his bank loan and send money home to his family, he applied for several credit cards and began to gamble on credit. All the time, he hoped for a big win so that all of his troubles would be solved.

Finally, Sakngea's financial problems became so bad that he regularly began to miss the payments to his family. He was spending so much time trying to win back what he had lost that he had little sleep on the weekends, and was too stressed to sleep even if he stayed away from the casino. His work was affected, and eventually he had to tell his boss about his situation.

His boss knew that gambling was a problem for other workers in the mining industry, and put Sakngea in touch with a counsellor through Gambling Help WA. The counsellor began working with Sakngea to deal with his gambling behaviour, and provided access to financial advice to take some of the pressure off his finances. The first step was getting Sakngea to recognise that his gambling had become an addiction, and that a variety of strategies would be needed to help him deal with it.

One of the first steps to help Sakngea to restrict and then stop his gambling was to identify the things that triggered gambling, and to change or control some of those triggers (stimulus control). Since Sakngea did not have many other activities to fill his weekends and cope with his isolation, he was put in touch with a local Cambodian community group. This group gave him a social network, involved him in projects that would fill his time and gave him a sense of self-worth through helping others. With his counsellor, he worked on developing strategies to stay away from the casino and other gambling situations. He developed a plan of easy steps to deal with the emotional loss he felt from not being able to gamble. This consisted of a series of rewards (reinforcements)—mainly self-administered—when he managed to accomplish each step. Financial planning allowed him to postpone some debts, and this allowed him to resume full payments to his family. This again gave Sakngea the feeling that he could contribute, and his sense of self-efficacy improved.

He also decided to recruit support from his workmates, by admitting that he had a gambling problem and asking them to help him stay away from at-work gambling situations. They decided to move their usual lunchtime card games to out-of-work hours, and to include Sakngea in alternative social activities at lunchtime instead. As the boss had been trying for some time to improve the workers' fitness, together they developed a lunchtime exercise program.

Because Sakngea occasionally found himself drawn back to the casino, his counsellor helped him to develop a relapse management plan, so that if he did slip it was only a small one. It was also not seen as a failure of his behaviour change, but as a momentary hitch in his progress. Over time, Sakngea found that his involvement in the workplace social network and in the Cambodian community met all his social needs. He had little time and no desire to return to gambling.

1   Voluntary pre-commitment schemes, where gamblers are required to identify up front how much they are prepared to lose, are a topic of ongoing debate. How would these schemes be classified as behaviour change strategies?

2   Can opponent–process theory be used to explain Sakngea's excitement and pleasure in gambling?

3   Many smokers have 'given up' smoking many times, only to return to the habit. How could relapse management help them quit permanently?

4   How does the slogan 'Never give up giving up' fit with theories of relapse management?

Points to consider

The first step in dealing with problem gambling is to get the person to recognise that their gambling has become an addiction, and that a variety of strategies are needed to help them deal with it. This involves helping the person to identify the things that triggered gambling, and changing or controlling some of those triggers (stimulus control). These can include alternative activities and providing for social needs. With counselling support, the person could develop strategies to stay away from the casino and other gambling situations. A plan of easy steps to deal with the emotional loss would involve a series of rewards (reinforcements), mainly self-administered. Financial planning is often needed to postpone or refinance debts. Social support is also important. If the person is able to admit to having a gambling problem, social contacts can be helpful in changing conditions that involve gambling. A relapse management plan is very useful, so that any slip is only small and is seen not as a failure of the behaviour change but as only a momentary hitch.

Learn more
Access additional resources to broaden your understanding of this chapter. See the Guided Tour for access details.

CHAPTER SUMMARY

- Understanding motivation—the factors that arouse, sustain and direct behaviour—is important in changing behaviour. Motivation has genetic, biological and cognitive components, but is also strongly influenced by learning.

- Primary drives are based on the biological needs of the organism. Acquired drives arise out of experience with the environment.

- Opponent–process theory and optimal level theories suggest that the organism is motivated to maintain balance as well as to satisfy needs.

- Successful strategies for behaviour change involve picking appropriate behaviours and methods, not expecting too much, giving methods a chance to work, and recognising that methods may be failures but people are not.

- Awareness of antecedents and reinforcements of behaviour are necessary before change can occur. Stimulus control techniques involve modifying the effects of antecedents.

- Low-awareness habits require the behaviour to be made more salient before it can be changed.

- Reinforcement, particularly if it is controlled by the individual, needs to be part of behaviour change strategies. The schedule of reinforcement that will be most effective differs at different stages of the change process.

- The use of good behaviour bonds is a method for increasing the costs of not changing a behaviour and increasing the gains of changing it. Lapses are common, so planning ahead to deal with them is an important part of behaviour change.

FURTHER READING

Carver CS & Scheier MF (1999) *On the Self-regulation of Behavior.* Cambridge University Press.

Fishbein M (2008) A reasoned action approach to health promotion. *Medical Decision Making* 28, 834–44.

Martin LR, Haskard-Zolnierek KB & DiMatteo MR (2010) *Health Behavior Change and Treatment Adherence: Evidence-based Guidelines for Improving Healthcare.* Oxford University Press.

Morabia A (2020) Editorial: JUMBO, MRFIT, and the making of public health epidemiology. *American Journal of Epidemiology* 189(6), 487–90. https://doi.org/10.1093/aje/kwz271

Ornish D & Ornish A (2019) *Undo It! How Simple Lifestyle Changes can Reverse Most Chronic Diseases.* Penguin Random House.

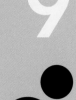

9

A Complex Example: Activity, Eating and Body

Activity and eating as behavioural health issues

The aim of this chapter is to bring together many of the ideas from the previous chapters and examine a particularly complex combination of health behaviours. It addresses the nature of these behaviours, the motivations for them and the risks and gains associated with them, and how the general principles of behaviour change might be utilised.

Much of the world is experiencing what has been called an epidemic of obesity (Friedrich, 2017; Pozza & Isidori, 2018; Mitchell et al., 2011). It has been noted that two-thirds of adults in Australia are classified as overweight or obese and, more disturbingly, that the rate of obesity in adults has roughly doubled over the last 20 years (ABS, 2018a). It has been estimated that **overweight** and **obesity** have replaced smoking as the number-one modifiable health risk in developed countries. As one author put it:

> The table fork is by far the deadliest weapon created by humans. Each year, this humble utensil abets the deaths of millions of people by conveying into their bodies all kinds of fatty foodstuffs known to cause heart attacks, cancers, strokes, diabetes and other diseases.

This extreme statement was intended to make a point, but the health risks associated with obesity are real and significant (Kinlen et al., 2017).

PAUSE & REFLECT

Think about the people around you, such as family and friends. Also think about university students— research has shown that they are generally less likely to be obese than other people of the same age.

Do your family and friends seem to you to be generally overweight?

Do you frequently discuss weight with other people?

Why might university students be less likely to be obese than others in their age cohort?

MEASUREMENT OF BODY MASS

The most common way of estimating body fat—due mostly to its ease of calculation—is the **body mass index (BMI)**. This is recognised as a good estimator of whether someone's weight is healthy for their height (Keys et al., 1972) and is frequently used in determining the extent of overweight and obesity in an individual or group. The measure involves dividing the individual's weight (measured in kilograms) by the square of their height (measured in metres).

Common suggestions are that the healthy range of BMI for adults is 18.5–25. Both overweight and underweight have been shown to have negative health consequences. Overweight is commonly defined as a BMI between the top of the healthy range and 30, while a BMI over 30 is categorised as obese. Use of the BMI with children is not considered to be appropriate unless corrections for the age of the child are used (CDCP, 2011). There are also national differences in how BMI is applied. Lower BMIs are regarded as healthy in many Asian countries, due to differences in body structure between Asians and Caucasians.

Overweight
The label for a range of weight that is above what is considered to be healthy.

Obesity
The label for a range of weight that is significantly above what is considered to be healthy, and documented as presenting a serious risk to health.

Body mass index (BMI)
An approximate measure of an individual's amount of body fat, frequently used by health professionals because it is easy to calculate.

While important at population level, there are problems with using this simple measure at the individual level—a thing that should be well understood by health professionals. For example, many elite athletes, such as football players, have BMIs well above 26 largely due to the high levels of (relatively heavy) muscle mass for their height. There is even some evidence that the mildly overweight range (26–30) may not result in higher mortality than the defined healthy range (Flegal et al., 2005). However, BMI is extremely useful in considering the general health status of particular populations; that is, when looking at how weight can affect the health of people within a particular group (NCD Risk Factor Collaboration, 2019).

9.1 CASE STUDY

FANASINA AND EXERCISE

This case study looks at the elements involved in changing a health-related behaviour: physical activity.

Fanasina is a 19-year-old university student who lives with her parents. When she was in high school, she played several sports and got plenty of other exercise by walking to and from school. She notices that she is not exercising any more. She drives her car everywhere, even down to the shops. She is aware that she is feeling unfit and is beginning to gain weight. She feels tired much more often than she used to, and is not sleeping as well. She does not like the changes that have happened to her appearance, particularly the 'spare tire' developing around her middle. She decides to examine the antecedents for her exercise behaviour as a first step to increasing her activity levels.

1   Why do you think Fanasina got so much exercise during her school years?
2   Why do you think Fanasina's exercise behaviour has changed so much in a relatively short time?

HEALTH ISSUES IN OVERWEIGHT AND OBESITY

The most obvious evidence of a concern with overweight in the media in recent years has been the frequency with which weight and weight loss are discussed. Even during the COVID-19 pandemic, the amount of media attention to, and stigmatising of, obesity increased (Flint, 2020). Researchers have started to explore connections between pandemics such as COVID-19 and obesity and this area is likely to be of interest to health professionals in the future (Flint, 2020; Clemmensen et al., 2020). Interest in overweight and obesity is particularly common in media directed at women: virtually every issue of women's magazines, every lifestyle television program and every newspaper section devoted to health discusses weight loss and methods for achieving it.

Australian data on the proportion of each gender that is overweight (75% of men and 60% of women; AIHW, 2021e) and on the health consequences of overweight suggests that media aimed at men should be even more focused on weight loss, but this is not the case. The reason usually offered for the discrepancy is that other people, such as partners and health professionals, worry about men's overweight primarily because of its impact on health, while women worry about their own, primarily because of its impact on appearance. Surveys in many countries have shown a particularly troubling increase in overweight and obesity in children, even the very young. The rates of overweight and obesity in Australian children are worryingly high, although there may be some evidence that they have reached a plateau (AIHW, 2017). It is possible that this is linked to media attention given to the problem. With high rates of overweight and obesity have come worrying increases in risk factors such as high blood pressure, raised blood sugar levels and type 2 diabetes among children (Daniels et al., 2005). Obesity and overweight have also been linked to poorer quality of life in adolescents (Keating et al., 2011).

Reductions in the rates of overweight would result in greatly increased disease-free years later in life, due to reductions in the rates of coronary heart disease, bowel cancer, diabetes, strokes and even arthritis. Changes to energy balance (Ravussin & Ryan, 2018)—that is, modification of diet and exercise patterns—in children and young adults (Katzmarzyk et al., 2019) could have an enormous impact on the costs of health care, and extend the healthy and active years of life for each person.

The issues involved in this idea of energy balance are extremely complex, however, and this complexity is often overlooked. There is a tendency to confuse behaviours (e.g. "I will walk for 20 minutes" or "I will eat smaller portions"), where intentions are reasonably good predictors, with outcomes (e.g. "I will get fit" or "I will lose weight"), where intentions are much poorer predictors (Fishbein, 2008).

Most of the attention on energy balance tends to focus on restriction of intake: limiting the amount or the kind of food that the individual eats. This is often unpleasant for the individual and may have social, emotional and even serious health consequences. Another consequence has been the search for a 'magic bullet': a simple, quick and painless way of restricting intake. The major result of this has been a massive increase in weight reduction products. Many are based on the idea of replacing normal meals with filling but low-kilojoule shakes, soups or bars. Although these products are improving in terms of dietary balance, fibre, vitamins and minerals, it is likely that their main value is short-term (Egger, 2006). Few of them offer anything that could not be achieved by choosing lower-kilojoule foods. One of the main objections to them is that the individual does not learn a great deal about long-term eating behaviour.

Many of the magic bullets are totally fraudulent, offering no-pain weight loss through untested, unproven and even dangerous methods in exchange for large amounts of money. One such product—SensaSlim, an oral weight-loss spray—had its approval by the Australian Therapeutic Goods Administration withdrawn on the grounds that its claimed research support was faked (Medew, 2011). The claims for this product were supposedly backed by a Geneva-based research group. Investigation showed that the pictures of the group's executives had actually been copied from the website of a US lung clinic, which had nothing to do with SensaSlim or even with weight loss. Sadly, the product (and its supposed 'scientific' support) is still available on the internet. The US Federal Trade Commission (FTC, 2004) states that ads which claim a person can lose large amounts of weight quickly by taking a pill, putting on a patch or rubbing in a cream "are almost always false".

A different type of rapid weight loss treatment involves **bariatric surgery**, such as bypass operations or lap-band surgery (where the size of the stomach is reduced by placing a band around the stomach to restrict the amount of food that can be eaten). Such surgical procedures can have dramatic effects (O'Brien et al., 2019). Surgery is considered a last-choice option after other

Bariatric surgery
Surgery aimed at weight loss in the obese that works by reducing the size of the stomach, either by insertion of a mechanical device (e.g. lap-band) or removal of part of the stomach.

approaches to weight control have failed and it is used only with moderate to severe obesity. It can place the patient at serious risk of after-effects such as infections and surgical complications, and side effects such as gastric upset and ongoing heartburn. Surgery is only suitable in extreme cases of clinical obesity where the health risks of doing nothing are immediate and severe. If a person has surgery to reverse their lap-band procedure, they tend to quickly regain weight. Surgery needs to be combined with long-term changes in eating behaviours if long-term weight loss is to be achieved and maintained.

Ecological model
A model which proposes that overweight and obesity include biological, behavioural and environmental factors in addition to food intake.

In reality, overweight is not just about how much food is taken in. It is also highly dependent on the kind of food—and other intakes such as alcohol—as well as the output side of the balance, such as work and exercise (Scarborough et al., 2011). Environmental and biological factors also play a role in this complex system. Figure 9.1 presents an **ecological model** for understanding obesity (Swinburn et al., 1999).

Since part of the complexity comes from misunderstanding the contributors (to the obesity problem and solutions), topics are discussed separately in more detail later in this chapter. As activity is in many ways the simpler side of the intake–output equation, it will be looked at first.

FIGURE 9.1 An ecological model for understanding obesity

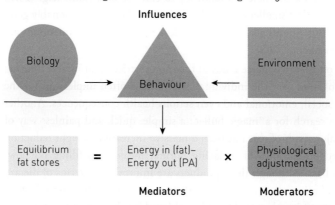

Swinburn et al. (1999)

9.2 CASE STUDY

FANASINA (CONT.)

Fanasina decides that part of the difference is that several things that used to trigger exercise—a school requirement that she play sport, the fact that her friends played sport, and special times during the day set aside for exercise—no longer happen. Now she has a part-time job and her studies take up a lot of time. When she is not studying, she likes to talk to her friends on the phone or meet them at the pub or coffee shop to talk. She also notes that exercise makes her feel tired now, that there never seems to be enough time and that she does not particularly like to get sweaty.

Fanasina realises that the antecedents for her behaviour need to be changed. Apart from triggers, there used to be a number of stimuli that no longer occur: having someone tell her that it was time to exercise, having exercise clothes with her, having easy access to a place to exercise, and remembering to exercise. Fanasina decides that she will set aside specific times for exercise each week. She will make it hard to forget these by marking them in her calendar and leaving herself notes and reminders on her desk and phone. She asks her parents to remind her to exercise, washes her exercise clothes as soon as she finishes exercising, and places the clean clothes in her sports bag ready for the next scheduled exercise. On days when exercise is scheduled, she leaves the sports bag at the front door as a reminder. These are all examples of stimulus control.

1   Can you think of any other ways Fanasina might control the stimuli that trigger exercise behaviour?

2   How might Fanasina use reinforcements to modify her behaviour?

Physical activity

Messages encouraging increased physical activity are everywhere. Schools and worksites frequently run programs explaining the benefits of activity and the risks associated with a sedentary lifestyle. One Australian city—Rockhampton—undertook a government-funded program to encourage everyone to take 10 000 steps each day (Brown et al., 2006). This program led to several similar programs and organisations such as 10 000 Steps, which claims to have had almost half a million members. A lot of the attention being given to exercise, however, fails to explain the differences and similarities of incidental exercise (effortful work, and exercise involved in daily activities such as walking, stair-climbing and house or garden work) and intentional exercise (effortful activity undertaken solely for the purpose of improving fitness). Even the latter needs to be subdivided by purpose, as individuals may exercise for goals related to the three Fs: fatness (or size), fitness (or function) and figure (or fashion).

Size (fatness)

Evidence suggests that adding exercise to diet can be faster, more effective and have greater health benefits than dieting alone (Cox, 2017). The debates about the merits of eating less versus exercising more are complicated by the fact that eating less on its own only removes weight (with health benefits primarily limited to areas where risks arise from too much body fat), while exercise changes the nature of the weight (with health benefits that can arise from better cardiovascular, respiratory and musculoskeletal fitness). However, exercise has several drawbacks when the aim is to decrease body size, and these are increased when the individual is already obese. For the morbidly obese individual, even limited exercise may be very difficult, extremely uncomfortable and even seriously dangerous.

Media presentations focusing purely on weight loss, such as *The Biggest Loser*, may present a very biased view of how effective exercise (and dieting) can be in reducing body size (Bissell & Mocarski, 2016). First, contestants are selected to have generally good health (other than being obese) so that risks of acute health problems occurring during the program are limited. When injuries or cardiovascular or respiratory problems do occur, they tend to be edited out of the program, or at least minimised in the presentation. Contestants devote all their time to losing weight: a luxury that very few people can afford either in time or loss of earnings. The payoffs—monetary prizes, fame and publicity—are very great motivators (in the short term), and these payoffs are not available to the average obese individual. Finally, the duration of benefit is not considered. What do the biggest losers look like, and how is their health, a year after the program, or two years? Without a full consideration of all the issues that led to their serious obesity in the first place, it is difficult to determine whether any long-term benefit has resulted from the program.

Motivation is discussed in Chapter 8.

Such media representations, known as 'fattertainment', include TV shows such as *My 600 lb Life* and films such as *Shallow Hal*.

A problem that is often encountered by people who increase their exercise purely as a way of losing weight is that they may initially convert fat weight to heavier muscle weight, meaning that they initially gain rather than lose weight. This can be discouraging in the short term and needs to be recognised as a benefit rather than a disappointment. Clearly, the best outcome occurs when the individual begins to enjoy the exercise for its own sake. This becomes a much more straightforward motivation than potential weight loss, and is more likely to lead to long-term sustainable exercise patterns.

PAUSE & REFLECT

Have your exercise and physical activities changed over the past few years?
If so, why do you think this has happened? If not, what has maintained your behaviour?

Function (fitness)

Physical activity
Bodily movement produced by skeletal muscles that requires energy expenditure.

The least discussed, but in health terms often the most significant, effect of **physical activity** is improved function. The term **fitness** is mostly used when the benefits are spread across a number of body systems. Increased activity, even at low levels, has been shown to help cardiovascular and respiratory function, increase tolerance to effort and make individuals feel better (Su et al., 2019). Benefits may be seen in several body systems (Dias et al., 2018; Miguet et al., 2020; Buckinx et al., 2020). For example, even limited activity such as regular walking may reduce high blood pressure, reduce the occurrence of chest pain in patients with existing cardiovascular problems and reduce the occurrence of asthma attacks, headaches, muscular pain, depression and anxiety.

Fitness
A condition of health or physical soundness, which may be general or related to the ability to meet a specific demand ('fit for purpose').

What is often overlooked is that activity can be specifically targeted towards the particular health outcomes that are most important to the individual. Gentle movement activities, such as stretching, tai chi, yoga and Pilates, may produce major benefits in flexibility and mitigate problems such as muscular or joint pain, movement restriction, headache and negative emotions. However, they may do little for cardiovascular and respiratory function or strength. Weightlifting may build muscle mass, increasing strength and flexibility, but do little for general fitness. Vigorous, high-impact exercise such as running, dance-based exercises (e.g. Zumba), tennis, football or some martial arts may produce great benefit in terms of cardiovascular and respiratory function and the effectiveness of specific muscle groups, but can place individuals at greater risk of injury or **acute illness** events. This is particularly true of older people or those with pre-existing health conditions. It is always wise to consult a doctor before beginning any strenuous exercise program or significantly changing activity patterns.

Acute illness
A single episode of illness or disease, generally severe and over a limited period of time.

Figure (fashion)

It has been noted that men often exercise primarily for issues related to body shape; that is, to build up muscle and to reduce body fat levels so that muscle is more evident. At the same time, the majority of men, regardless of their weight and shape, are satisfied with their appearance. This seeming contradiction underlines the significant gender issues in the energy–balance equation. The majority of women are dissatisfied with their shape, and yet are not nearly as concerned with musculature as with size. Where most men would like to convert fat to muscle, women are most concerned with simply getting rid of the fat and having a thinner shape (Sattler et al., 2018). Some women may even avoid strenuous exercise out of a fear of becoming too muscular rather than fashionably thin.

Health promotion is discussed in Chapter 16.

Focus on body acceptance is a health-promoting way to address an individual's dissatisfaction with their body shape (Van Zutven et al., 2015).

9.3 CASE STUDY

FANASINA (CONT.)

Fanasina decides that she can increase the gains and reduce the costs of exercise by making an effort to change the way she thinks about exercise. Although she does not like getting sweaty and tired, she recognises that these are short-term costs. So she focuses on the gains. After she has exercised and showered, she feels 'tingly' and relaxed. Being tired has a positive side, in that she sleeps better and feels more awake during the day. This allows her to get more done in less time, and because she is becoming fitter she has more energy to bring to all her tasks. The increase in exercise also changes her thinking about her fitness and figure, and she finds this very rewarding. Finally, because she is enjoying the change to her activities, she persuades her friend Rachel to exercise with her. They join a netball team that plays once a week. Exercising with a friend makes it a social activity as well as a physical one, and replaces some of the lost social time. The amount of time that Fanasina now spends on study and work appeared to be a significant factor in her decreased exercise. She notes, however, that there is a lot of wasted time in her typical day, and this is where she can fit her exercise without losing out on more valuable activities.

1 The costs of exercise are often immediate, while the gains are long-term. How could this problem be overcome?
2 Can you think of some ways that Fanasina could better organise her time to make room for exercise?

EATING

One well-known weight loss program (Noom) uses the phrase "It's simple psychology" in its advertising. However, the determinants of what we eat, when we eat, how much we eat and why we eat are extremely variable. They include childhood learning and developmental factors (Fleischer et al., 2021), social and cultural influences and many psychological factors. The variety of these influences can be seen in 'food porn': television, online and print media presentations of the most exotic, delicious and attractive foods that can be produced by expert chefs and duplicated in your own home.

The huge number of sources of information about food indicates that we clearly do not just eat to survive. Hunger is only one small part of our motivation to eat. We also eat for pleasure, for social interaction, for our own emotional reasons (comfort, relaxation and stress reduction) and even to impress others. Have you ever bragged about what, where or how much you have eaten?

One easy way to think about the complexity of the issues is to separate what we eat from how much we eat, and why we eat.

What we eat

The Australian government, like those of many other countries, provides guidelines for healthy eating (eatforhealth.gov.au). It offers resources for specific groups, such as children, older adults and First Peoples, who have a variety of special issues related to eating behaviour. School programs in many countries teach children about **food pyramids** or 'food pies'. These indicate the various food groups and how much of each we should eat for health reasons. The smallest section of these graphic representations is always the section for fat. In developed countries, people's diet generally includes too much fat, and much of the health-related information about diet is focused on reducing the amount of fat as a proportion of food intake. This can have the unfortunate consequence of making some people fat-phobic, and extremely low-fat diets can be hazardous to children's health because fat has a role in growth and development. Further, the fact that many of the favoured childhood foods are classed in the fat category can make children simply tune out messages about a balanced diet.

Food pyramid
A triangular figure divided into segments to indicate what proportion of the diet each food group should comprise.

The reality is that what children eat is usually not within the children's control at all (Scaglioni et al., 2018). The decisions about what food to buy and prepare are commonly made by their parents or other carers.

Stimulus control
Changing a behaviour by changing its antecedents.

As the above discussion suggests, what we eat is under a great deal of **stimulus control**. Because of prior experience, we find certain types of food attractive and others unattractive. Salty, sweet and fatty foods tend to be very attractive to most people. Other stimulus characteristics of food (e.g. colour, texture, shape or thoughts about the source) can be highly important in determining attractiveness. For example, a person may have no problems with eating beef, lamb or pork because the meat comes in large, anonymous chunks, but be unable to eat chicken or fish because they are smaller and therefore look more like animals.

Children quite often have aversions to certain kinds of food, such as vegetables. Research has shown that they can be brought to increase their intake of these foods simply by exposing them to other people, including peers, role models or even unknown adults, who eat those foods (Ogden, 2007). Food that is strange in colour, texture or flavour may be less desirable than familiar foods. 'Picky eating' is more common in children, but restricted willingness to eat novel foods can often be found in adults as well.

Have you, or someone in your family, ever had a food aversion? Or a fad for eating a particular kind of food very frequently?

Did your family have an explanation for this that you shared with one another?

Did this aversion or fad influence what the other family members ate?

Culture and media are very important in educating people about new foods. Many novel ingredients—including Asian staple foods such as lemongrass, bok choy and varieties of chillies—are available in supermarkets in Western countries. Australasian customers have access to a very diverse range of foods because of their multicultural populations and the dramatic changes in the sources of immigrants and refugees over the past few decades. Cookery shows are useful in introducing viewers to a wide range of ingredients and preparation methods.

How much we eat

Another learnt component of the food intake equation is how much food is appropriate. Many older people were raised on the principle that they 'should' eat everything on their plate. This ethical requirement to avoid wasting food made sense during a depression or war, when the amount or kind of food available was limited. However, in most of the developed world, food is easily available, and quantities are seldom limited by any factor other than affordability. For most people in Western countries, affordability of healthy food is not a major problem.

Learning to identify appropriate portion and meal sizes follows similar patterns as learning what to eat. During childhood, parents make available what they believe are appropriately sized meals, and children are expected to eat those meals. If the child asks for more food or a particular kind of food, it is seen as appropriate to provide it. There is an ethical dimension, in that depriving a growing child of 'enough' food is frowned upon. There is also the contrary issue: it is quite common for a family, or restaurant goer, to keep eating until all the food is gone, even if this leads to a feeling of being overfull or bloated. Hunger is clearly not motivating this eating. If people are regularly presented with overly large portion sizes, they may (mistakenly) learn to think that it is an appropriate size. Travellers to the US often note that meal sizes in restaurants seem intended to satisfy the largest eaters, not the average, and that they have to leave a significant portion of their meal uneaten.

An important part of helping both children and adults to maintain a healthy weight or body shape is stimulus control; in this case, portion control (Hetherington et al., 2018). Instructions that an appropriate size for a meat portion is 'the size of a deck of cards' gives an individual more immediately accessible information than saying 'about 200 grams'. Reducing portion sizes, even without changing any other aspect of a meal, can be a very effective strategy for helping maintain a healthy weight or lose unwanted weight.

Why we eat

The most important, and complex, issue with regard to eating is motivation. The easiest assumption to make about eating is that people eat when they are hungry and stop when they are not. This is not a very accurate description of the eating patterns of most people.

Motivation is discussed in Chapter 8.

Eating tends to take place at mealtimes, in places where food is available even when it is not mealtime, and in the presence of attractive food in the environment. Stimulus control may be as important as, or more important than, needs and drives where eating behaviour is concerned.

An interesting—and perhaps counterintuitive—finding regarding stimulus control of eating is that overweight people are less likely than underweight or normal weight people to eat because they are hungry. The overweight person may be more likely to be triggered to eat by the presence of food, by the approach of a mealtime or by an emotional state (Schachter, 1971). This may happen because of early experience with food, which becomes associated with certain times, with social interaction or with comfort. As a result, some people may fail to regulate their eating by sensations of hunger. Instead, they eat when they are lonely, when they are stressed or simply when they are in the presence of food.

Food restriction diets fail to take these factors into account. They lead dieters to feel unsatisfied—not because they are still hungry but because they have not had their usual diet. They may also feel isolated because they cannot eat as others are eating or stressed because they have not eaten things that have been associated with pleasant tastes or emotional comfort. Such **comfort food** is typically high in sugar and fat, and although it can relieve some stress it also tends to add to abdominal fat stores (Spence, 2017). Overeating among dieters is quite common and has been connected with theories of disinhibition (the 'what the hell' effect) in the presence of food cues, along with regulation of mood by eating, escape from stress or the relapse violation effect (Davis, 2017).

Comfort food
Food, often with traditional or nostalgic connections, that is eaten primarily for positive emotional reasons rather than because of hunger.

Ogden (2007) discusses how control influences eating or overeating. An individual may believe, for a wide variety of reasons, that they cannot control their eating. They may, for example, believe that their weight is genetically determined, so efforts to change eating will not work. Alternatively, if they feel that many elements of their life (e.g. stress, other people's behaviour or work) are out of their control, they may believe that eating is one thing that they do have direct control over. Our beliefs about where control of our eating lies may have a quite significant effect on how we go about trying to change, or whether we make the effort to change at all.

Locus of control is discussed in more detail in Chapter 13.

Focusing simply on the individual and their motivation ignores a range of other very important factors. Swinburn and colleagues (1999) have referred to living conditions in developed countries as **obesogenic environments**. Many elements of the environment tend to encourage behaviours that lead to excess intake and inadequate outputs and there are far fewer elements that encourage healthier behaviours. Dealing with these elements requires making changes to the environment, perhaps through education, restrictions on advertising, better labelling of food or regulations about availability (Townshend & Lake, 2017). One example of the latter is limiting unhealthy choices in school canteens.

Obesogenic environment
An environment (including culture, physical structures and other elements) that encourages overeating and/or inadequate physical activity.

There may also be biological or genetic influences that exert some control over eating. **Set point theory** suggests that there may be brain mechanisms that 'defend' our current body fat content, so that if we eat too little—as in a restriction diet—our body tries to defend our current fat levels by making us hungrier. It also suggests that if we eat too much, our body will make us less hungry (Kennedy, 1953). In a major review, Müller et al. (2018) identify some basic problems with this theory. It does not really account for the environmental controls on eating discussed above, or explain why there is an obesity epidemic. They discuss some alternative balance models.

Set point theory
A theory that suggests that the body 'defends' a certain set weight against changes.

Settling point theory
A theory that changes in energy balance become habitual, and remain at the new level.

Settling point theory suggests that when either inputs (eating) or outputs (activity) change, the balance may settle at a new equilibrium point, then remain relatively stable at that point until either the inputs or the outputs change again. This agrees with the idea of the obesogenic environment: any obesity epidemic could result from either increased accessibility to food or a decrease in the need for physical activity, as a result of societal change. There are problems with this model, however. Probably the biggest one is simply the question, "Why don't we all get fat?"

Dual intervention point theory suggests that there may be two set points that define a range, with settling points in between. Overall, the evidence of purely biological control of weight is poor, and ignores the environmental factors noted above (Davis et al., 2018; Hall, 2018).

In Chapter 6, we discussed person–environment interactions as basic to understanding human behaviour. What is needed is a theory that takes account of both environmental influences and individual predispositions or vulnerabilities. Such models exist (Speakman et al., 2011) but are beyond the scope of the current discussion. Regulation of eating and activity behaviours is quite complex as they rely on a variety of systems at a variety of levels, and it is clear that any approach needs to involve both psychological and biological aspects.

Body image as a health issue

Given that overweight and obesity have become such a health pandemic (ABS, 2018a), it is informative to look at what people think about their bodies. Sadly, there are extremely high levels of body dissatisfaction, and substantial evidence that this dissatisfaction is causally linked to a wide range of psychological and physical health problems.

Learning is discussed in Chapter 6.

The strongest evidence is that there is a definite link between dissatisfaction with one's body and disordered eating (Brytek-Matera & Czepczor, 2017). Disordered eating includes, but is not restricted to, clinical eating disorders such as anorexia and bulimia nervosa. It also includes crash dieting, yoyo dieting (where weight gain and loss alternate) and eating a severely unbalanced diet that results in dietary deficiencies.

PAUSE & REFLECT

Are you satisfied or dissatisfied with your body?

What factors do you think contribute to your satisfaction or dissatisfaction with your body?

Research has linked numerous influences to the development and maintenance of weight-related problems. These include teasing (by peers, parents or others), early physical maturation, negative emotions, stress, developmental challenges, academic pressures, social comparison and, particularly, images in the media (Aparicio-Martinez et al., 2019; Jarman et al., 2021). This includes not only the presentation of fashion models and media stars who are uniformly abnormally thin, but also the relative scarcity not only of obese but also of normal, healthy-weight people. These skewed depictions can mean that girls learn to correlate attractiveness with thinness, while boys tend to correlate attractiveness with strength and low body fat levels as well (Engeln et al., 2020).

Periodically, media sources attempt to avert criticism that they are contributing to a society-wide body image problem, and run special features on 'normal' size models or restrict their use of very thin or very young models. These defensive activities are often short-lived or undermined by other media which continues to use unhealthy models or retouch pictures to increase market share at the expense of the more responsible media. However, use of the media to increase knowledge that there is a healthy weight range and that attractiveness is not limited to a single body type, should not be overlooked.

Intervention

With the issues being as complex as they are, it would be unreasonable to expect simple solutions. Clearly, behavioural interventions at the individual level have an important part to play. These interventions—either on their own or together with pharmacological treatments, dietary substitutes and even surgery—can be effective in many cases. Other approaches include meal replacement programs, online and phone-based interventions, and a more active role for health professionals in supporting the individual in their pursuit of a healthy weight. However, as overweight and obesity are issues for society as well as for the individual, it is important not to neglect intervention at the family, community and even global levels (Swinburn et al. 1999).

Behavioural change is discussed in Chapter 8.

9.4 CASE STUDY

DONALD AND OBESITY

This case study looks at factors that may be involved in encouraging and maintaining obesity in an individual.

Donald is a 43-year-old security guard at a suburban shopping centre in Adelaide. He was born in a town camp outside Alice Springs to a young Indigenous woman who was clinically obese. When Donald was 18 months old, his mother was hospitalised with complications of respiratory disease, and Donald was fostered to a white family in Adelaide. This family discouraged members of his mother's family from having any contact with Donald, and when his mother died in hospital they ceased all communication. The foster parents were overweight and Donald was raised on a diet that was heavy on potatoes, bread and other carbohydrates, and large portions of fried food. He received little attention from his foster parents, who were caring for four children, and most of that attention was at mealtimes.

When Donald was six, the foster parents decided that they could no longer care for so many children, and for the next four years Donald was shuttled from institution to foster home to institution. Food was always plentiful, and sweets and fatty foods were often given as treats. At age 10, he was placed with an aunty living in a small Indigenous community in western Queensland. She tried to ensure that Donald had enough food, but as fresh fruit and vegetables were hard to get and very expensive his diet was high in carbohydrates and processed food. Children at school made fun of him for being so fat, and he gradually found that his only friends were other overweight children.

When he reached high school, Donald started associating with other marginalised kids, and was introduced to beer. Food and beer gradually became his primary source of comfort against the teasing that he received, and the pressure from teachers and some other adults that he should lose weight for his own health. Donald did not finish high school. Because he was big and strong, he was able to get labouring jobs. However, labouring—particularly in hot weather—was very stressful for him and he got out of breath easily. It was common for him and other labourers on building sites to eat large fatty lunches, and to wind down at the end of the day at the pub with more fatty food and beer. As his weight continued to increase, he had to leave several labouring jobs due to physical issues with the work. He began to drift from place to place.

Eventually, Donald returned to Adelaide and obtained a job as a security guard at a shopping centre. He lives alone in a rented room, so he eats at the shopping centre or in the pub on the way home. His job involves little physical activity other than walking, and considerable time sitting. Because he was always thirsty and had to take increasingly frequent breaks to urinate, his boss sent him for a medical evaluation. Donald was discovered to have type 2 diabetes. The doctor gave him a printed diet to control his symptoms, but Donald could not find the time or energy to follow the diet very often. He found it hard not to just eat whatever looked good at the shopping centre's food court. He did manage to cut out drinking, but seemed to be hungrier after giving up alcohol. In the last month, Donald has developed increasingly severe chest pain when he climbs stairs at work, and has started to use escalators and lifts instead.

1   What biological and social elements may be contributing to Donald's obesity?
2   Why do you think Donald's weight received so little attention as a behavioural problem during his childhood?
3   What are some of the reasons why giving up alcohol has had so little effect on Donald's obesity?
4   What factors make a typical suburban shopping centre an obesogenic environment? What might be done to make it less so?

Points to consider

Many components are involved when an individual has developed a pattern of excess eating behaviour. In this case study there were cultural and social class factors: Donald's removal from his mother, family and culture at an early age, the instability of his early life, the lack of educational success, and a variety of other issues linked to deprivation and discrimination. There are also several individual behavioural issues, such as a lack of self-efficacy and the fact that the now-established health problems might have been avoided with early interventions. Behaviour change can be vital at any stage, but community development, education, government programs and basic help for the disadvantaged are also needed.

Learn more
Access additional
resources to broaden
your understanding
of this chapter. See
the Guided Tour for
access details.

CHAPTER SUMMARY

- The relationship between weight and health has become a major focus of attention in the area of health behaviour. High rates of overweight and obesity, and low levels of physical activity, have been identified as significant public health issues, particularly in developed countries.

- Although the health problems associated with overweight and lack of activity are greater for men, concern with body weight and shape are greater for women.

- The issues are complicated, and a focus on just one aspect of the physical activity–eating interaction can produce an unbalanced picture and incomplete solutions.

- Reduction in physical activity has been related to an increase in the number of sedentary jobs and sedentary leisure pursuits, such as use of online media.

- The behavioural issues in eating are complex, as consideration needs to be given to what we eat, how much we eat and why we eat. Various theories have been advanced regarding how individual eating is regulated and why overeating occurs even when the individual is consciously attempting to eat less.

- Elements of the environment and society contribute independently to the problem of overweight in society, and a broader ecological model helps with understanding this issue.

- Body image is an important part of the equation. High levels of body dissatisfaction make the activity–eating interaction even more difficult to understand, and create a need for more comprehensive solutions to the public health problem.

FURTHER READING

Clark A, Franklin J, Pratt I & McGrice M (2010) Overweight and obesity: Use of portion control in management. *Australian Family Physician* 39(6), 407–11.

DoH [Department of Health] (n.d.) *Overweight and Obesity.*
https://www.health.gov.au/health-topics/overweight-and-obesity

Gaesser G & Angadi S (2021) Obesity treatment: Weight loss versus increasing fitness and physical activity for reducing health risks. *iScience* 24(10), 102995. https://doi.org/10.1016/j.isci.2021.102995.

Lewin E (2019) '*We Can Really Call This an Epidemic*': Obesity Rates Double in 10 Years.
https://www1.racgp.org.au/newsgp/clinical/'we-can-really-call-this-an-epidemic'/obesity-rate

Ogden J (2007) Eating behaviour. In J Ogden *Health Psychology: A Textbook* (4th edn), Ch. 6. Open University Press.

Pool R (2001) *Fat: Fighting the Obesity Epidemic.* Oxford University Press.

PART III

PSYCHOPHYSIOLOGICAL ASPECTS OF HEALTH

» Chapter 10: Understanding Mind and Body Interactions 178
» Chapter 11: A Complex Example: Understanding Pain 194
» Chapter 12: Stress and Trauma 206
» Chapter 13: Coping: How to Deal with Stress 222

IS IT ALL IN YOUR MIND?

So far, the focus of this book has largely been on behavioural and cognitive factors as they impact on health, while the issue of emotion has hovered somewhere in the background. Emotion has been mentioned frequently, but up to now has not been dealt with directly or in depth. Yet anyone who thinks about what health means will be aware that emotions are a critical component. To take one example, the media is full of stories about stress: effects of stress on how people feel and behave, and effects of stress on their health. Invariably, stress is thought of as existing within the emotional domain of the individual. Part III examines this domain and how it is linked to the concepts that have been discussed up to this point.

So, why is it titled 'psychophysiological aspects'? It is intended to get you to think of the psychological (mental) and the physiological (bodily) elements of the person as inseparably connected. Western patterns of thinking have often tried to separate the mind from the body, as if the two could operate in isolation from one another. One of the main aims of Part III is to challenge those patterns of thinking. What needs to be considered, particularly when we think about health and illness, is the whole person. In Chapters 4 and 5, we discussed in some detail how illness affects the whole person, not just limited elements of them. In the next few chapters, we focus on how the whole person, with a mind and a body, experiences their emotional world.

OXFORD UNIVERSITY PRESS

The first place to start is an understanding of what emotion is and how it works. Chapter 10 examines the interactions between the elements of the whole person that give rise to the experiences we call emotion. It looks at the importance of the brain and nervous system, along with other systems of the body, as well as at the importance of thought processes on the operations of these systems. It considers the role of faulty regulation of emotions in mental illnesses such as anxiety disorders and depression. An integrated perspective is vital to the understanding of how emotional states can produce health effects in key systems of the body, such as the cardiovascular and immune systems; these are also considered.

Pain is often thought to be a condition of the body. Chapter 11 examines how this most common of all symptoms is also an emotional and cognitive condition. The diagnosis and management of pain constitutes a large part of the work of health professionals, but is often based on incomplete understandings of where pain comes from, why it persists as it does, and what can be done about it.

Chapter 12 shifts the focus to stress. Again, this is a very common concept in discussions of health, but frequently is poorly understood. The total process that we refer to as stress involves elements of stimulus and response. Whether we experience our situation as stressful is dependent on judgments that we make about the significance of several aspects of that situation, such as our appraisal of how much the situation demands of us and whether we have capabilities or the resources to meet those demands. The effects of the most extreme level of demand—traumatic events—are also considered.

Fortunately, stress is neither inevitable nor irresistible. Chapter 13 looks at coping strategies that we can adopt to deal with the experience of stress, including naturally occurring ways that we cope with stress. It also introduces some strategies that can help with stress management.

In Part III, the idea of the individual as a whole person is more of a focus than it has been in Parts I and II. We encourage you to think back to earlier chapters from this holistic viewpoint, as this will make it easier for you to understand all the links between health and human behaviour.

OXFORD UNIVERSITY PRESS

10 Understanding Mind and Body Interactions

CHAPTER OBJECTIVES

By the end of this chapter, you should be able to:

» understand interactions between psychological and physical states

» understand the functions of different areas of the brain and the role the autonomic nervous system plays in emotion

» apply the principles of emotion to explain interactions between mind and body, and how these impact on health

» apply an integrated understanding of health to issues such as cardiovascular disease, cancer, mental illness and functioning of the immune system

KEYWORDS

» attribution theory of emotion

» cytokines

» dysregulation of emotions

» emotions

» holism

» psychoneuroimmunology

» psychophysiology

» psychosomatic illness

» type A (coronary prone) behaviour pattern

» type C (or cancer prone) behaviour pattern

» type D (distressed) personality

Introduction

Even though the link between feeling bad in a psychological sense and feeling bad in a physical sense is well recognised, Western philosophy has traditionally regarded the mind (psyche) and body (soma) as separate domains (known as mind–body dualism). Traditionally, the mind and body were viewed as parallel and independent; only some disease states were thought to involve both. The discipline of psychology challenged mind–body dualism. Sigmund Freud (1856–1939) suggested that individuals could convert unconscious psychological conflicts into physical symptoms, and in so doing reduce the anxiety associated with the conflict. Indeed, in response to highly stressful events, there are reported cases of individuals suddenly losing their ability to speak or hear, or developing some form of paralysis. In the late 19th and early 20th centuries, such cases were labelled 'conversion hysteria'.

Subsequently, the personality, rather than a single specific unconscious conflict, was proposed as a contributing factor to the development of ill health. Researchers such as Flanders Dunbar (1947) and Alexander (1943) argued that psychological conflicts produce anxiety and, over time, prompt associated physiological changes to take place via the autonomic nervous system. It was proposed, for example, that repressed anger associated with a frustrated need for love and attention increased the secretion of digestive acids that eroded the stomach lining and produced an ulcer.

The term **psychosomatic illness** was reserved for a few specific conditions (e.g. bronchial asthma, neurodermatitis and gastric ulcers) that were regarded as being caused by worry. Over time, other diseases were added to the list, including hypertension (high blood pressure) and arthritis. However, there was no genuine consensus about what constituted a psychosomatic illness.

Psychosomatic illness An outdated term reserved for a few specific conditions (e.g. bronchial asthma, neurodermatitis and gastric ulcers) that were regarded as being caused by worry.

Ideas proposed during the early psychosomatic movement are still popular today, despite widespread criticism (associated with the poor methodological rigour of earlier experiments and its applicability to a very restricted range of conditions). Medical advances have proven some of these earlier notions to be incorrect and further shaped our thinking. In contrast to psychosomatic models of the role of worry as the single cause in the development of gastric ulcers, for example, two Australians, Barry Marshall and Robin Warren, received the Nobel Prize in 2005 for their discovery that the *Helicobacter pylori* bacterium was the cause of most stomach ulcers and gastritis. This does not mean, however, that emotions such as worry play no part in the development or aggravation of ulcers. We now know that the onset of disease is associated with a variety of factors, including genetic predisposition, environmental factors, early learning experiences, current stressors, cognitions and coping strategies, all of which add to oxidative stress—a build-up of toxins that the body's protective systems can't overcome (Zeliger, 2016).

PAUSE & REFLECT

Some people are reluctant to accept that the mind and body interact in health and illness. Why do you think this might be the case? What arguments could you make for a more integrated approach?

Holism
A word derived from Greek, meaning entire or total.

Holism, or holistic health care, is a broad, integrating concept that takes into account cognitions, emotions, and social and spiritual awareness, in addition to traditional physical or biomedical knowledge. Holism attempts to bridge the gap between the physical and mental aspects of patients' suffering. In a health sense, it means that all the properties of health or illness cannot be explained by adding up each element. Complementary and alternative health practitioners have subscribed to this idea for hundreds of years and have sought to understand health and illness in the wider context of an individual's life (Russell, 2016).

This chapter explores interactions between the mind and body, with particular emphasis on the role of emotion and physiological functioning in health. We investigate the interplay between emotion and different areas of the brain, arousal states and cognitions, as well as factors influencing the expression of emotion. The chapter also discusses how poor regulation of emotion is linked to adverse mental and social consequences for individuals. We apply our understanding of psychology and physiology (psychophysiology) to cardiovascular conditions, cancer, mental illness and immune responses.

Emotion

Emotions
Positive or negative responses to external stimuli (situations, events, things and people) and/or internal mental representations (thoughts, dreams and ideas).

Emotions are such a common component of our experience that it is difficult to imagine life without them. Because an understanding of emotion is critical to an understanding of so many aspects of health and illness, the following section examines emotion in detail.

Emotion is an adaptive, goal-defining aspect of experience, associated with changes across multiple response systems (APA, 2021a). An emotion may, for example, influence decision-making, produce behaviour such as crying or smiling, and generate automatic bodily changes such as sweating or a pounding heart. Emotions can be natural (unlearnt) responses to stimuli that have affective (feeling-producing) properties, such as when an individual accidentally burns their hand on the stove and screams out in response to the pain. Emotions can also be learnt responses to stimuli that have personal value, such as feeling a surge of happiness when you see a loved one after time apart. As such, emotions involve multiple appraisal processes that judge or assess the significance of stimuli in terms of what it means to the individual, with responses modified accordingly.

10.1 CASE STUDY

MARTIN AND IRRITABLE BOWEL SYNDROME

This case study examines the experience of an individual with a physical problem that is closely linked with psychological experience.

Martin is a 17-year-old student completing Year 12. As the year has gone on, he has coped well with schoolwork by studying harder than ever, but has begun to experience a range of uncomfortable abdominal symptoms. Some days he will be constipated, but feel his bowels are full and bloated. He has sensations of nausea at times, while at others he just has rumblings in his stomach, accompanied by feelings of bloating and pressure. The following day, he is frequently awakened early in the morning by an urgent need to have a bowel movement, and when he does, he is likely to experience strong pain followed by a rush of diarrhoea. On these days, he tends to have additional attacks of diarrhoea all day—often he has to leave class to rush to the toilet. He also has a lot of wind on these days, which he finds very embarrassing.

1   What emotional experiences are likely to be linked to Martin's condition?

2   How do physical and mental factors interact in these emotions?

PHYSIOLOGY OF EMOTION

The physical side of our experience of emotion is basically under the control of the autonomic nervous system, which regulates the body's internal environment. The autonomic nervous system has two divisions: sympathetic and parasympathetic. The sympathetic division operates to promote energy expenditure when the body is under demand. This happens when, for example, we are startled or find ourselves in a dangerous situation. Sympathetic nervous system activation produces the 'fight or flight' response. Activation of the sympathetic division is associated with the experience of strong emotion. Characteristics of sympathetic nervous system activation are:

- increased heart rate, speeding delivery of oxygen and nutrients to skeletal muscle;

- deeper and more rapid breathing to increase available oxygen, with the pancreas secreting glucagons to increase sugar release into the bloodstream and to muscles;

- constriction of blood vessels leading to the gastrointestinal tract so as to shut down digestion, and dilation of blood vessels leading to muscles;

- secretion by adrenal glands of the hormone adrenaline to sustain a number of reactions, resulting in tremor (butterflies in stomach), dilation of pupils (increasing visual acuity), shutdown of salivary glands (causing dry mouth), increased sweating (better heat dissipation) and contraction of surface muscles (goosebumps).

In contrast, the parasympathetic division of the autonomic nervous system operates during relaxation to promote energy conservation. Once the emergency is over, the parasympathetic nervous system takes over to reduce energy loss and provide appropriate conditions for acquisition of energy (e.g. digestion).

The physiological responses described above are fairly easy to measure with electronic or chemical sensors, and many efforts have been made to try to understand emotion by studying physiology. Our understanding of emotional control entered a new phase with the advent of functional magnetic resonance imaging (fMRI) studies (Gu et al., 2019), which enabled higher mental processes in humans to be detected. Cognitive neuroscientists continue to investigate the 'hot' control of emotions as well as the 'cold' control of attention and memory. However, fMRI studies can only tell us part of the story. For example, we know that some individuals can manipulate the results of lie detector tests. The polygraph measures small changes in a number of physiological variables, such as heart rate and sweating, but people can change their test results by changing their thought patterns.

The influence of the brain and cognition on emotions is discussed in the next section.

EMOTION AND THE BRAIN

Vulnerability and capability are discussed in Chapter 4.

Emotional reactions may be most easily observed in the body's responses to sympathetic activation, but overall coordination of emotion is conducted by the brain, in particular the cortex, hypothalamus and limbic system, including the amygdala. Electrical stimulation of parts of the hypothalamus, for example, can lead to sympathetic activation and emotional behaviour (e.g. rage or terror) in laboratory animals.

The role of the limbic system in emotions, particularly violence, has raised the possibility that psychosurgery can alter behaviour, though the ethics of such operations are highly questionable. In laboratory studies with animals, destruction of tissue in a part of the limbic system called the amygdala produced docile behaviour. Any alterations to the brain tend to result in widespread behaviour effects and the use of psychosurgery in humans remains highly controversial.

Emotions are regulated by a range of cognitive processes that vary from attentional mechanisms (e.g. ignoring emotional stimuli and choosing to focus on something else) to cognitive change (e.g. reinterpreting the meaning of stimuli). When this happens, the behavioural and neural processes that normally accompany an emotion are also inhibited. It seems that paying less attention to emotional stimuli affects emotional appraisal systems in the amygdala, although research evidence on this is mixed. In terms of cognitive change strategies to control emotions, studies have shown that emotional appraisal is related to neural control systems in the cortex, and to cingulate control systems (LeDoux & Brown, 2017).

Some research has indicated that the dominant hemisphere of the brain is associated with positive emotions, while the non-dominant hemisphere involves negative ones (valence theory). Gainotti (2019) found that evidence from research on ageing supports the view that the non-dominant hemisphere is associated with all emotions. Clearly, the cortex plays a significant role in emotion.

AROUSAL AND EMOTION

Links between arousal and emotion are well recognised. James (1890) proposed that an exciting event leads to physical arousal, and our perception of this arousal is emotion. It was assumed that different emotions resulted from the perception of different patterns of arousal. This theory, elaborated by Lange and called the James–Lange theory, placed emphasis on arousal, which preceded the experience of emotion, determined the nature of the emotion experienced and, when it faded, led to the disappearance of the emotional experience.

Cannon (1932), in his critique of the James–Lange theory, proposed several limitations. He suggested the following.

1 Separation of the brain from sensations in the body (in the case of spinal lesions) did not eliminate emotional behaviour.

2 The same bodily changes appear to occur in response to a range of emotions, making it difficult to see how we could perceive one emotion over another.

3 There is a poor correlation between bodily changes and changes in emotional experience.

4 Bodily changes are fairly slow compared with the speed of emotional experience.

5 Artificial induction of bodily changes (e.g. by an injection of epinephrine [synthetic adrenaline]) does not produce emotion.

Although some of these criticisms, such as points two and four, have not been completely supported by subsequent research, the other points reveal crucial flaws in the James–Lange theory.

Cannon (1932) offered an alternative view of emotion, called activation theory (now known as the Cannon–Bard theory). This theory proposed that the perception of an exciting stimulus leads to disinhibition of the midbrain and results in a general sympathetic nervous system discharge, which produces the physiological arousal and experience of emotion. Unfortunately for Cannon, this theory did not actually meet all of his own criticisms of the James–Lange theory. First, measures of physiological arousal do not compare well with one another. The presentation of a stimulus, for example, may produce an increase in heart rate and a particular emotion, but a repeat presentation of the same stimulus may produce the same emotion but with a decrease in heart rate. Activation theory still does not explain why artificial induction of physiological arousal does not produce emotion. It also fails to explain the richness or variety of emotions we experience. It took another 30 years for the next step to be taken in unravelling the puzzle of emotion.

COGNITION AND EMOTION

Schachter (1964) proposed a two-factor theory of emotion. Although he agreed that arousal was basic to emotion, he proposed that cognitions about arousal are the other element on which emotions are based. For individuals to really experience emotion, they must have both a state of arousal and an appropriate set of cognitions that label the experience as emotional. This was demonstrated in a classic experiment by Schachter and Singer (1962), which is worth describing in detail. (It should be noted that this study involved deception of participants. It would almost certainly be regarded as unethical within our current understanding of the ethics of psychological research.)

Participants were male university students recruited to a study of 'the effects of vitamins on vision', which enabled the experimenter to give participants an injection without telling them either that the experiment concerned emotion, or that they might be receiving an injection of epinephrine. When participants arrived for the experiment, they were given a description of a fictitious vitamin compound called Suproxin, with which they were to be injected. They were given an injection of epinephrine and one of three sets of instructions. The 'Informed' participants were told, correctly, that the Suproxin might produce shaking of the hands, pounding of the heart, and a warm and flushed feeling. The 'Ignorant' participants were told nothing about side effects. To determine whether mentioning side effects alone might alter response, 'Misinformed' participants were told, incorrectly, that the Suproxin might produce numbness of the feet, itching and slight headache. As a control condition, a group of different participants was given a placebo (a saline injection) and either Informed or left Ignorant. It was expected that Informed participants would have a good explanation (the injection) for their experienced state and would not report emotion. The Ignorant and Misinformed participants would not have a good explanation for their experienced internal state, and so would begin looking for one. The researchers arranged to give them an emotional explanation.

Participants were placed in a waiting room with someone they were told was another participant in the vision experiment, but who was actually a stooge: a paid confederate of the researcher. This stooge then proceeded to act either euphorically or angrily. The results showed that physiological arousal was not sufficient to produce emotional experience.

1   The Informed group did not indicate feeling euphoric or angry, nor did they act as if they were. They showed that cognitions were not sufficient on their own to produce emotion.

2   The Placebo group reported little emotion in the presence of the stooge (although enough to suggest that the experience of receiving an injection was in itself arousing).

3   Both the Ignorant and, to an even greater extent, the Misinformed participants reported feeling either euphoric in the presence of a euphoric stooge or angry in the presence of an angry stooge, and proceeded to act emotionally as well.

Attribution theory of emotion
The idea that emotion results when physiological arousal and emotion-related cognitions about that arousal exist at the same time.

Schachter (1964) proposed that participants attributed their arousal to emotion in the presence of appropriate cognitions, which he called the **attribution theory of emotion**. Attribution theory suggests some interesting possibilities. It should be possible, for example, to begin an emotional experience with either physiological arousal and have emotional cognitions follow, or with appropriate cognitions and have arousal follow. The theory underlying this research was that arousal (excitation) from one source ought to be transferable to another emotion if appropriate cognitions were present. One study looked at athletes who had just finished exercising and had some residual physical arousal. If they were angered, they became angrier than when they did not have that residual arousal. This would suggest that arousal produced by another emotion, such as fear, might also transfer to anger. In line with this, studies of police officers found they were more likely to use weapons against both offenders and innocent bystanders when their arousal levels were high.

Another influential two-factor (physiological arousal plus cognitions) theory of emotion is Arnold's appraisal theory (1960). She proposed that it is not the events (situational or physical) that produce emotional responses, but the individual's appraisal of those events. Consider the effect of walking round a corner and coming face to face with a lion. An initial reaction might be a startled response, but before you experience a true emotional response you would be influenced by whether the lion was in a cage or out, whether it was alive or stuffed, and whether it was a picture or genuine. Genuine experience of emotion, therefore, depends on our appraisal of events: their meaning, their relationship to us as individuals, and our needs and wants.

PAUSE & REFLECT

What is the role of appraisal in the experience of emotion?
How could this explain why we like to watch things in movies that we would hate to watch in real life, such as a kind person dying slowly from disease?

The importance of appraisal regarding stress is considered again in Chapter 12.

Consider what your reaction would be to a film that showed a boy undergoing a tribal initiation rite that involved having the underside of his penis slit open. Lazarus and Alfert (1964) found that people who saw this as a silent film appraised it as real and reacted with high levels of arousal and expressed emotion. Others, who heard the soundtrack that told them that the film was staged using special effects and that the boy was not really being operated on or hurt, experienced much less physiological arousal in the face of the same scenes. Individuals who heard the soundtrack before they saw the film were even less aroused. Apparently, their appraisal had been completed before the events started, and could exert greater control over their responses. Thus, appraisal about what we might encounter in the future allows us to predict, and even exert control over, what we will experience when we encounter the expected events.

10.2 CASE STUDY

MARTIN (CONT.)

Emotions are likely to be both a cause and an outcome in Martin's condition. While it is not clear what might have caused Martin to develop this particular condition at this particular time, there are nervous system connections between the brain and the bowel. During times of strong emotion, sensory signals from the bowel may be interpreted differently by the brain, and signals from the brain may cause the bowel to squeeze more, leading to both pain and changes to bowel habits. Martin's symptoms are not constant—sometimes he will go for a week without a bad episode—but as the year progresses, the constipation and diarrhoea become more frequent. Martin makes an appointment to see his doctor. His doctor suspects that Martin has Irritable Bowel Syndrome (IBS). However, there is really no test that can diagnose IBS. The tests the doctor is running are to eliminate the possibility of conditions with similar symptoms, such as coeliac disease, Crohn's disease or intolerance of dairy products. In this case, all the tests indicate no other condition. When Martin learns about IBS from his doctor, he is not at all happy to hear that the cause of his problems is not clear, but much happier to learn that there are things that can be done to help him.

1 Is there any illness or disease that is not affected by emotional issues?
2 How does understanding and managing emotions affect the kind of illness that an individual may experience?

EXPRESSION OF EMOTION

The most widely studied medium of emotional communication is facial expression. Charles Darwin proposed that much of our facial communication is innate: the communication of emotions by facial expression has evolutionary value. By warning others of our intention to act in a particular way, we enable them to respond to an intention without the need for the act itself. A fearful expression may signal to friends that they should prepare for flight. An expression of sadness signals the need for support.

Similar expressions are universal; that is, found across all cultures. A study showed that New Guinea highlanders, who had experienced little contact with Westerners, were easily able to recognise and label emotional expressions on the faces of Westerners they encountered (Ekman, 1980). When asked to express the same emotions, they were able to display them in a way that was understood by Westerners. Other evidence for the generality of expression has come from studies of emotional expressions of infants.

In general, facial expressions play an important role in emotions. One small body of research suggests that socially anxious individuals show negative biases in interpreting the facial expressions of others. Anxious patients may interpret a facial expression as angry when in fact it is neutral. This finding suggests that helping patients to develop a more accurate interpretation of facial expressions could be a useful intervention in dealing with excess anxiety (Ferguson et al., 2021; Leleu et al., 2014).

EMOTION AND HEALTH

Emotion is a complex phenomenon. It involves internal state, mental activity, survival value and other physical and psychological elements, all of which can affect our health or our appraisal of our health, or can be affected by our health.

Being ill may arouse our emotional experience by creating internal biochemical conditions characteristic of emotion (e.g. increasing circulating adrenaline, or endorphins), by mimicking arousal (increasing heart rate, or sweating) or simply by producing negative cognitions. Such experiences are commonly recognised. Someone who is, say, overactive or irrational may be described as 'feverish'. This is not surprising, since very high temperatures can cause delirium. Diseases that depress the body's processes, such as the common cold or glandular fever, may make people feel emotionally flat or depressed. A number of physical illnesses are known to cause mood change: AIDS (Clucas et al., 2011) and cancer (Banks et al., 2010) are just two examples. Both COVID-19 (Pfefferbaum & North, 2020) and restrictions associated with it (Terry et al., 2020) have been shown to affect emotions. Similarly, drugs taken for physical conditions can produce or modify some of the physiological or mental characteristics of emotional states. It is known, for example, that treatment for hepatitis B can lead to depression, and that a class of drugs prescribed for hypertension (beta-blockers) are sometimes taken by musicians to reduce symptoms of stage fright without interfering with dexterity. The use of drug side effects to modify emotion or its consequences can, however, be quite dangerous.

In contrast, emotions may create sensations we interpret as illness. Consider the example of emergency workers at a major disaster. They may experience long periods of physiological arousal during the rescue. After the rescue, the threat is removed and they may expect to feel relieved, but because they have depleted bodily resources from the constant state of high alertness, they feel emotionally flat and physically unwell. Any prolonged stressful experience can produce similar effects. Conversely, happy experiences or the experience of support from those around us can lead to positive health outcomes. This might operate through facial feedback, biochemical means and many other pathways. There is clear and substantial evidence that links optimism, social support and even an aggressive fighting attitude with improved outcomes for various health situations such as recovery from surgery, response to infection and cancer (Corn et al., 2020). One study of over 1000 patients showed that hope (positive emotion) was associated with lower chances of developing disease (e.g. hypertension, diabetes or respiratory tract infection) and curiosity with lower likelihood of hypertension and diabetes (Smart Richman et al., 2005). Improvements of physical and mental health have also resulted from treatment aimed at increasing self-confidence, assertiveness and optimism.

REGULATION OF EMOTION AND MENTAL ILLNESS

Various aspects of emotion play a role in different mental disorders. Individuals suffering from a major depressive or anxiety disorder demonstrate difficulty managing their emotions. One variable of interest is overall emotionality, which involves feeling intense positive or negative emotions. In anxiety and depressive disorders, there may be low levels of positive emotion such as happiness and/or high levels of negative emotion such as fear and sadness. Intense emotions are not dysfunctional in themselves; it is the overall greater occurrence and strength that can render them pathological.

Another variable of interest is the **dysregulation of emotions** (poor management of emotions). Dysregulation involves three elements:

1 poor understanding or insight;

2 negative reactivity;

3 ineffective or maladaptive coping intelligence (APA, 2021a).

It is more difficult for individuals to regulate their emotions if they do not recognise or understand what they are feeling, or if they have negative reactions to what they are feeling. Such individuals may fear their emotions, or believe they are powerless to control their emotions. Poor coping or maladaptive management means not being able to take action to soothe anxiety, calm down anger or use other regulation strategies to control impulses. To a certain extent, emotional dysregulation is the opposite of emotional intelligence. It appears that emotional dysregulation is directly connected to mental health symptoms independent of our negative emotions; that is, symptoms are not just being reported because people feel bad (Deutz et al., 2020).

Emotions can also have an indirect influence on our mental well-being and daily functioning. Possessing an optimistic or pessimistic outlook on life, for example, affects our perception of the likelihood of a good outcome. It therefore alters the way we make decisions, the kind of risks we feel are worth taking and the amount of effort we will expend to achieve a certain goal. Emotion can also affect health-related behaviours such as drinking alcohol, smoking cigarettes, exercise, diet and even the way we drive our car.

> **Dysregulation of emotions**
> Poor understanding or insight, negative reactivity and ineffective or maladaptive coping intelligence.

> *Emotional intelligence is discussed in Chapter 2.*

10.3 CASE STUDY

MARTIN (CONT.)

The recommendations that Martin receives from his doctor are about treating his symptoms. For example, he is advised that he can add fibre to his diet if constipation is the main problem, and that there are over-the-counter medications to relieve constipation and reduce attacks of diarrhoea. To help him deal with the causes, he is also given lifestyle advice, such as avoiding caffeine (limiting coffee, tea and cola drinks), not eating large meals, and noting if there are any specific foods that trigger his attacks and then limiting those. However, as IBS tends to differ between individuals, the doctor tells Martin that the best general advice tends to revolve around psychophysiological triggers such as stress. Martin is advised that regular exercise and sleeping patterns—both the timing of sleep and the amount of sleep (at least eight hours per night)—are really important. Martin has been neglecting both exercise and sleep during Year 12 because he felt it was more important to spend his time studying. Importantly, Martin was also told that while IBS can be upsetting, it does not cause permanent damage to the intestines or lead to more serious disease.

1 How could the principles of behaviour change (see Chapter 8) benefit Martin?

2 How important is good time management to maintaining health during stressful periods of life?

Psychophysiology

Psychophysiology
The study of the interactions between the physiological and psychological aspects of a situation as experienced by an individual.

Psychophysiology enables us to better to understand individual experiences at both physiological and psychological levels. Often, they arise from the same underlying causes and occur together in response to the same stimuli. The combined response is important.

There are specific areas in which knowledge gained from psychophysiology has made an enormous difference to the way health and illnesses are considered, and subsequently the way in which health professionals assess and care for patients (Andreassi, 2006). These differences are primarily, but not exclusively, related to emotion. The following sections examine psychophysiology in regards to cardiovascular function, cancer and immune function.

CARDIOVASCULAR PSYCHOPHYSIOLOGY

Heart disease and stroke—diseases of the cardiovascular system—are two major causes of death. Though there is a traditional belief in the link between the heart and emotions, it appears that the heart is more a victim of emotions than the seat of emotions.

There are many studies of short-term physiological responses to behavioural demands that include physiological responses. These include changes in adrenaline and noradrenaline levels that affect cardiovascular function and alter heart rate, rhythm and electrical activity, blood pressure and cardiac output (how much blood is being pumped). People who, for example, are involved in a problem-solving task show faster heart rates and higher blood pressure when working under time pressure than when working at their preferred pace. Similarly, students display striking elevations of cortisol (a physiological measure of stress) when sitting a major exam (Jones et al., 1986) and in other stressful situations (Suh, 2018).

The type A behaviour pattern is also discussed in Chapter 4.

Long-term responses—including changes in blood pressure, heart rate and rhythm; cholesterol levels in the blood, blood coagulation and platelet aggregation; and adaptation patterns such as hyper-reactivity—have been noted in response to severe or prolonged stress. High stress periods at work are accompanied by increases in serum cholesterol, a risk factor for heart disease due to an increased likelihood of blocked arteries. Even minor stresses (hassles) that continue over a long time have been shown to result in relatively enduring changes in cardiovascular functioning. Other research has linked characteristics of the individual to heart disease. Sahoo et al. (2018) reviewed the literature and found strong and consistent evidence for links with depression, isolation and a lack of quality social support. There are established relationships with social factors such as education, social class and job type, but there is some debate about whether these differences might be related to lack of control or other psychosocial factors.

Type A (coronary prone) behaviour pattern
The idea that individuals who show a pattern of competitive achievement, an exaggerated sense of time urgency, and aggressiveness and hostility are at greatly increased risk of heart attack.

Research has attempted to link personality and heart disease, including seemingly stable personality characteristics such as anger or hostility, competitiveness, stoicism or optimism. The **type A (coronary prone) behaviour pattern** was proposed as an independent risk factor for heart disease as far back as the 1950s, but there has been much criticism of the complexity of the concept, and little research to support it in more recent times. However, a tendency to become angry often, particularly if that anger is directed at the self, has been predictive of clinical events such as a heart attack (Chida & Steptoe, 2009). It is likely, though, that these relationships are mediated by arousal changes over a long period of time and the physiological effects of arousal damage on the body.

The **type D (distressed) personality** is an emerging construct to help explain links between behaviour and disease. Individuals with type D personality have a tendency to feel negative emotions (e.g. depression and anxiety) combined with a reluctance to discuss these feelings with others (negative affectivity combined with social inhibition) to avoid social disapproval (Smith et al., 2018). A man may, for example, feel anxious or depressed about a lack of meaningful satisfaction in his highly paid position, but deliberately choose not to tell his wife, friends or work colleagues about it. Mols and Denollet (2010) reported that type D represents a general vulnerability for both mental and physical health.

A similar concept, alexithymia, has received a lot of attention in relation to health, but it is not clear how much overlap there is with type D (Epifanio et al., 2018). The likely conclusion is that experiencing negative emotion with difficulty in expressing those emotions is a health risk.

Some studies have examined life events as causes of acute cardiovascular events. There is an apparent link between bereavement and death from pre-existing heart problems. For many people, the most likely time for death from heart attack is Monday morning—the beginning of the work week. An interesting line of research has shown that deaths from all causes are lower than expected in the month before important events such as birthdays and anniversaries, and higher than expected in the month following them. Again, such results could possibly be explained by short-term physiological responses.

Depression worsens the risks and outcomes for a wide variety of health conditions (Stubbs et al., 2017). After taking other risk factors into account, depression is an independent risk factor for heart disease (Glozier et al., 2013; Ai & Caretta, 2021). Linking disease-specific physical symptoms with a patient's underlying depression and anxiety may avoid unnecessary treatment. A patient with a cardiovascular condition, say, may have continuing chest pain due to anxiety rather than the physical symptoms caused by the condition. In response to the reported symptoms, health care providers may escalate the cardiovascular disease medication regime and order more invasive tests, without realising that anxiety may be a contributing cause (Katon et al., 2007).

Type D (distressed) personality
A tendency to feel negative emotions combined with a reluctance to discuss those feelings with others, that increases the probability of disease.

PAUSE & REFLECT

As a future health professional, how might you distinguish between disease-specific physical symptoms and those engendered by emotion?

CANCER PSYCHOPHYSIOLOGY

Some researchers proposed a **type C (cancer prone) behaviour pattern** linked to cancer (Eskelinen & Ollonen, 2011). Although several studies have shown that a passive and emotionally repressed personality style is associated with higher rates of occurrence and death from cancer, serious questions exist about type C research. It is likely that passivity and emotional repression come with, or after, a diagnosis of cancer. These traits are just as likely to be the result of the diagnosis as to be present before diagnosis. Other studies have shown that a passive coping style can lead to shorter survival times for cancer patients, while an aggressive coping style is associated with longer survival. How much this has to do with behavioural differences—such as aggressive patients getting more or better care

Type C (cancer prone) behaviour pattern
The idea that a passive and emotionally repressed personality style is associated with higher rates of cancer occurrence and death from cancer.

as a result of demanding it, while passive patients ignore symptoms until it is too late—is not clear. The idea that psychological factors can cause cancer is not well supported by the research, but in some cases such factors can be related to differences in cancer survival rates, or how distressing the experience is for individuals (Aschwanden et al., 2019). Exactly how to conceptualise type C to make it more useful for research and intervention is still under discussion (Rymarczyk et al., 2020).

PSYCHONEUROIMMUNOLOGY

Psychoneuroimmunology
The study of communications between the brain and the immune system.

Psychoneuroimmunology (PNI) is concerned with communication between the brain and immune system (Segerstrom, 2012). At first, the idea that there was crosstalk between the brain and the immune system was rejected by many immunologists, who regarded the immune system as autonomous. It is now known not only that people are more susceptible to infections and other illness at times of stress, but also that stress measurably alters immune functioning.

Molecular and cellular systems in the brain are geared to represent dangers occurring in various parts of the body monitored by the immune system. The immune system provides immediate and short-term defence against infectious agents in the blood and body tissues. When pathogens trigger the immune system, **cytokines** are produced.

Cytokines
A group of proteins and peptides that work as signalling compounds, enabling cells to communicate with each other; they regulate the body's response to infection, inflammation and trauma.

Pro-inflammatory cytokines fight disease by producing fever, inflammation and tissue destruction, and eliciting behaviours such as nausea and tiredness as well as symptoms of depression, requiring the person to rest. Anti-inflammatory cytokines have healing effects. Stress in patients predicts a range of adverse clinical outcomes, such as slower wound healing, lower production of antibodies to flu vaccine, and more rapid progression of immune disorders (Segerstrom, 2010; Kany et al., 2019).

On the other hand, positive emotions have also been shown to have a variety of health benefits (Kok et al., 2013). Positive emotions may improve immune function, and psychological interventions of various sorts have been shown to lessen the risk of infection, reduce the need for antibiotic treatment and even double survival times in individuals with cancer. Interestingly, laughter is linked to immune function, with a number of reports showing reduction in clinical symptoms and improvement in immune markers in a variety of conditions (Park et al., 2016). These health consequences of prolonged stress and ways of coping with the consequences are discussed in more detail in following chapters.

PAUSE & REFLECT

Think about how the mind communicates with the immune system.

What are the implications of this in terms of strong or prolonged emotion and the risk of disease?

10.4 CASE STUDY

SIXUE AND ANXIETY

Sixue is a 37-year-old mother of three children. As long as she can remember, she has had problems with anxiety. At school, she used to feel sick to the stomach, sweaty and trembling any time that she had to speak in class. During recess periods, she tended to stay on the edge of play—sitting with one or two friends and talking rather than actively being involved in games. She came to feel that she was awkward and unskilled, and finally asked her parents to have her excused from physical education on medical grounds: that she was prone to palpitations, shortness of breath and headaches if required to exercise. Outside of school, however, she was quite active. Since she lived on the edge of a small rural town, she could easily ride her bicycle into the countryside, and enjoyed the experience of hard physical exercise. Although she was very shy in class, she studied hard and did very well. It was only speaking in class that caused her problems. She knew she was smart and hard-working, but also thought that there was something wrong with her body or her mind because she always felt so frightened in social situations.

She found puberty very difficult because she experienced bodily changes later than most of the girls in her class. She felt like a child around the more physically developed girls, and this contributed to her being embarrassed in classroom situations. Even though there were less-developed girls and she caught up with most of the others a year later, she continued to feel immature and out of things. Her anxiety became worse in social situations outside of school, and she became more of a loner.

During high school, she became interested in how the brain and body worked, and did extremely well in science subjects. She began to see that there were some patterns to her own anxiety. First of all, a lot of her relatives, including her parents, had problems with anxiety or depression. One of her uncles drank heavily and was unable to keep a job. Sixue realised that he was not bad, but that he drank to deal with his anxiety. Although nobody in the family talked about anxiety, there were a number of other signs that it was a problem for many of her family members. Her younger sister, two years her junior, became depressed during high school. The sister was placed on antidepressant medication and started to see a counsellor. Sixue considered seeing someone about her own anxiety, but did not do so because she thought she should be able to handle things by herself. She thought that being smart and physically fit should give her enough resources to handle things.

Because her high school required her to do some kind of sport, she took up tennis, worked hard at it and became quite skilled. However, she became very anxious before any kind of competition, so she never did well in those. It became common for her to be physically sick before any competition, and while playing she would feel dizzy and uncoordinated. However, she met a boy who, like her, enjoyed playing tennis but not competing. After more than a year of being friends, they started dating—not so much because they were strongly attracted to one another, but just to have someone to be with in social situations.

During university, her anxiety problems became somewhat worse, and she missed a lot of lectures because of anxiety attacks. Her boyfriend had chosen the same university and they were doing the same science subjects, so he helped her with notes and they worked together at studying and assignments. Even though she had a lot of trouble at exam time—she always seemed to catch cold or injure herself, and would be sick before and sometimes during tests—she completed her degree.

Sixue felt very relieved when her boyfriend asked her to marry him, as that took the pressure off her to work full-time. They decided to postpone having children until they could set themselves up financially, and she took a job working in a laboratory for a pharmaceutical company. It was very routine work and didn't pay much but it allowed her to work on her own, and the company was understanding about her frequent sick days.

As soon as Sixue fell pregnant, she stopped work and began to spend almost all of her time at home. She took a lot of pride in keeping her house clean and in preparing meals for her husband, but hated entertaining because it made her feel shaky and unwell. Gradually, they stopped socialising with other people.

After the birth of Sixue's third child, her doctor suggested that she might be suffering from an anxiety disorder, and referred her to a psychiatrist. Sixue has begun taking medication to limit the physiological symptoms, and is seeing a psychologist to help her with the psychological and social impacts.

1   What genetic, biological and social factors might have contributed to Sixue's family being subject to anxiety problems?

2   How did Sixue's cognitions about her physiological states during her school years contribute to her emotional difficulties in young adulthood?

3   What were some of the interactions between her emotions and her choices about her lifestyle?

Points to consider

Social phobias are the most common type of phobia; many people suffer to a greater or lesser degree from anxiety related to social situations. This can range from mild nervousness in stressful interactions—something we all experience—to inability to leave home under any conditions. People with extreme social phobias are often undiagnosed, partly because they don't leave home and so are not observed by other people. This can make the process of treatment difficult, as patients often miss appointments or find excuses to avoid seeking treatment at all.

CHAPTER SUMMARY

Learn more
Access additional resources to broaden your understanding of this chapter. See the Guided Tour for access details.

- The separation of mind and body in Western philosophy has affected our thinking about health, how illness arises and approaches to treatment.

- A more integrated view has highlighted the importance of emotion to health and well-being. Emotion results from the combination of physiological arousal and emotion-relevant cognition.

- The appraisal that the individual makes of their situation determines what, and how much, emotion they will experience. The close integration of physiological and psychological factors in health has led to a large body of research linking the two.

- Cardiovascular psychophysiology looks at interactions between psychological events and the workings of the heart and circulation. The psychophysiology of cancer is less researched, but significant links have been found with occurrence and progression of cancer.

- Psychoneuroimmunology examines the connections between psychological experience, the operations of the nervous system and immune functioning. The integration of physiological and psychological factors provides a background for the understanding of stress and coping.

- It is now recognised that emotional health is relevant to maintaining good physical health and to recovering from physical illness. Emotional health also enhances an individual's capacity to lead a fulfilling life, study, work, pursue leisure interests and optimise day-to-day functioning.

- Disturbances to emotional well-being, such as anxiety and depression, compromise these capacities, often in debilitating and ongoing ways.

- Conceptualising health and illness in a holistic way has produced different approaches to understanding, assessing and treating illness.

FURTHER READING

Danese A, Lewis SJ (2017) Psychoneuroimmunology of early-life stress: The hidden wounds of childhood trauma? *Neuropsychopharmacology* 42, 99–114. https://doi.org/10.1038/npp.2016.198

Kautz M (2021) Applications of psychoneuroimmunology models of toxic stress in prevention and intervention efforts across early development. *Brain, Behavior & Immunity – Health*, 16, 100322. https://doi.org/10.1016/j.bbih.2021.100322

Lutgendorf SK & Costanzo ES (2003) Psychoneuroimmunology and health psychology: An integrative model (invited review). *Brain, Behavior and Immunity – Health*, 17, 225–32.

Schachter S (1964) The interaction of cognitive and physiological determinants of emotional state. In L Berkowitz (Ed.) *Advances in Experimental Social Psychology* (vol. 1, pp. 49–80). Academic Press.

11 A Complex Example: Understanding Pain

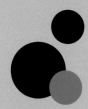

A broader understanding of pain

We live with minor pain all the time; indeed, low-level pain is critical to our survival. Low-level pain provides feedback about the functioning of our bodily systems and informs the unconscious adjustments we make to our posture and body position. An extremely small number of individuals are born with insensitivity to pain, which is known as congenital analgesia (Mouraux & Iannetti, 2018). Not only are they at risk from accidents but they may also unknowingly damage themselves through an inability to recognise when they are hurt. Pain that is more intense gains our attention but is usually acute and the experience disappears in hours, days or weeks. Other forms of pain may persist for several months, worsen over time and become chronic. Pain is the most common reason why people seek medical care. The Cochrane Pain, Palliative and Supportive Care Group (CPPSCG, 2021) for example, lists 713 systematic reviews on pain management on its website. Interestingly, the prospect of uncontrolled pain is an aspect of illness that is feared by individuals at end of life (Seow et al., 2021).

It is usually assumed that pain arises in predictable and measurable ways from tissue damage, but attempts to determine a precise relationship between the extent of tissue damage and pain have been only partly successful. Further, many people experience pain in the absence of any observable physical damage. There is no evidence that pain without physical damage (psychogenic) or unclear origin (idiopathic) is any less real to the sufferer than pain with associated tissue damage (organic).

Unfortunately, some health professionals may make assumptions about a person with pain symptoms. If a physical cause (e.g. a bulging disc, arthritic condition of the spine or neuropathy) cannot be found for the pain, there is an overwhelming tendency to assign psychological causes (Lee et al., 2020). This judgment leads to treating people with psychogenic pain differently from those with organic pain, particularly when the pain is reported to persist over a long period of time. Judgments by health professionals may result in not providing narcotic medication for someone complaining of migraine pain, for example—a decision that could be medically and ethically unsafe.

Given the propensity of health professionals to misjudge the pain experience, it is essential for you to develop a good understanding of this issue. This chapter explores how pain is reported or expressed, the physiology and neurochemical basis of pain, and how the body works to inhibit perceptions of pain. Psychological factors that increase pain sensations (e.g. anxiety, stress, depression and focusing attention on the pain) are discussed, along with recent developments in pain control and management of chronic pain.

The interplay of physical symptoms and emotion is discussed in Chapter 10.

11.1 CASE STUDY

AZEM AND AMPUTATION

Azem is a 44-year-old motor mechanic who loves riding his motorcycle. He belongs to a recreational motorcycle club, where he enjoys the social side as well as hands-on maintenance and design of motorcycles. He recently built his own model of motorcycle, specifically designed to be comfortable for him personally on long rides.

Sadly, as a result of a serious accident in which he was speeding and lost control on a slippery road surface and slid underneath a car, he had his right leg amputated just above the knee. All of his other injuries were minor, and after being fitted with an artificial limb he was able to return to his normal work and family commitments. However, the loss of his leg meant that he could no longer safely ride a motorcycle.

Azem's reactions are on several levels: physical (immediate severe pain), behavioural (changes to his lifestyle), cognitive and emotional. He experiences many and varied emotions, which are to some extent dependent on his cognitions about his loss. As he realises that his careless riding was responsible for the loss of his leg, he directs his anger inward. Frequently, he feels churned up about the unfairness of his situation, but he also feels guilty and stupid. He can't blame the driver of the car but wishes he could, because this would give him a direct target for his anger.

1   What factors would determine the severity and nature of Azem's pain?
2   How would being able to blame someone else make Azem feel differently about his pain?

Reporting pain

Pain is fundamentally a psychophysiological experience. The International Association for the Study of Pain (IASP, 2020) defines pain as "an unpleasant sensory and emotional experience associated with, or resembling that associated with, actual or potential tissue damage". The IASP emphasises that "pain is always subjective". This means that it is internal to the specific individual and cannot be linked to external judgments about what is causing it, how bad it is or what it feels like. The extent of pain and level of incapacity caused by pain in daily life depend in large part on how it is interpreted and the context in which in occurs (Sonneborn & Williams, 2020). Natural labour and childbirth, for example, are associated with a great deal of physical pain and yet women are often able to cope without analgesia because of the release of natural endorphins, the joy attached to the experience, knowledge that it is acute and will be of (relatively) short duration, and the support offered by others. Similarly, some players in contact sports such as football codes have diminished pain sensitivity and continue playing a game despite grievous injuries. These joyful or challenging contexts differ from those of an office worker who is under stress to meet a deadline and suffering lower back pain. In this situation, stress aggravates the experience of pain, narrows the individual's focus and intensifies the pain experience.

Pain is an imprecise science, which means there are challenges associated with providing an accurate description of it. There are many common words used to describe pain—words and terms that can be a useful source of information for health professionals attempting to understand the complaint. The nature of pain may be described as throbbing, shooting or a constant dull ache. It is important, too, to determine the intensity of pain. This is often achieved by asking the person to describe their pain on a scale of 0 (no pain) to 10 (worst pain imaginable). When assessing pain in young children, simple diagrams of the body can be used to locate the pain and line drawings of faces showing different expressions can be used to rate pain intensity. There are also verbal scales for assessing pain, the emotions produced by pain, and a number of other pain-associated dimensions (Jaaniste et al., 2021).

Pain can also be conveyed by observing behaviour. People demonstrate pain through facial expressions or groans, by protecting the tender area, or by limiting movement that may provoke pain. When pain has persisted for some time (e.g. in the case of lower back pain), people change the way they stand or walk. Observation and analysis of physiological, psychological and behavioural elements of pain behaviour are important to define the characteristics of different kinds of pain.

Part of the complexity of measuring pain is simply due to differences in what the individual perceives as being the most important *to them*. Often this importance is tied to the impact on their own life: the losses they experience as a result of their pain. These usually include thoughts about what their pain prevents them from doing. This could include social activities, sports and leisure, work and employment, self-care and day-to-day living, but also the meaning of these activities for the individual. Chronic pain might mean loss of enjoyment, social networks or a sense of self-worth. It may also mean the occurrence of emotional distress such as depression, frustration, anger, anxiety or fear. If the individual's pain requires them to use a visible support (e.g. walking stick or frame) or noticeable supports (e.g. pain-relieving medications that may cause sleepiness, inability to operate machinery, unusual amounts of resting), the individual may experience **stigma** from others about their disability. In many senses, chronic pain shares these characteristics with other chronic conditions (see Chapter 5).

Stigma
A mark of disapproval that may be attached to an individual who differs from social or cultural norms.

PAUSE & REFLECT

Think about the worst pain you have experienced, and what caused it.

What words would you use to describe that pain?

How did the experience differ from pain generated by other causes?

Factors affecting the experience and reporting of pain

The reporting of pain is influenced by many factors, such as age, gender, context, attention, fatigue, previous experience of pain, and coping style (Boring et al., 2021). Of particular importance to the delivery of effective health care to our diverse communities is an understanding of how culture can influence differences in the meaning attached to pain and how it is experienced and expressed. Although there are no racial differences in the ability to discriminate painful stimuli, **culture** may influence pain tolerance and how intensely pain is reported. Culture also influences the extent to which it is appropriate (or inappropriate) to express pain. Failure to groan, cry out, grimace or thrash does not mean that the person is pain-free; it may reflect cultural values. People from different cultures who have difficulty speaking and understanding English report miscommunication and a lack of information sharing by health professionals. A systematic review (Santos-Salas et al., 2016) of cancer sufferers from different ethnic minority groups reported that, compared with standard information on controlling pain, individualised education and coaching increased knowledge of pain self-management, redressed personal misconceptions about pain treatment and reduced racial or ethnic disparities in pain control.

Culture
The way of life and beliefs shared by members of a group.

Individuals may be reluctant to ask for pain relief for different reasons. As identified by Santos-Salas et al. (2016), individuals from culturally and linguistically diverse backgrounds may have difficulty communicating their needs. Some may not know the options available to them for pain relief, and so attempt to tolerate the pain or suffer in silence. People from some Asian cultures may place the needs of others before their own, believe that the needs of others are more important, or not wish to disturb the person in authority (i.e. the doctor or nurse) by making a request for pain relief. Some people may hold strong views about their innate ability to cope without pain-relieving drugs. Others may be afraid to take drugs because of adverse side effects or a fear of becoming dependent on medication.

Physiology of acute pain

Nociceptors
Nerve endings in the peripheral nerves that identify injury and release chemical messengers that pass to the spinal cord and into the cerebral cortex.

Acute pain sensations generally arise when injured tissues release chemicals that activate nerve endings called **nociceptors** to send pain signals through the spinal cord to the brain. The cerebral cortex identifies the site of injury and acts to block the pain (muscle contractions) or change bodily functions (e.g. blood flow or breathing).

There are three kinds of stimuli that can activate pain perception: mechanical (tissue damage), thermal (exposure to temperature) and polymodal (which triggers chemical reactions from tissue damage). Two major types of peripheral nerve fibres are involved in nociception. A-delta fibres are small, myelinated fibres that transmit sharp pain in response to mechanical or thermal pain. C-fibres are unmyelinated nerve fibres involved in multimodal pain that transmit dull or aching pain. Myelination increases the speed of transmission, so sudden and intense pain is rapidly conducted to the cerebral cortex. The difference in conduction speed explains why pain seems to occur in two distinct waves. A painful stimulus first causes a sharp localised pain, followed by a dull diffuse pain.

Sensory aspects of pain are determined by A-delta fibre activity in the thalamus and sensory areas of the cerebral cortex. The motivational and affective elements of pain are influenced more strongly by C-fibres. Processes in the cerebral cortex are involved in cognitive judgments about pain, such as the evaluation of its meaning. Pain sensation, intensity and duration interact to influence pain perception, its negative consequences and related emotions through a central network of pathways in the limbic structures and thalamus to the cortex. The affective dimension of pain (or secondary affect) relates to feelings of unpleasantness, negative emotions and concern for the future (Yam et al., 2018).

Gate-control theory
The idea that that the brain controls the experience of pain by influencing the amount of pain stimulation that is allowed to pass a sensory gate at the level of the spinal cord.

An important advance in our understanding of pain resulted from the **gate-control theory** of Melzack and Wall (2003). This theory proposed that the brain exerts 'downward' control over the experience of pain by influencing the amount of pain stimulation that is allowed to pass a sensory 'gate' at the level of the spinal cord. The amount of pain experienced by the individual is related to the amount of information that gets through the gate to the brain.

This, in turn, depends on:

- the amount of activity in the peripheral pain fibres (i.e. where the pain starts);
- the amount of activity in other peripheral fibres (that carry non-pain information and may compete with pain information to get through the gate);
- messages coming from the brain.

This theory helps to explain why pain experiences can vary according to the physical, emotional or mental conditions at a given time. Inappropriate physical activity, anxiety or boredom could open the gate, while medication, relaxation and interesting life events could close it. This theory is supported by continuing evidence that the brain exerts downward control over other sensory information as well (Sandweiss, 2019). Paying close attention to only one kind of input inhibits the reception of other kinds of input.

11.2 CASE STUDY

AZEM (CONT.)

As well as the immediate damage to tissue and nerves, Azem has experienced a sense of loss after his accident. He was initially very depressed by the amputation, and retreated into social isolation. He lives alone, and felt less embarrassed and different if he was by himself. To make matters worse, Azem feels pain and itching in the missing foot. He finds this very distressing, especially as it is genuinely an itch he can't scratch. His doctor explains the experience to him. Some of the long nerve cells in Azem's leg were damaged, but not destroyed, by the amputation. These nerves formerly carried information from the foot and lower leg to the brain via the spinal cord, and input from these cells are still being interpreted by Azem's brain as coming from the foot. Some of these signals are pain signals, so, as far as Azem's brain is concerned, he has pain in the foot. This phenomenon is known as phantom pain.

Much depends on how Azem experiences pain in the short and long term. Loss of activities, and negative emotions associated with loss, may lead Azem to focus attention on his bodily sensations. Even boredom is associated with increased awareness of, and sensitivity to, pain.

1   What kinds of experiences might change Azem's pain experience, including his phantom pain?
2   How could the concept of self-efficacy help in understanding how Azem feels about the loss of his leg and his pain?

Neurochemical basis of acute pain

Pain motivates us to take quick action to relieve an injury. As discussed, the brain can control the amount of pain experienced by blocking transmission of pain signals. A landmark study by Reynolds (1969) pursued a different line of thinking and demonstrated that electrical stimulation in a rat brain produced such a high level of analgesia that abdominal surgery could be performed on the animal without anaesthetic. Akil et al. (1984) discovered that the neurochemical basis for this effect was related to **endogenous opioid peptides**. These peptides, known as endorphins, are a group of amino acids that function as neurotransmitters that suppress pain when they are released.

Opiates (e.g. morphine and heroin) are plant-based drugs that help control pain. Endogenous opioid peptides are opiate-like substances produced by the body as part of its internal pain regulation system. There are several forms of opioid peptides, such as beta-

Endogenous opioid peptides
Opiate-like neurochemical substances, produced in the body, that act as an internal pain regulation system.

endorphins, which vary in potency, receptive action and other characteristics. Endogenous opioid peptides are found in the adrenal glands, pituitary gland and hypothalamus, and are released in response to stress. Opioids, which have a powerful analgesic effect, are used to treat chronic pain.

Unfortunately, opioids have several serious drawbacks. In the short term, they cause drowsiness, interfere with mental function and cause changes to other bodily processes (e.g. constipation). If used for any length of time, opioids are physically addictive and produce psychological dependence. Their use needs to be carefully considered, and detailed guidelines have been issued by pain experts to guide clinical practice (Wyse et al., 2019).

Since 2010, prescriptions for opioids in Australia have increased from 10 million to 14 million every year (TGA, 2019). One of the main factors contributing to increased usage is their prescription for chronic non-cancer pain, despite limited evidence of the safety or effectiveness of opioids for many patients. Opioids also produce an increased sensitivity to pain, so that over time greater amounts are needed to achieve the same effect (James & Jowza, 2019) (see Chapter 8 for discussion of opponent–process theory). They also play a role in depressing immune functioning and cardiovascular control, but we are yet to understand their full function.

Psychological responses

Acute pain
Pain that is more intense and gains the individual's immediate attention, but usually disappears within hours, days or weeks.

Chronic pain, in comparison to **acute pain**, involves complex interactions between physiological, psychological, social and behavioural components. Chronic pain interferes with activities of daily living and persists despite the best efforts of the individual to control it. A systematic review of 30 randomised controlled trials identified that depression and anxiety were common among chronic pain sufferers (Jandaghi et al., 2020).

Depression reflects the feelings of despair that often accompany chronic pain. When pain persists for a long time, depressed pain patients are more likely to be preoccupied with the pain, believe that the pain will never stop and, indeed, will get worse (Jandaghi et al., 2020). Maladaptive coping strategies such as catastrophising or wishful thinking about the condition can magnify the distress, complicate treatment and contribute to illness behaviour. Chronic pain requires individualised, multiple techniques for its management.

Illness behaviour is discussed in Chapter 4.

When an individual experiences pain over a lengthy period of time, it is not uncommon for some fairly dramatic behavioural changes to occur (see Chapter 4). These include protecting the injury site out of fear of aggravating the pain, using medication (painkillers), feeling unhappy and helpless, and complaining about the pain. All these behaviours are predictable in the short term but may become habitual, leading to a subtype of abnormal illness behaviour called **persistent (chronic) pain syndrome** (Addison, 1984). Peck (1982) defined four traps in this syndrome: the "Take it Easy Trap", "Medication Trap", "Depression Trap" and "Complaint–Resentment–Guilt Trap". Back pain sufferers are urged to avoid the first of these by increasing their levels of activity. Medication can be a serious problem for sufferers of long-term pain because the drugs used are either addictive (e.g. opioids) or have other serious side effects. Depression needs to be managed as a psychological illness, whether it occurs in reaction to an obvious loss or without a visible cause. Complaining is a natural behaviour when an individual is in pain but it can develop into a habit, which causes resentment in others if it goes on too long. This, in turn, can lead to others feeling guilty for not being supportive. It can also lead the complaining individual to feel guilty about

Persistent (chronic) pain syndrome
A subtype of abnormal illness behaviour that can occur if an individual experiences pain over a lengthy period of time.

the burden they place on those around them. These characteristic traps of persistent pain syndrome may produce secondary gains and exacerbate the behaviour. The individual may be excused from normal duties and responsibilities, receive drugs, and be served by family and/or professionals.

The process of learning to cope with persistent pain involves a wide range of behavioural techniques, not just medication. Perhaps the most basic of these is simply the provision of information about pain. If the pain is understood only in terms of tissue damage, then logic suggests that rest, avoidance of activity and pursuit of healing are the only appropriate responses. Over an extended time, the similarity of this list of suggestions to the persistent pain syndrome should be obvious. Alternative ways of thinking about pain are required. These are frequently based on the idea of accepting chronic pain and responding to it as a changed (but not sinister or dangerous) condition (Thompson et al., 2020). Control of the pain—that is, learning ways to live with it instead of chasing ways to get rid of it—then becomes possible.

11.3 CASE STUDY

AZEM (CONT.)

Azem has experienced an initial period of time when he feels overwhelmed by his pain and loss. His doctor is concerned that he may be developing persistent pain syndrome. However, Azem finds that the phantom pain in his right foot is less severe after he is fitted with a prosthesis (artificial leg). About the same time, some members of his motorcycle club decide to seek him out. They drop by his house to talk, and specifically to ask for his advice about design issues. Azem gradually becomes interested in design and returns to the club for meetings; however, he still remains very unhappy about his inability to ride. One of his friends offers to take him for a ride as a passenger, and after the ride Azem reports to the doctor that his pain has reduced. He designs and builds a motorcycle which doesn't require the use of a right foot, and rides it everywhere.

The provision of a prosthesis for his leg and a new motorbike have enabled Azem to regain something approaching his former image of himself, as well as recover favoured activities and friends who may have drifted away while he was not able to walk or ride. These changes have enabled him to experience more positive emotion and less negative emotion. The result is an improvement not only in his mental health but also in his acceptance of and adaptation to any residual pain.

1   What is the difference between tolerating pain and accepting pain?
2   How do theories of grieving (see Chapter 3) help in understanding a loss of function such as Azem's loss of his leg?

Pain control techniques

This section briefly introduces several **pain control** techniques (Flynn, 2020; Jensen et al., 2020). Controlling pain can mean different things. Treatment could result in the person no

Pain control
The ability to reduce the experience of pain, report of pain, emotional concern about pain, inability to tolerate pain or presence of pain-related behaviours.

longer feeling anything in the injured area (e.g. by inserting drugs into the spinal cord to block sensation), feeling sensation but not pain (e.g. through sensory control techniques), feeling pain but not being concerned by it, or still feeling pain but being able to cope with it.

The most common form of pain control is through drugs that affect neural transmissions locally, to the spinal cord, or to higher brain regions. Antidepressants, for example, aim to improve mood and reduce anxiety, but also affect the downward pathways from the brain that modulate pain. Medication is usually sufficient and successful in managing acute pain, but may not be effective in the longer term.

PAUSE & REFLECT

Cancer pain management guidelines are concerned that pain may be undertreated by health professionals because of fear of addiction.

If fears of addiction are emerging, how can health professionals monitor a patient's response to pain and intervene?

Biofeedback
The control of internal processes through conditioning, using mechanical devices to make those internal processes perceptible.

Biofeedback training provides biophysiological information to a person about a bodily process such as heart rate or blood pressure. The bodily function is tracked by a machine and converted to a tone. While listening to the tone, the individual is taught how to modify the function through techniques such as concentration, relaxation and slow breathing. Eventually, some individuals can become proficient at slowing their heart rate or increasing circulation in an area without feedback from the machine (Moss, 2020). There is growing evidence on the effectiveness of biofeedback techniques, even though the specific method of action is unclear. It could be, for example, that effects are largely a result of relaxation, enhanced self-control or a placebo effect rather than the biofeedback technique per se.

Relaxation
Placing the body into a low state of arousal by progressively relaxing sections of the body and taking deeper and longer breaths.

Relaxation training is widely used. It enables individuals to put their body into a low state of arousal by progressively relaxing sections of the body and taking deeper and longer breaths. Such techniques are very useful during labour and childbirth. Similarly, meditation can be used to achieve relaxation by focusing attention on a simple and unchanging stimulus. Relaxation is relatively successful in cases of acute pain and can be useful in managing chronic pain in conjunction with other treatment.

Hypnosis
A deep, trance-like state of relaxation.

Hypnosis requires the person to enter a deep state of relaxation. Once in a trance-like state, the individual is told that their pain will reduce and is instructed to think differently about the pain (altering the meaning attached to the pain). The exact mechanism by which hypnosis works is unclear, but several studies have used it successfully for pain associated with different injuries, illnesses and conditions.

PAUSE & REFLECT

Many case studies and several controlled clinical trials have indicated the effectiveness of hypnotherapy for some medical conditions; however, because of the inadequacy of some research designs, hypnotherapy, like many complementary therapies, is still criticised for not having strong scientific evidence to support its claims.

Would you recommend hypnotherapy to pain sufferers? Why or why not?

Behavioural activation

An increasingly common approach focuses on behavioural activation; that is, getting the individual to gradually return to 'lost' activities that produce enjoyment. As the enjoyable activities are regained, the individual often discovers that pain doesn't increase, and that gains in enjoyment and function are worth the costs of pain (Lorenzo-Luaces & Dobson, 2019).

Pacing is an approach that aims to achieve specific staged goals of behavioural activation. It has a considerable appeal to individuals with chronic pain due to osteoarthritis (Wantonoro, 2020). Pacing enables goals to be perceived as sensible and achievable. However, pacing is really more of a cognitive perspective than a single method, and therefore evidence for pacing per se is difficult to separate from other associated interventions.

Pain management programs primarily address concerns associated with chronic pain. These programs include many of the techniques outlined previously, with a heavy emphasis on patient education, cognitions and close attention to all aspects of living such as sleep, diet, exercise and social and family engagement, as well as specific goal-setting. A systematic review of 85 studies with 15 255 participants found that inpatient programs with these characteristics were most effective for individuals suffering severe chronic pain and that benefits were maintained into the future (Lewis & Bean, 2021).

Cognitive techniques assist people to control pain by thinking positively about their experience and ability to manage. With the use of coaching strategies, individuals develop an expectation of success and reconceptualise their role as competent and resourceful, which promotes feelings of self-efficacy. Individuals also learn to monitor negative, maladaptive thoughts, feelings and behaviours. Through positive self-talk and skills training (e.g. relaxation), people begin to attribute their success to their own efforts and thus minimise the likelihood of relapse into maladaptive patterns of behaviour. It is increasingly recognised that an important component of cognitive approaches is acceptance that pain is not a danger signal, but a part of a person's normal life experience.

Pain management programs
Programs that address concerns associated with chronic pain, with strong emphasis on patient education, cognitive components and a physical therapy component.

11.4 CASE STUDY

JUNE AND LUNG CANCER PAIN

June is a 59-year-old Chinese woman born in Hong Kong. When she completed her commerce degree, June was employed by an Australian import/export company and eventually became regional manager for its Asian division. June's position was demanding: she often worked to a tight schedule, travelled a great deal and regularly entertained potential clients for business development. She found cigarette smoking relaxing. Her father and older brother had smoked when she was growing up, and many of her Asian clients smoked.

June is at high risk for lung cancer because of her gender, her history of smoking and (more currently) her exposure to secondary smoke from being around people who smoke (both in her family of origin and in her business life). Furthermore, her lifestyle is stressful and sedentary.

When she was in her mid-40s, June was feeling the consequences of smoking (e.g. breathlessness when walking quickly) and decided to quit. Life continued to go well for her, but six months ago June contracted the flu and had respiratory distress. She was in bed for three days and found it difficult to fully recover. After two months, she was still experiencing fatigue, had a persistent dry cough and one night started to cough up blood. She spoke to her doctor, who ordered a chest CT scan. This revealed moderate emphysema and dark spots on June's left lung. A biopsy determined she had lung cancer. June was referred to an oncologist and commenced chemotherapy. Over time June experienced considerable neuropathic pain, which is a common consequence of chemotherapy. She took extended sick leave from work.

A year later, June was diagnosed with secondary cancer (metastases) in her spine. She continued to experience neuropathic pain. Neuropathic pain as a result of nerve damage from a tumour is usually less responsive to opioids (e.g. morphine) or requires higher doses. June suffered many side effects from taking the medication over a long period of time. She went online and found some useful information about coping with pain. She read that people have certain coping predispositions that they use when faced with a stressor such as pain. An individual's coping style not only influenced the specific coping strategies they might use to deal with stress, but also their responses to that stress (e.g. increased pain or depression). Information on the website prompted June to reflect on how she tends to cope with stress.

June believed that she could tolerate the cancer pain. She realised that she tended to stay in command of her feelings and rarely expressed negative feelings. This belief in being stoic and coping silently was taught to her from a very young age by her Chinese father and grandmother. Out of interest, June decided to complete an online questionnaire on coping styles (see below).

1   What factors placed June at risk of developing lung cancer?
2   How might June have reacted to her experience of persistent pain and its impact on her work and lifestyle?
3   What might be the benefits of a repressive coping style in coping with cancer pain?

Points to consider

When faced with persistent cancer pain, individuals show varied responses. Some people seem to cope well, report low to moderate pain, and appear to show little psychological distress. In contrast, others cope poorly, report high levels of pain and feel depressed. Given June's international lifestyle and work demands, she is likely to grieve the loss of these activities, and negative emotions associated with loss may lead her to focus attention on her pain. As noted previously, even boredom is associated with increased awareness of, and sensitivity to, pain.

The Coping Strategies Questionnaire has 50 items and responses are made on a seven-point Likert scale (0 = never, 6 = always). The items assess five cognitive and two behavioural strategies for coping with pain (Wilkie & Keefe, 1991). The cognitive strategies include coping self-statements, catastrophising, diverting attention, reinterpreting pain sensation and ignoring pain sensations. The behavioural strategies include praying/hoping and increasing behavioural activities. June's score indicated that she had a repressive coping style. People with this coping style are particularly prone to rely on two specific strategies: intentionally not paying attention to their pain, and engaging in active behaviours or thoughts to maintain a positive mood or distract themselves from a negative mood.

A repressive coping style is potentially adaptive. It may allow June to develop a high pain tolerance through her belief that she can cope, and minimise sensitivity to her pain by diverting her attention to other things. She is likely to reinterpret her pain sensations to be positive messages from her body to take care, and ignore pain sensations. Consequently, she is less likely to experience anxiety and depression as a result of the pain. She is also less likely to perceive the pain as a catastrophe than someone who is highly anxious. Catastrophising is a maladaptive cognitive coping strategy as the person tends to think the worst about their condition and their ability to cope.

CHAPTER SUMMARY

Learn more
Access additional resources to broaden your understanding of this chapter. See the Guided Tour for access details.

- Pain is a significant and complex aspect of illness that involves an interplay of physiological, psychological, social and behavioural factors.

- There is greater understanding about the transmission of pain and the role of neurochemicals such as endogenous opioid peptides in regulating pain.

- In contrast to acute pain, chronic pain is long-term and not necessarily related to a specific disease or injury.

- Chronic pain is difficult to treat because of adverse and pervasive effects on daily activities and the development of maladaptive coping strategies. Treatments can involve pharmaceutical drugs and alterations to the sensory pathways involved in pain transmission.

- Increasingly, psychological interventions such as biofeedback, relaxation, hypnosis and cognitive–behavioural strategies are having some success. Nevertheless, chronic pain requires a comprehensive program to minimise pain and enhance the likelihood of adaptive coping strategies.

FURTHER READING

Dydyk AM & Conermann T (2021) Chronic pain. StatPearls [online]. PMID: 31971706.

Lee R, Rashid A, Thomson W & Cordingley L (2020) Reluctant to assess pain: A qualitative study of health care professionals' beliefs about the role of pain in juvenile idiopathic arthritis. *Arthritis Care & Research* 72(1), 69–77.

Wall PD & Melzack R (1996) *The Challenge of Pain*. Penguin Books.

Yam M, Loh Y, Tan C, Khadijah S, Manan A & Basir R (2018) General pathways of pain sensation and the major neurotransmitters involved in pain regulation. *International Journal of Molecular Science* 19, 2164. doi:10.3390/ijms19082164

12 Stress and Trauma

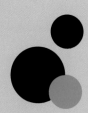

CHAPTER OBJECTIVES

By the end of this chapter, you should be able to:

» understand the differences between viewing stress as a stimulus and a response, and a process that links the two

» know how concepts of stress, appraisal and coping are linked

» describe and compare demands and resources, and describe how these affect the experience of stress

» use a goodness of fit model to explain differences in individual responses to stress and coping

» understand the effects of traumatic events as an extreme form of the stress process

KEYWORDS

» allostasis
» allostatic load
» catastrophising
» chronic strain
» fight or flight response

» goodness of fit
» hassles
» post-traumatic stress disorder
» primary appraisal

» secondary appraisal
» stress
» stress response
» stressor
» tend and befriend

What is stress?

Stress has been a popular topic in the media over the past few decades. Much has been made of whether the stresses of everyday life are greater now than in the past, and whether stress is the disease of the 21st century. It is widely accepted that stress has a significant negative impact on health (Garfin et al., 2018) and that the successful management of stress will prevent that negative impact. One major German insurance company offers lower rates for people who regularly practise meditation, based on the premise that those people will make fewer claims based on stress. To evaluate whether stress affects health and, if so, how much, it is necessary to clarify what stress is. Such clarification is complicated by the fact that stress is often thought of as an event, and often as a response of an individual to events (Dich et al., 2020).

Stress as a stimulus

When describing stress, many people tend to think of specific events (stimuli) that have produced the experience for them or for others. Examples include examinations, bereavements, natural disasters, illness, relationship breakdown, accidents and so forth. Holmes and Rahe (1967) developed a life events scale that attempted to classify how stressful certain events were for people by assigning the events a weighting based on a survey of a large sample of people. Not surprisingly, the events rated as most stressful were major personal losses such as the death of a child or long-time spouse or partner. More surprisingly, positive events—such as being promoted, getting married or buying a new car—were also weighted as producing stress.

PAUSE & REFLECT

Think of a positive event in your own life that was stressful for you.

What were the characteristics of that event that made it stressful?

Would everyone else in that situation have felt the same amount of stress that you did?

12.1 CASE STUDY

EDUARDO AND HARD WORK

This case study examines an individual's experience of stress and some of the consequences that may arise from it.

Eduardo is a 28-year-old male working as the manager of a paper products company. Eduardo enjoys his work and would very much like to continue to move upward in his career. Due to difficulties in the industry, he has been working up to 18 hours a day during the week and additional hours on weekends. He has been eating irregular meals, often does not see his wife for more than a few hours each day, and sometimes does not see his two children except for short times on the weekends. Although his wife understands why Eduardo works as hard as he does, she still complains from time to time about his absence from home.

In recent years, Eduardo has found it necessary to make some significant changes to his life. He does very little exercise, partly due to lack of time, and partly because he and his wife gave up their gym memberships to save money. After the birth of their second child, they moved to a larger house, which meant taking on a substantially larger mortgage. It also meant moving further from the city where Eduardo works, which means that he has to spend more time commuting. He drives to and from work, and often spends considerable amounts of time stuck in traffic.

1   Is Eduardo experiencing stress?

2   What things in your life produce stress for you?

There are major problems with the view that some stimuli are inherently stressful. Events that are stressful for some (e.g. jumping out of a plane) can be recreational for others. It is hard to imagine that a woman who was brutalised by an abusive husband would have the same level of reaction to his death as a woman who loved her kind husband. Another problem arises from the observation that some people may not perceive major life events as being relevant to stress at all, or being relevant only sometimes. This suggests there is a threshold for stress, and that a particular stimulus must register above that threshold before it is perceived as standing out from background stimuli. Consider the individual who makes a career out of performing in public. If there is a lot at stake in a particular performance, that person may experience stress, but if the performance is simple and routine, they may not.

Just looking at the events themselves does not make it possible to understand the difference between a stress and a challenge. We often seek out activities that produce excitement or that make us feel elation when we have successfully completed them, and this is very difficult to explain using a stimulus definition of stress. The stimulus should always be stressful or not stressful. The impact of any given stimulus is based on the fact that it requires adaptation on the part of the individual. Stress could be thought of as "an extreme level of everyday life" (Fisher, 1986, p. 7). Adaptation to any extreme event requires mobilisation of resources by the individual, and this changes the individual's internal physiological state.

Stressor
An event that appears likely to an observer to produce stress.

It is generally more productive to refer to events as **stressors**, which may vary in terms of their likelihood of producing a response within the individual.

STRESS AS A RESPONSE

When stress is conceptualised as a response of the individual, the focus is placed on the physical and mental reactions that result. The mental component includes thoughts, ideas and beliefs. Most of the research in this area has focused on physical arousal and how it relates to outcomes such as performance, coping and health, rather than on the mental component.

A well-known principle in psychology is the curvilinear or inverted-U relationship between arousal and performance (see Figure 12.1). This Yerkes–Dodson Law (based on Yerkes & Dodson, 1908) indicates that there will be an optimal level of arousal for performance of any task. If arousal is too low, the person will be unmotivated to perform. As arousal increases, motivation will increase to a point where the individual is focused

FIGURE 12.1 The arousal–performance curve

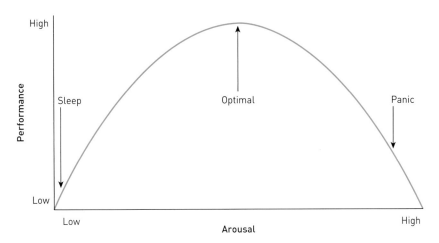

and energised. As arousal increases past that point, errors will increase until ultimately the person's behaviour becomes panicky and disorganised. The arousal–performance curve will be different for each task and each person. It has been established that well-known tasks are much less prone to breakdown than novel ones. This is why we practise skills. The presence of arousal increases the occurrence of dominant (i.e. more probable) responses. For a new task, these will be errors; for a well-known one, these responses will be correct.

Sometimes, the term 'eustress' (Selye, 1978) is used to describe arousal that is at the optimal level for performance and that provides motivation and direction for the individual's behaviour. The word 'eustress' means good stress, and can be distinguished from distress (bad stress) by its effects on how the individual acts and feels. It is likely, however, that an individual will not really think of an optimal level of arousal in terms of stress at all. For most people, the concept of stress implies 'bad', so the idea that it can be good is confusing.

The nature of the **stress response**, a pattern of physiological and/or cognitive reactions to a situation that is experienced by an individual, is quite variable. Ninety years ago, Cannon (1932) described the **fight or flight response** based on the release of catecholamines, which prepare the individual for action. But whether the individual will fight or turn and run cannot be explained by what is going on in the body. Although the release of catecholamines may be similar, if not exactly the same, for every individual, their cognitions that go with running and those that go with standing to fight are very different. It is now generally recognised that there is not a single generalised response to environmental demand. Not only do individuals differ in the likelihood that they will be flooded with catecholamines, but also in the effects that those hormones will have on their behavioural and physical responses.

Optimal level theories of motivation are also discussed in Chapter 6.

Stress response
A pattern of physiological and cognitive reactions experienced by an individual in relation to a situation.

Fight or flight response
The release of catecholamines, which prepare the body for action.

PAUSE & REFLECT

How do you know when you are under stress?

Do you respond to stressors in your life in a typical way?

Is your response primarily physical or mental?

STRESS AS A PROCESS

It is much more useful to conceptualise stress as a process involving a complex interaction between the individual and the situation. Figure 12.2 shows a biopsychosocial model of **stress** (Frankenhaeuser, 1991). Because the process takes place within the individual, stress is a subjective experience. It is impossible for an observer to look at the situation and the person, and determine exactly what is going to happen.

The key element of interactive stress models is the balance between the individual's appraisals of the environmental demand and their resources for dealing with the demand. Lazarus and Folkman (1984) presented a detailed model of how these appraisals take place, and their impact on the experience of stress.

Typically, in the presence of an environmental demand, people first assess or appraise the severity of the demand. This is referred to as **primary appraisal**. With everyday demands, with which the resources of individuals are more than adequate to cope, the demand is appraised as being not a significant threat to well-being; that is, as something that can be dealt with routinely. In the case of severe demand, where either the harm or loss already experienced or the threat of future loss is great, individuals may need to make additional, non-routine resources available to deal with it. Then the primary appraisal will be that the situation is stressful. The primary appraisal could even be that the demand is irrelevant and can safely be ignored. This might be the case if, for instance, we heard a dog barking viciously but could see that it was locked up.

The next appraisal that individuals make is about their own resources; this is called **secondary appraisal**. This appraisal can range from no resources (time to panic) to plenty of resources (no

Stress
A perceived imbalance between demands and resources.

Primary appraisal
The idea that, in the presence of an environmental demand, individuals first assess or appraise the severity of the demand.

Secondary appraisal
The appraisal that individuals make about their own resources.

FIGURE 12.2 A biopsychosocial model of stress

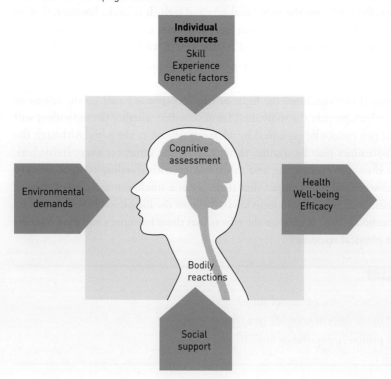

Frankenhaeuser (1991)

sweat). It could even be that no resources are needed; it is safe to ignore the demand completely. Primary and secondary appraisals don't necessarily occur at the same time, and each of them can change over time. Even so, they are usually very closely linked. In an emergency, we may make an instantaneous appraisal of demand and react. Later, when we have time to do the secondary appraisal, we might be surprised at the outcome. For example, a person who has reacted quickly and managed to avoid an accident may think, "How did I get out of that?"

The process of appraisal is highly individual. Not only do the resources of individuals differ, but so do the appraisals they make of those resources. We are often surprised by which individuals cope with a severe stress and which do not. A physically strong person may be less able to deal with a prolonged physical demand than a weak person, not because their resources are depleted more rapidly but because they appraise them as inadequate and therefore give up sooner. The individual may **catastrophise**, telling themselves that the situation is impossible for them to cope with when in fact it is not. People also differ in their ability to adopt new roles in the face of demands. Many victims of Nazi concentration camps during the Second World War died during their first days in the camp because their resources were not adaptable to such extreme demands. Those who survived—often for amazingly long periods of time—were able to divert resources towards survival by redefining themselves, or living for each day, or living for the single goal of being a witness to the atrocities at the end of the war. So, there is another way of defining stress: the individual's appraisals that the resources they can call on are not sufficient to deal with the demands placed on them.

> **Catastrophising**
> The appraisal by an individual that a situation is impossible for them to cope with when in fact it is not.

PAUSE & REFLECT

What are some advantages of thinking about stress as a process rather than as a series of events or responses to events?

How would this be helpful in thinking about why a teacher might experience burnout from their workload?

When stressors are being appraised by individuals, there are several important characteristics that affect their impact.

1   *Clear vs ambiguous.* If we know exactly what the demand is and how to deal with it, it will have a different effect than if the demand is ambiguous. Research by one of the authors of this book (Jones, 1970) with industrial foremen showed that major conflicts with superiors were less stressful when there were clear conflict resolution procedures, than minor conflicts in the absence of those procedures.

2   *Acute vs chronic.* Time-limited events, such as a physical assault, will have different effects from ongoing chronic stressors such as disability or unemployment.

3   *Intermittent vs continuous.* University examinations, which occur in regular, predictable cycles, will have different effects from a continuously occurring stress, such as pain following an injury or surgery. This is independent of whether the stressor occurs over a long or short period of time.

4   *Random vs personally relevant.* Being the victim of a natural disaster, such as a bridge collapse, would have quite a different impact from an event that we felt had relevance to our self-image or esteem, such as being fired from a job for incompetence.

5   *Limited vs pervasive.* Some events affect limited areas of life (e.g. breaking your non-dominant arm), while others affect every aspect. Becoming a quadriplegic, for example,

means the loss of far more than mobility: it may also mean the loss of sexuality and employment, and a complete change of lifestyle.

6   *Controllable vs uncontrollable.* Many theorists, such as Fisher (1986) and Thompson et al. (2018), believe that this is the most important appraisal of all. The more controllable a stressor is, the less likely it is to produce stress (Limbachia et al., 2021) (see Figure 12.3).

FIGURE 12.3 Demands and resources

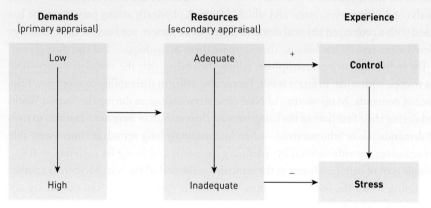

Fisher (1986)

12.2 CASE STUDY

EDUARDO (CONT.)

Eduardo is exposed to a number of stressors, including working long hours, not being able to see his family and not eating regular meals. Whether this means he is experiencing stress is not clear, however, because we don't know how his situation looks to him. Whether another person would also experience those same responses in the face of the same stressors would depend on various factors; a single person, for example, might find the lack of contact with family less of a problem. Someone who was less attached to their career might find the events less challenging. Whether Eduardo feels stressed depends on his appraisal of his situation.

However, he suffers from indigestion and has trouble both getting to sleep and staying asleep. This means that he is showing stress responses. These symptoms may be related to his experience of stress, but they might also be due to purely physical causes. Eduardo complains to his wife that he feels pressured at work, and that one of his superiors has been making negative comments about the quality of his work. He can't understand why he is being singled out by this person, and finds it uncomfortable to attend meetings when that person is present. These meetings always make his indigestion worse, and he can't sleep the night before a meeting.

1   How can you use a biopsychosocial model to understand what Eduardo is experiencing?

2   What factors would be relevant to Eduardo's appraisal of his situation?

3   Would Eduardo's appraisal be the same if he were Chief Executive Officer of his firm, with salary and bonuses of several million dollars a year?

DAILY HASSLES

Not all the stresses that face individuals are major. Researchers have also looked at the effects of minor stressful events on health (Charles et al., 2013; Sin et al., 2020). Such events, or **hassles**, can include being put on hold during a phone call, finding that you have run out of toilet paper or have to make a small decision. Not only can these small hassles produce irritation, but they can also aggravate physical and mental health in several ways. The cumulative impact of small hassles can wear the individual down. They can also exaggerate the effects of a concurrent major life event, sometimes by being the straw that breaks the individual's back. Research has shown that daily hassles can predict health outcomes for secondary and tertiary students (Pascoe et al., 2020) even where (or possibly *especially* where) an individual has not experienced any major life events.

COVID-19 and the quarantine and lockdown periods associated with it obviously produced a lot of unique hassles. At the time of writing, research is beginning to consider COVID-19 related stress and coping (Neff et al., 2021; Yang et al., 2021).

One special case of minor hassle that can have particularly strong effects is **chronic strain**, the repeated or constant occurrence of a minor stressor. Usually, people become habituated to a minor stressor and so it fades as a source of stress. However, if prolonged, exposure may have the same effect as many daily stressors. Examples include background noise at work, a personality conflict with someone who you constantly come into contact with and cannot avoid, financial problems, a poor living environment and family problems. One kind of chronic strain that has been shown to have health consequences is having a job that is high in demands but low in control. Such job situations have been demonstrated to predict psychological and cardiovascular problems (Norberg et al., 2020).

Hassles
Apparently minor events that can cause irritation, aggravate existing health problems or (in large numbers or over a prolonged period of time) affect an individual's health.

Chronic strain
The repeated or constant occurrence of a minor stressor.

PAUSE & REFLECT

What daily hassles bother you the most? Do any of them produce chronic strain for you? If so, why do you think this happens? If not, why not?

It is a good idea to keep in mind that daily life provides uplifts as well as hassles (Pascoe et al., 2020). Uplifts are small victories or pleasing moments that indicate that things are going well. They include a successful interaction with someone, a completed job or finding a way to solve a problem. Uplifts have not always shown as large a relationship to health as hassles.

ANXIETY

It is not uncommon for people to confuse the concepts of stress and anxiety. Clearly, there is a high degree of relationship between them and they often occur together, but it is important to distinguish some of the differences. Anxiety is an emotional state and, like other emotions, consists of somatic (physiological), cognitive and behavioural components. The somatic effects often include an accelerated heartbeat, stomach symptoms (e.g. nausea or pain), sweating and trembling. Cognitive components can include feelings of dread, trouble concentrating or having your mind go blank, feeling irritable or jumpy, or thinking about things that might go wrong. Behavioural components include withdrawing from the situation, seeking out comfort or doing things to damp down the feelings (e.g. drinking or using drugs).

Unlike fear, which is usually attached to a particular object, anxiety may occur with or without a specific focus. Students frequently experience examination anxiety, for example, not because they are unprepared or because they have appraised the demands as being greater than their resources, but because of the importance of the examinations for their future progress. Anxiety might also occur because everyone else is (or appears to be) anxious, or simply from past learning. Spielberger (1975) differentiated between state anxiety (a temporary condition) and trait anxiety (a more generalised and long-term condition of the individual). Anxiety may result from stress appraisals and may serve to focus and activate the individual to cope. However, too much anxiety (see the Yerkes–Dodson Law above) can be disruptive, and lead to avoidance or disorganised behaviour. The occurrence of anxiety is a highly individual thing. It may be the result of a generalised biological (and possibly inherited) vulnerability, a generalised psychological vulnerability (based on early experiences of control) or a specific psychological vulnerability (where the individual learns to focus anxiety on certain events) (Barlow, 2000). If anxiety becomes a common experience, the individual may have an anxiety disorder and need to seek professional help.

Different kinds of anxiety disorders have been distinguished by mental health professionals. The usual categorisation (APA, 2013) includes generalised anxiety disorder (GAD), panic disorder (PD), social phobia, obsessive compulsive disorder (OCD) and post-traumatic stress disorder (PTSD).

GAD is a long-lasting state of anxiety not related to a particular object or event. It typically involves continual worry about everyday matters, with ongoing symptoms of anxiety. PD is diagnosed when the individual has sudden and intense attacks of apprehension—often marked by considerable somatic components such as rapid heartbeat, nausea, trembling or breathlessness—accompanied by cognitions; these somatic symptoms have long-term and serious meaning for the individual's health. Phobias refer to anxiety that is aroused by specific objects or events, such as public speaking or spiders.

Phobias are discussed in Chapter 6.

In OCD, the anxiety involves ongoing and intrusive thoughts (obsessions) that can only be relieved by the carrying out of specific acts or rituals (compulsions). The relationship between the obsessions and the compulsions is not necessarily a rational one, and in severe cases the carrying out of the compulsions can interfere with normal activities of living or affect the health of the individual. PTSD is discussed in more detail in the trauma section later in this chapter.

THE INDIVIDUAL'S RESPONSE TO STRESS

The way in which the individual reacts to a demand will depend on a number of factors, but one useful way to think about this is **goodness of fit** between the individual and the demand (Jones, 2001). We talked about individual vulnerability and capability in Chapter 4, and these are aspects of goodness of fit. Individuals differ in physical strength, immune competence, genetic predispositions, mental resilience, networks of social supports, financial resources and so on. When a demand occurs, the individual may have the right resources—or they may not. If they have a good fit, they will cope even if the demand is severe. In the absence of a good fit, even a minor demand can be catastrophic.

Goodness of fit
The appropriateness of the individual's resources to the specific demands that they face.

In some cases, the individual may be able to substitute one resource for another. They may, for example, want to have a nice garden but not have the time or interest to work on it. If they have enough money, they can hire someone else to do the work. To take another example, if we do not know how to make two parts fit together easily, we may be inclined to use brute strength to force them together.

Vulnerability and capability are discussed in Chapter 4.

It has been suggested that there are gender differences in response to stress: that women use different resources from men. Although it has been traditional to talk about the fight or flight response as a general one, Evetts (2017) supported earlier research that proposed this was primarily a male response and that women are more likely to **tend and befriend** when stressed, by looking after their children or seeking social support. This theory offers interesting directions for future research.

Tend and befriend
The idea that women, when stressed, look after their children or seek out social support in order to deal with their stress.

HEALTH EFFECTS OF STRESS

Much has been written about the health effects of stress (Garfin et al., 2018), including increased susceptibility to infections, an increased likelihood of clinical events at the same level of risk, and a decreased rate of healing. It has even been shown that stress in pregnant women affects the health outcomes of the children in later life. We won't include a survey of the literature about the negative effects of stress at this point. What is more useful is a model for how the health effects may come about. Figure 12.4, which can be seen as an elaboration of Figure 12.3, shows pathways to the development of physical and psychiatric illness. The fact that physiological responses to stress lead to both seems logical enough, but many authors have almost entirely overlooked the behavioural consequences. People use a variety of behavioural coping strategies that negatively affect health outcomes. These include substance abuse (e.g. smoking, drinking and drug use) which results in increased exposures to toxins. They may divert time away from healthy activities such as exercise and relaxation to task-focused activities, and divert attention from symptoms and self-care activities. The all-too-common strategy of substituting increased effort for increased skill leads to higher risks of accident and injury.

FIGURE 12.4 Effects of stress on health

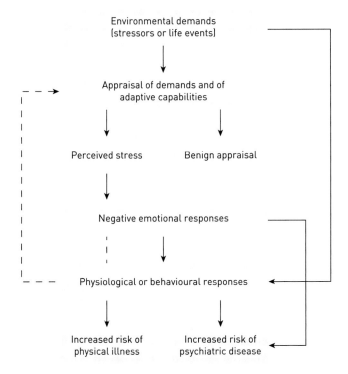

Cohen et al. (1995)

ALLOSTASIS

One theoretical approach that aims to explain individual differences in responses to stress and how they interact with health involves the concept of allostasis (Guidi et al., 2021). When faced with a situation that is interpreted by the individual as a stress or challenge, various systems of the body are activated to protect functioning and enable the organism to operate with greatest effect and least damage. This is called **allostasis** (McEwen, 2005). This concept relates to homeostasis; that is, when the organism attempts to keep physiological states (e.g. body temperature) at an optimal level. Allostasis differs in that it is seen as a specific type of homeostasis, with the aim not of maintaining one level but of finding the best level to cope with the perceived demands of a situation. Several systems have been identified as being part of the allostatic processes, including hormonal, cardiovascular, neural and immune systems. When the process of allostasis works, then adaptation to the stressors or challenges is effective.

In some circumstances, allostatic systems can be overused, not perform normally, or fail to switch off once the demands have been dealt with. This has been called **allostatic load**. McEwen (1998) described three types of allostatic load: frequent activation of the allostatic systems, failure to shut off allostatic activity after stress, and inadequate response of allostatic systems, which can throw excess demand on other systems that may lead to negative effects rather than adaptation. Any of these types of allostatic load can lead to problems with health (Fava et al., 2019). This may occur by aggravating wear and tear, by misdirecting bodily resources in such a way that the overall effect is negative for health, or by interfering with normal operations of bodily systems.

The concept of allostasis is useful in generating research ideas, but the similarity between the proposed mechanisms and other stress theories (e.g. chronic strain) makes it difficult to determine the independent contribution of the concepts. Traditionally, research has treated socio-economic and demographic characteristics (e.g. ethnicity, gender and age) as independent, additive influences on health. However, a rigorous population-based study by Rodriguez et al., (2019) revealed that allostatic load is strongly associated with social class.

Allostasis
The process of maintaining balance in bodily systems, through physiological or behavioural means, in the face of a demand.

Allostatic load
The cumulative cost to the body of allostasis.

Homeostasis is discussed in Chapter 8.

PAUSE & REFLECT

A friend tells you that too much stress can cause cancer.

What kinds of issues would you need to think about before you decided whether this could be true?

How could stress affect the structure of cells so that they become cancerous?

12.3 CASE STUDY

EDUARDO (CONT.)

Eduardo wants to succeed in his career and believes that he can do so. As a result, he is motivated to continue putting in long hours and expending extra effort. Although he feels that he has the support of his wife and family, the fact that he is not home as much as they would like bothers him. Eduardo keeps reminding himself that it will all be worth it when he has a secure career. He has apparently appraised the demands as being within his resources to manage. Those resources include some that are within himself (the ability to work hard and cope with long hours) and some that are outside (support from his wife and family). His motivation to do well encourages him to continue to try to meet the demands of his situation.

However, he and his wife decide that additional resources would help him. They decide that more exercise would help him to be more resilient, and that he needs to eat better. He visits his doctor to find out if the indigestion is an indication of disease or a response to his situation. He looks for more information about the effects of stress, and ways in which he might be better able to cope. Not much of this seems to be directly useful, and worrying about it actually makes him feel worse about his situation.

1   How have Eduardo's appraisals changed?
2   How would his experience of stress be different in the face of a single traumatic experience?

Trauma

Sometimes events unexpectedly intrude into an individual's life and threaten their physical or psychological safety or integrity (Schnurr & Green, 2004). The term 'trauma' is used to describe such events. These may include a natural disaster or an event such as war, violent personal assault such as rape or robbery, being taken captive or imprisoned, or being involved in an accident. Each of these places enormous demands on resources. Research has identified trauma associated with medical interventions during events such as childbirth (Crawley et al., 2018). This can be true even when individuals are not personally involved but witness such an occurrence (e.g. midwives) or hear about it happening to someone close to them (Toohill et al., 2019). Where numbers of people are affected by the same trauma, there are broader public mental health consequences (Kleber, 2019).

Sympathetic arousal is discussed in Chapter 10.

Events of these kinds produce very strong responses in individuals. As with illness, reactions may include physical, emotional, cognitive and behavioural aspects. Common physical reactions include nausea, shaking and sweating, which are all typical of extremely elevated levels of sympathetic nervous system arousal.

Common emotional reactions include fear and anxiety on the one hand, or numbness and detachment on the other. Cognitive reactions often include confusion and disorientation, poor attention or concentration, and thoughts or images of the traumatic event. Behavioural reactions can include avoidance or escape behaviours, and restlessness and searching for information. These are all normal, and usually occur most strongly during or immediately after the event.

The primary appraisals will vary quite a lot from one event to another. If a child of rich parents is kidnapped for ransom, for example, it may be a continuous and personally relevant trauma, while an individual's appraisal of an earthquake is likely to be that it is acute and random. The appraisal that most traumatic events have in common, however, is that they are uncontrollable. When events are appraised as uncontrollable, secondary appraisals are usually that resources are going to be insufficient. In both cases above, there is little that the individual can do to gain control over the initial event.

Normal reactions to illness are discussed in Chapter 4.

As with reactions to illness, individuals may have abnormal or normal reactions to trauma. It is the persistence of maladaptive symptoms and responses that identifies abnormal reactions. Norris et al. (2002) looked at studies involving 60 000 people who had been involved in disasters (mostly natural disasters) and found that the impact was greatest in the first 12 months. Only a minority of individuals remained significantly impaired after a year. Lynch and Lachman (2020) found that the age of first trauma can affect the impact the trauma has in adulthood.

The nature of the trauma and following events have a great effect on what proportion of people show abnormal reactions. If there is a significant aftermath to a traumatic event (e.g. the continuing radiation risk in Ukraine many years after the Chernobyl nuclear reactor meltdown), the proportion of individuals affected will be higher than if there is little aftermath (e.g. being a witness to a fatal automobile accident). The same is true if traumas are repeated, such as those faced by responders who face repeated bushfires (Harvey et al., 2016).

POST-TRAUMATIC STRESS DISORDER

Post-traumatic stress disorder
A persistent pattern of symptoms, including preoccupation, nightmares and flashbacks, that some individuals experience after a major stressful event.

When individuals have been exposed to a traumatic event and had an intense response to it, this can occasionally lead to later psychological problems. **Post-traumatic stress disorder** (PTSD) is a condition that has received a fair amount of attention in the media. The important thing to remember about PTSD is that it is a response that persists, or reappears, long after the event. PTSD is considered to involve re-experiencing the traumatic event, continuing avoidance of stimuli that remind the individual of the event, and/or numbing of general responsiveness to everyday life, resulting in significant distress or impairment of functioning. Often, sufferers experience nightmares or intrusive thoughts about the event (cognitive), relive the fear and anxiety of the event (emotional), have sudden flashes of physical arousal (physical) and experience interference with work and social life (behavioural). PTSD is more likely to occur if experiences are clearly life-threatening (particularly horrific) or result in injury and death to family and close friends, separation from family, and loss of property or dislocation (Lancaster et al., 2016). The 2004 Asian tsunami and the 2010 Japanese tsunami and subsequent nuclear accident, for instance, have had—and will continue to have for some time—all these effects for many of the people involved.

PTSD can have significant impacts on ongoing cognitive functions (Sumner et al., 2017), such as depression and anxiety. It is not surprising that PTSD can affect not only mental but also physical health (Ryder et al., 2018). Factors about the individual that also have an influence on long-term adjustment include cultural differences, psychological preparedness and coping styles. While there is little that can be done to change the first, disaster managers are learning new ways to influence the others. Strategies include having good warning systems and public knowledge of the possibility of an event, good immediate and long-term support programs after an event, and helping people with coping. The availability of coping strategies with beneficial health outcomes is commonly overlooked. Chapter 13 examines this, and focuses on stress management and coping behaviours.

12.4 CASE STUDY

ALIZIA AND AN EARTHQUAKE

Alizia is a 53-year-old academic who is attending a conference on an island in Indonesia. She has been enjoying the conference discussions, lying on the beach at the end of the day and dining with colleagues in the evening. One evening at dinner, the ground begins to shake, the ceiling in her hotel begins to crack and fall, and the people around her begin to scream and run. When a piece of concrete lands on the chair next to her, shattering it to pieces, she jumps out of a broken window into the street. The air is filled with a sound like thunder, there is dust everywhere and the ground is still shaking. She is thrown to the ground, grabs hold of a lamp post with one arm and covers her head with the other.

All around her, people are running and shouting or screaming. Her own heart has begun to race, she feels sick to her stomach and suddenly realises that she is screaming too. She begins to think about the possibility that the wall of the hotel may fall and kill her, but she is too terrified to move to get out of the way. She finds that it is difficult to breathe because of all the dust in the air, and that she has begun to shake all over. She closes her eyes—more to avoid seeing what is going on around her than to keep the dust out of them—and desperately wishes to be somewhere, anywhere else.

Gradually, after what seems to her to be hours, things begin to quieten down and the ground stops shaking. She can smell burning as well as dust, but can't bring herself to open her eyes or let go of the lamp post. She slides down closer to the base of the post and curls herself into a ball, but still can't get rid of the thought that the hotel is going to fall on her. She hears sirens, people screaming and crying. Although she stops screaming, she can't stop crying. She begins to think about moving to a safer place where the hotel can't fall on her, but just then there is another tremor—although it is only a small one. It makes her freeze, and she continues crying.

After several minutes, she realises that one of the voices she hears is crying for help. This makes her open her eyes and look around. It is hard to see for all the dust, which she is terrified to realise is now mixed with smoke. However, she can see that the woman calling for help is sitting in the road and has blood streaming down her face. Alizia begins to crawl towards the woman, but then thinks that this is stupid as it will take ages to reach the injured woman. Standing up, she crosses to the injured woman and uses the tail of her shirt to wipe away some of the blood. She knows from experience that scalp wounds tend to bleed profusely, so she concentrates on compressing the wound to reduce the bleeding. Because she can still smell smoke, she looks around to see if she can find the source. It seems to be limited to a small area at the back of the hotel and she can see that several people are working to put it out, so she turns her attention back to the injured woman. Remembering some basic first aid, she helps the woman to lie down and checks her for other injuries, which seem to be limited to small cuts, scrapes and bruises. Only then does she realise that she is also badly scratched, and has a few bits of broken glass embedded in her leg from a broken window. However, none of her injuries are serious, and the other woman's head wound is. She keeps the compression on the head wound, as this seems to be helping, and looks around for possible sources of help.

Every few minutes, there are additional small aftershocks. Each time, Alizia feels her heart leap in terror and wants to grab hold of the ground. Eventually, emergency services arrive and take over tending the injured woman. Alizia is too frightened to go back into the hotel and luckily was holding her handbag, containing her passport and wallet, when she jumped out of the window. She seeks help for herself, getting her wounds cleaned, some bottled water to drink and a sheltered place to lie down. The next morning, she is evacuated to a safe area and can contact the consulate to arrange for transport to the airport and a flight home.

For the next two years, Alizia seems to experience no impact from the earthquake. However, over time, she begins to have flashbacks to the experience, with vivid images of blood and a re-experience of her initial feelings of panic. Alizia is now receiving treatment for PTSD.

1   What are the somatic, cognitive and behavioural reactions that Alizia experienced during the earthquake?

2   How would her reactions to this situation differ from her usual stress responses?

3   Once Alizia has begun to help someone else, her reactions appear to have changed dramatically. Why might this be the case?

Points to consider

It is virtually impossible to predict whether or not a given person will experience PTSD. Key factors include age, gender, nationality, social supports, acceptance of the reality of the symptoms by other people and prior life experiences, as well as all the variables discussed above. Hundreds of studies have been carried out but, given the difficulties of defining a trauma and defining normal or abnormal reactions to trauma, it is not surprising that PTSD is quite controversial. Studies may show rates as low as 1% or as high as 100%, and it is impossible to compare the conditions under which the rates were obtained. The most important factor must be the person's perception of the event and their well-being.

Learn more
Access additional resources to broaden your understanding of this chapter. See the Guided Tour for access details.

CHAPTER SUMMARY

- The topic of stress has received a great deal of attention.

- Stressors are events that have the potential to produce stress. Stress responses describe the ways that individuals experience stress. The term 'stress' should be reserved for the process by which the individual and the situation interact to produce a response that is experienced as stressful.

- A critical part of this process is the individual's appraisal that the demands of the situation exceed their resources for dealing with the demand.

- Daily hassles, as well as major life events, can produce stress for an individual.

- The goodness of fit between the individual's resources and the demands they face influences their appraisal. Stress leads to health effects through negative emotional states and/or physiological or behavioural responses. Trauma—extreme events that threaten physical or psychological safety—may produce particularly strong stress responses.

FURTHER READING

Harkness E & Hayden E (Eds) (2020) *The Oxford Handbook of Stress and Mental Health.* Oxford University Press.

Schiraldi G (2016) *The Post-traumatic Stress Disorder Sourcebook: A Guide to Healing, Recovery and Growth* (2nd rev. edn). McGraw-Hill Education.

Schulkin J (Ed.) (2012) *Allostasis, Homeostasis, and the Costs of Physiological Adaptation.* MIT Press.

Taylor SE & Stanton A (2021) *Health Psychology: Stress and Coping* (11th edn). McGraw-Hill.

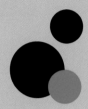

13 Coping: How to Deal with Stress

Introduction

Because stress is such a common experience, it is not surprising that a lot of attention has been given to managing it. The evidence is good (Dolan et al., 2021) that a number of skills and behaviours are helpful in dealing with stress. Most people who experience stress in the short term can find some technique that suits them and improves well-being. There is also considerable evidence that reducing stress produces overall health benefits as well. Attempting to manage stress is called coping. Management does not necessarily guarantee complete—or any—success in controlling stress. Different strategies can be used by different individuals at different times with good effect. Sometimes we are not even aware that we are behaving strategically; we just react to circumstances we find ourselves in, but an outside observer can see the strategy if they are looking for it.

Types of coping

Coping strategies can be classified into two groups—problem-focused (or task-focused) and emotion focused (Lazarus & Folkman, 1984). Deciding which type of strategy to use depends on the desired outcome.

PROBLEM-FOCUSED COPING

The aim is to modify the balance between demands and resources in a particular situation, which will clearly be more useful the more control the individual has over the situation. **Problem-focused coping** can involve decreasing or eliminating the demand or increasing the resources available to meet that demand (Lazarus & Folkman, 1984).

If the individual is hungry, they can reduce the demand of the situation by eating. If they have a large amount of work to do, they can complete it. If they are attacked, they can run away or fight. These are attempts to modify the demand. Problem-focused coping aimed at the demand commonly involves increased effort, fuelled by increased **arousal**. It can involve problem-solving that leads to meeting tasks more efficiently. It can also involve a variety of other strategies, such as modifying the task, learning new skills, deflecting the responsibility for the task onto someone else, or leaving the situation so that the demand is avoided.

Resources can also be addressed. When we know a task is coming, we prepare for it. The athlete builds their stamina prior to a competition. Patients are encouraged to build up their strength and mentally prepare for surgery. Getting help from others is a very common and useful way of increasing our resources.

EMOTION-FOCUSED COPING

Coping is sometimes aimed at dealing with the way that the demand makes us feel. The parent who gives their share of food to their child remains hungry, but may feel good that they are doing a worthwhile thing. If we have too much work and cannot possibly do it all, we may acknowledge that fact and manage the emotion (worry) that the situation causes. If we are attacked and can neither run nor fight, we can still cope with the emotion of fear. These approaches are referred to as **emotion-focused coping**.

Coping
Any strategy by which an individual attempts to manage the perceived discrepancy between demands and resources.

Problem-focused coping
Behaviour, such as problem-solving or increased effort, aimed at modifying the balance between demands and resources in a particular situation by reducing the demand or increasing resources.

Arousal
The activation of the sympathetic nervous system, which produces visceral changes and provides energy for behaviour.

Emotion-focused coping
Behaviour, such as relaxation, distraction or prayer, aimed not at dealing with situational demands but with the way the demands make an individual feel.

Emotion-focused coping approaches to stress management can be put into three groups. The first includes approaches that tap into an individual's existing positive emotional experiences. These experiences can vary considerably. Things such as humour and laughter, music and hobbies can be useful for some people. Humour can work by distracting the person from situations producing stress, but also produce more direct effects on physiological and cognitive processes (Zander-Schellenberg, 2020). The same holds true for music, art and dance. Spirituality is attracting more attention as a moderator of stress, with some evidence that religious commitment is protective of physical and mental health (Lorenz et al., 2019). Many people report using prayer as a stress management technique. The good feelings associated with these pleasurable experiences become a buffer against stress and reduce its effects on health.

The second group contains techniques aimed principally at modifying physiological arousal. These include deep breathing, muscle relaxation and exercise, which can help individuals deal with stress that arises from illness and stress that makes illness worse.

The third group includes techniques aimed at modifying the cognitions associated with the experience of stress. This can include various kinds of psychotherapy, such as psychoanalysis, and a variety of cognitive behavioural approaches. The latter are often combined with relaxation and exercise programs to address both the physiological and cognitive aspects of negative emotions that are characteristic of stress responses. Attention is being paid to the role of positive cognitions in general, and optimism has been found to predict positive health outcomes (Scheier & Carver, 2018). Techniques to replace cognitive distortions with optimistic cognitions are a significant part of stress management.

Which is better?

Much research has been devoted to trying to determine which is more effective: problem- or emotion-focused coping. Although some research indicates that problem-focused is better, the most important factor is control. The more control the individual has in a situation, the more likely it is that problem-focused coping will be effective. Imagine that you are presented with a small ball and asked to place it in a hole that is several times its diameter. This should be an easy task: hold the ball in your hand and just put it in the hole. Now, imagine that you are playing golf and the rules take away some control. You can't pick up, or even touch, the ball with your hand. You must leave it on the ground and try to roll it into the hole with a club. The rules have taken away control and the task has become much more difficult and frustrating—as anyone who has played golf will testify.

The concept of goodness of fit between demands and resources was introduced in the discussion of stress appraisals. Another goodness of fit hypothesis (Vitaliano et al., 1990) suggests that if there is a good match between the nature of the demand and the selected coping strategy, coping will be more effective; goodness of fit is more important than which coping strategy has been selected. In reality, we usually use both kinds of coping in any given situation. If there is an examination coming up, students will almost certainly use problem-focused strategies (e.g. studying) as well as emotion-focused strategies (e.g. getting enough sleep, talking to friends).

Individuals differ in their beliefs about control. **Locus of control** theory (Rotter, 1966) suggests that these broad beliefs about the main causes of events are important in the choices people make about how to behave and how they feel. People who tend to believe that they can direct their own outcomes by their own choices and actions are described as having

Stress appraisals are discussed in Chapter 12.

Locus of control
The degree to which an individual attributes the cause of events to internal factors or external forces.

an internal locus of control (LoC I). People who feel that their outcomes are not under their own control are described as having an external locus of control (LoC E). They are sometimes further divided into those who believe that their life outcomes are the result of the actions of powerful other people, or the result of fate, luck or chance. Locus of control can be useful in thinking about how individuals deal with their health. Those who have an internal locus of control regarding health have been shown to be more likely to adopt positive health behaviours than those with an external locus. However, these are not the ends of a single continuum; in situations where little control is possible, an external locus can produce better health outcomes (Gore et al., 2016).

Stress management techniques

The experience of being stressed is an emotional one. This means that the stress response is composed of physiological arousal and cognitions that are stress-relevant (two-factor theory of emotion). Approaches to managing stress may begin with either of these components, and often involve both (Can et al., 2020). The model by Cohen et al. (1995) (Figure 12.4) indicated that the critical link between stress and risks to health is physiological or behavioural responses. This is the step for which coping may be of most use.

The two-factor theory of emotion is discussed in Chapter 10.

It is often valuable to get professional help when learning how to manage stress. Such help can be obtained through books, classes, online, government or NGO bodies, or individual consultation with a trained counsellor, psychologist or other health practitioner. However, many people are able to pick up stress management techniques from a brief description, or can make up their own. There is no magic involved in any one technique, and it is a good idea to be critical of 'miracle cures' for stress. This chapter briefly talks about physical relaxation, meditation and some cognitive behavioural approaches.

The basic principles of behaviour change are vital in an individual's attempts to deal with stress using psychological techniques. For major problems, professional help should always be sought. An appropriate aim and method need to be selected, a realistic target set, and the method must be given time and practice to work. It is important to remember that if a method does not work this does not mean that the individual is a failure. A different approach may be quite successful.

STRESS MANAGEMENT BASED ON RELAXATION

Almost all behavioural approaches to stress management revolve around the very simple fact that most of us are not very good at relaxing our bodies or our minds. Therefore, the first step in dealing with stress involves learning and practising relaxation (Norelli et al., 2021). Several techniques are known to work and produce a range of positive benefits (Toussaint et al., 2021). An individual may need to try a variety of approaches before finding one that suits them.

The word 'relaxation' is sometimes used to describe anything we do that is not work. It can include exercise, watching sports, hobbies, being with friends or even using or abusing so-called recreational drugs. Although these may lead to the individual feeling more relaxed, they may not lower stress. In fact, recreational activities can be sources of stress.

What does relaxation mean to you?

When do you feel most relaxed?

Clench your fist as tightly as you can for about 10 seconds and then relax it completely.

How does the feeling in your hand compare to your previous thoughts about relaxation?

While almost everyone can remember having had a wonderful feeling of complete relaxation at some time, the trick is to develop the skill to create that feeling at will—not simply wait for it to occur. Many psychologists and psychiatrists view relaxation as so central to recovery that they encourage many (or all) of their patients to learn and use relaxation as an adjunct to medication and counselling.

Generally, relaxation is a pleasurable state, one that includes physical and mental components. At the physical level, the pleasure is primarily related to the activation of the parasympathetic nervous system, aimed at restoring resources that have been used up by activation of the sympathetic system. There is a fair degree of commonality in individuals' descriptions of it. At the cognitive level, there is more variability. Some people talk about relaxation as the absence of events, using terms such as 'peaceful', 'quiet', 'at rest' or 'unworried'. Others focus on the presence of signs, using terms such as 'focus', 'well-being' or 'happiness'.

For many people, learning how to relax is the end in itself. With regular practice, relaxation can improve physical and mental well-being (Unger et al., 2017). Almost everyone who learns how to relax finds benefits in other areas of their life. It is often reported, for example, that relaxation helps people to concentrate, communicate with others and deal with difficult situations. Certainly, mental relaxation feeds into physical and vice versa. As with anything else in life, if an individual wants to be good at relaxation, they need to practise.

13.1 CASE STUDY

EDUARDO AND HARD WORK

Eduardo, who we first discussed in Chapter 12, finds that he is experiencing physical and mental signs of stress. He has butterflies in his stomach, headaches and lower back pain. He is so preoccupied in thinking about the job that he finds it difficult to concentrate. He cannot seem to turn off his mind, which keeps him awake at night. He can't seem to maintain the coping strategies he adopted (see Chapter 12). He is too tired and sore for regular exercise, his wife seems less supportive than she used to be, and eating a balanced diet seems to be just too hard. As his physical symptoms get worse, Eduardo begins to get irritable and sometimes yells at his children for being noisy when he is trying to work. Although he has never been a big drinker, he starts having four glasses of wine each night to help him relax and get to sleep.

His constant physical arousal and mental preoccupation, and his anger and drinking, are coping strategies that may well be effective during a difficult situation but clearly are now being overused. The thing he needs most for dealing with his stress symptoms is the ability to turn these coping strategies off until they are needed.

Remember that, in the physical world, threats tend to arise unexpectedly. Eduardo is wasting resources by responding to threats that haven't actually occurred.

1   What skills would enable Eduardo to conserve his resources until they are needed?

2   What other stress management approaches might he find easier to use on a regular basis without adding to his sense of being stressed?

Relaxation is closely related to the management of conditions associated with excess physiological arousal. Insomnia often comes from lying in bed worrying about not sleeping, and erectile impotence from worry about maintaining an erection. In such conditions, stimulus control methods can do a lot for an individual on their own, but they usually work better when combined with relaxation. Relaxation helps the individual to deal with the excess physiological arousal. A relaxation skill learnt for one purpose can be used for others as well. A variety of cognitive therapeutic techniques combine relaxation with other activities. One such technique, called systematic desensitisation, is discussed later in this chapter.

Breathing

A very simple and effective relaxation technique involves slow and regular breathing. People who are anxious or panicky frequently breathe rapidly, contributing to the experience of anxiety. Breathing exercises interrupt this process, are easy to explain and do, and can be an effective intervention even when used by individuals with little or no training. Practise taking deeper than usual breaths, breathing in for a slow count of five and out for the same. Most people find this breathing pattern is calming and incompatible with feeling anxious.

Exercise

Exercise builds physical resources such as strength and agility, lowers blood pressure and often produces physical relaxation. Everyone can gain from exercise, but each person needs to find an appropriate exercise program for their needs. Age, gender, body type and existing level of fitness, for example, can affect what is appropriate for the individual.

The **FITT principle** (Katsukawa, 2016) outlines four conditions that determine the appropriateness of an exercise program for an individual at a specific time. These are Frequency (how often to exercise), Intensity (how hard to exercise), Time (how long to exercise) and Type (what kind of exercise to adopt). Different sets of recommendations are available for each condition, to avoid injury.

FITT principle
Four conditions that determine the appropriateness of an exercise program for an individual at a specific time: frequency, intensity, time and type.

In addition to its obvious physical benefits, exercise is useful in the management of stress and mental health (Stubbs et al., 2016). This benefit occurs from many different types of exercise, for different levels and types of stress and mental health.

As with any other technique, what makes exercise effective is practice and participation. Many experts believe that maximum benefit from any kind of exercise requires participation for at least half an hour at least three times a week. This holds for gentle walking as much as it does for vigorous activity, such as playing tennis. Playing squash or running marathons can be good exercise, but they require a high pre-existing level of fitness and regular exercise to maintain that high level of fitness. Too many unfit people have suffered injuries, heart attacks or strokes during unaccustomed strenuous activity: it is unsafe to ignore the risks.

Yoga can be considered as exercise, meditation and a physical relaxation technique. It is known to be an effective technique for managing stress (Sahni et al., 2021).

OXFORD UNIVERSITY PRESS

PAUSE & REFLECT

How does exercise make you feel?

What are the good effects in the short term and long term?

Do you feel that you exercise enough? If not, try to determine why you don't exercise more.

Progressive relaxation

One of the simplest techniques aimed at achieving physical relaxation involves **progressive relaxation**, often combined with a program of thoughts or actions. The idea is simply to relax muscle groups one at a time so that the individual learns and remembers what relaxation feels like (Toussaint et al., 2021). As with all relaxation techniques, the key to progressive relaxation is practice and repetition. Like exercise, regular muscle relaxation creates and maintains the required skills and techniques.

The Jacobson method (Jacobson, 1938) uses tension and relaxation of muscles as the basis for progressive relaxation. Each group of muscles is tensed while the person becomes aware of the sensation of tension, and then relaxed while the sensation of relaxation is considered. The comparison of sensations increases the individual's understanding of what they are trying to avoid and what they are trying to achieve. As this kind of relaxation method is easy to describe and highly effective for many people, it will be used as an example.

To practise progressive relaxation, follow these steps.

1   Find a private, quiet place to practise. Some of the exercises will look a bit odd to others. Intrusions will not help you to relax. Wear comfortable clothing and loosen any constricting items, such as a tie or belt.

2   Sit upright in a comfortable straight chair or lie on a firm flat surface, such as carpet or an exercise mat. (As the idea is to learn relaxation, not fall asleep, it is best to not use your bed. Later, relaxation can be used to help with sleep.) It is not a good idea to practise relaxation if you are sunk too deeply into a padded chair. Close your eyes to make focusing on bodily sensations easier. Begin by breathing deeply and slowly.

3   Begin with the extremities of the body and work towards the top. Start with the toes and feet, move to the legs, then the arms, then the trunk, and finish with the neck and head.

4   Tense each group of muscles for a slow count of five and study the sensations of tension. The tighter you tense the muscles, the easier it will be to see what tension feels like (but if serious pain occurs—stop!). Then relax the muscles for a slow count of five and study the sensation of relaxation. This may include feelings of heat, coolness or heaviness, depending on the muscle group and the individual. It doesn't matter what you feel, only that you learn what relaxation of that muscle group feels like for you. When relaxing muscles that you usually keep tensed, you may even experience aches or twitches. For people who have a lot of headaches, this can occur with neck muscles; for people who have chronic back pain, with back muscles. Again, if these sensations are severe or if tension sets off a migraine or muscle spasm—stop! You may need to consult an expert.

5   Repeat that muscle group, tensing for a slow count of five and relaxing for a slow count of five, all the time studying the sensations.

6   Move on to another group. Groups may be further divided, such as working first on your lower back and then on the abdominal muscles. Face and head usually involve more than one exercise, such as forehead and scalp lifting, grimacing or scowling.

Progressive relaxation
A stress management strategy that involves relaxation of muscle groups one at a time so that the individual learns and remembers what relaxation feels like.

7   Some people find that images help with the tension of muscle groups. For the toes and feet, for example, you could imagine curling your toes down as if you were trying to touch your heels with them. For the back, press your spine into the floor as if you were trying to lift your legs, but don't actually lift them. For the face, try to move your eyebrows to the back of your head, then try to move them down to your chin.

8   It should take you at least 20 minutes to go through the whole procedure, and may take longer. Try to end each repetition with all muscle groups relaxed for a few minutes. Repeat as often as is useful. Many people do the exercises several times a day, every day; others only as needed when they feel physically tense or note a symptom coming on. To keep in practice, three times a week is probably the minimum.

Progressive relaxation techniques are easily found online, from free-access websites, podcasts and sponsored sources. They describe each step and provide good guides to the timing of each step. The sources may contain spoken instructions, or include soothing music or images as well. Once an individual has learnt and practised the method, they can choose to dispense with the recording or use it only occasionally.

Biofeedback

Biofeedback, logically enough, involves feeding back information to the individual about biological processes of which they are normally unaware. This requires the use of devices that might measure muscle tension, skin temperature, heart rate and blood pressure, or a number of other biological variables that are related to tension and anxiety. The aim of feeding back the biological signals using these mechanical devices is to help the individual gain voluntary control over them. This works by operant conditioning in that the individual is constantly reinforcing their relaxation, as indicated by a change in the biofeedback signal. Biofeedback has been used for an enormous range of problems, from incontinence to anxiety. Its use in clinical treatment is well established (Glick & Greco, 2010).

We use informal biofeedback when we weigh ourselves or take our temperature. A mechanical device is used to give us information we need to change the result through voluntary behaviour. Biofeedback as a stress management technique provides increased voluntary control of the physical manifestations of stress, such as relaxing tight forehead or neck muscles, reducing sweaty hands, and even lowering blood pressure without medication. It is important to remember that operant conditioning can also take place even if the organism is not aware that it is occurring. This principle is also true for biofeedback. It may work better for children than adults, possibly because children are more enthusiastic about the machines or have higher expectations of success.

Meditation/mindfulness

There are many approaches to meditation, ranging from highly structured programs to general guidelines. Some, such as yoga, tai chi and qigong (Abbott & Lavretsky, 2013) or transcendental meditation, were originally based on a philosophy or religion, but can also be practised without this component and still produce benefits. Individuals who are interested in the general approach of meditation can choose a form that best suits their own needs and interests. In general, the idea of meditation is to rid the mind of worries and concerns so that a peaceful state is achieved (Behan, 2020).

The similarities between meditation and physical relaxation are many. Whatever suits the individual, makes sense to them, and makes them feel comfortable is the appropriate

Biofeedback
The control of internal processes through conditioning, using mechanical devices to make those internal processes perceptible.

For a reminder about operant conditioning and how it works, see Chapter 6.

method for them. There is no reason why the individual cannot create a method based on personal experience and suggestions from others. Meditation approaches tend to fall into two categories: concentrative meditation, in which attention is concentrated on an image or sound to the exclusion of other stimuli; and mindfulness meditation, in which the individual allows thoughts and stimuli to pass without reacting to them and becomes more mindful of the present moment.

Mindfulness has become increasingly popular, and many people find it highly effective for managing stress (Querstret et al., 2020; Behan, 2020). An online search will locate a large number of sources. There are variations in what different sources include in their mindfulness techniques, but they share some common principles. These basically revolve around:

> Non-judging. Be an impartial witness to your own experience. Become aware of the constant stream of judging and reacting to inner and outer experience

> Patience. A form of wisdom, patience demonstrates that we accept the fact that things sometimes unfold in their own time. Allow for this

> Beginner's Mind. Remaining open and curious allows us to be receptive to new possibilities and prevents us from getting stuck in the rut of our own expertise

> Trust. Develop a basic trust with yourself and your feelings. Know it's OK to make mistakes

> Non-Striving. The goal is to be with yourself right here, right now. Pay attention to what is unfolding without trying to change anything

> Acceptance. See things as they are. This sets the stage for acting appropriately in your life no matter what is happening

> Letting Go. When we pay attention to our inner experience, we discover there are certain thoughts, emotions and situations the mind wants to hold onto. Let your experience be what it is right now (adapted from 'The Foundations of Mindfulness Practice: Attitudes and Commitment' in Kabat-Zinn 2013, pp. 19–38).

In general, meditation requires an individual to find a physical setting or position that facilitates meditation. In some approaches, particular postures are required; in others, the guidelines for progressive relaxation are appropriate.

Breathing is important to every meditation approach and is usually the first step. Slow, regular, deep breathing sets the tone for the mental side of meditation. From there, techniques are used to rid the mind of conscious thought. Concentrative meditation often uses images, such as "Imagine that you are in the middle of a cloud, nothing can be seen clearly and everything that comes to your mind is allowed to fade into the cloud." It can involve repetitive actions, such as repeatedly chanting or saying a sound or phrase (a mantra). Eyes may be closed, but in some concentrative meditation approaches the eyes are open and focused on an image, an object or a mandala (a geometric or pictorial design usually enclosed in a circle, representing the entire universe).

As with physical relaxation, techniques can be learnt from books, courses and online, or directly from experts. Studies of meditation approaches have shown physical benefits, including lower levels of stress hormones, decreased blood pressure and easier breathing, along with psychological benefits including decreases in negative emotions and improved learning ability and memory.

13.2 CASE STUDY

EDUARDO (CONT.)

As soon as Eduardo thinks about his work, he experiences a flash of panic, becomes tense and his symptoms return. His thoughts about his situation have now become the focus of his stress response. The only thing that seems to help him to switch off these thoughts is alcohol. His drinking has increased, not to help him sleep but to help him stop thinking. It also stops him thinking about more appropriate stress management techniques. He has stopped exercising, eats too much and, combined with the alcohol, has gained a lot of weight. He eats a lot of comfort food when he is drinking—chips, chocolate and pies. His wife has grown tired of his drinking and irritability, and particularly his level of anger. She forbids him from drinking at home, so he spends more time in pubs. He drives when he shouldn't because he does not think about the risks when he has been drinking. Through some people he met at the pub, he has begun experimenting with illegal drugs.

1   How could a two-factor theory about emotion explain the link between Eduardo's panicky feelings and his anger and irritability?

2   What can a biopsychosocial model of stress contribute to understanding why some techniques work for Eduardo, while others do not?

PHARMACOLOGICAL APPROACHES TO RELAXATION

Prescription drugs

Another way to achieve lower levels of physical arousal involves the use of drugs. Some are prescription drugs, some are freely available and are often used by people who are feeling tense or stressed (Garakani et al., 2020).

Probably the most familiar prescription drugs for lowering arousal levels are benzodiazepines (e.g. Ativan, Xanax and Rohypnol), which are minor tranquillisers that are usually prescribed for anxiety or sleep problems. Benzodiazepines can be very effective but have several negative effects, the worst of which is the risk of addiction or psychological dependence. Their use under a doctor's supervision for a short time for acute problems (e.g. reactions following a bereavement or trauma) is quite important, but because of the problem of dependence, abuse is common. Ideally, benzodiazepines are used in the short term to deal with anxiety until more permanent coping strategies can be learnt and become effective.

The other major class of drugs used for relaxation effects are beta-blockers. These block the receptor sites for a neurotransmitter and interfere with the physical effects of sympathetic nervous system activation. Beta-blockers are usually prescribed after a heart attack. They decrease the amount of strain put on the heart to pump blood, and eliminate symptoms such as angina (chest pain) and shortness of breath. While they have fewer negative effects than benzodiazepines, they can be used only under a doctor's supervision. Beta-blockers can produce physical dependence.

One problem of both classes of drugs is that stopping their use can produce rebound effects; that is, higher levels of the very symptoms that they were used to treat, such as increased anxiety or tension. While prescription drugs have a place in short-term treatment of anxiety and depression, they also have risks (Garakani et al., 2020).

Non-prescription drugs

Some common drugs used to deal with stress and anxiety don't need a doctor's prescription. At the top of the list is alcohol, which many people use to self-medicate their stress responses or anxiety. In small amounts, it produces relaxation. As with prescription drugs, however, it can result in addiction and even death. It also disinhibits behaviour, which means it reduces the amount of control that the individual usually exercises over their behaviour and makes it more likely that they will do things that they wouldn't if they were sober. Because of its easy availability, its effect on judgment and motor control, alcohol is implicated in a large proportion of car and other accidents. It also frequently contributes to violence and suicide.

The other common over-the-counter drug is nicotine. Nicotine is actually a stimulant, but the way in which smokers use cigarettes results in their perception that they are relaxing. As nicotine is extremely addictive, what is almost certainly being relieved is the craving for nicotine, rather than the stress itself.

Illegal drugs

Opponent–process theories of motivation are discussed in Chapter 6.

There are many illegal (sometimes called recreational) drugs, such as marijuana, cocaine, ecstasy and heroin, that produce strong physical and psychological effects that can reduce stress or anxiety. Their use is not primarily for stress management but for their other physical effects, such as changes in perception or a short rush of highly pleasurable sensation. These substances are prone to cause physical addiction and/or psychological dependence, and show the same kind of rebound effect as benzodiazepines. The effects of drugs are best understood using opponent–process theories of motivation.

PAUSE & REFLECT

Risky behaviours are also discussed in Chapter 6.

Some substances that are stimulants, such as the caffeine in coffee or energy drinks, are often taken when people say that they are relaxing or taking a break.

Why do you think people associate these stimulants with relaxation?

If you use a substance (e.g. caffeine) to regulate your stress levels, do you consider it helps?

COGNITIVE BEHAVIOURAL TECHNIQUES

The focus of techniques discussed so far is physical relaxation, but in meditation and progressive relaxation, emphasis is usually placed on thoughts and how to keep them from intruding into relaxation. Clearly, this is often easier said than done.

Cognitive behavioural therapy
Counselling therapies in which an individual can learn to control or modify worrying or intrusive thoughts, thereby improving their mental health.

The contribution of thoughts (cognitions) to the experience of stress is significant, and worrying thoughts are often the biggest barrier to coping with stress. A group of cognitive techniques based on this idea is broadly referred to as **cognitive behavioural therapy** (CBT). CBT techniques have been used in a wide range of mental health conditions and have shown excellent therapeutic outcomes (Fordham et al., 2021). CBT is now regarded as the "gold standard" of psychotherapies (David et al., 2018).

If worrying or intrusive cognitions can be controlled or modified, stress can be avoided much more easily. Although some of these techniques are simple and to some extent can be used by the individual without professional support, they were developed as therapeutic tools and the expertise of a psychologist or other trained health professional is important to their proper use. This chapter gives an overview of a few CBT techniques.

Systematic desensitisation

Once the individual has learnt what relaxation feels like and has practised a technique often enough to gain a sense of control over tension, strategies to deal with specific sources of stress can be utilised. One of the most common techniques is **systematic desensitisation** (Wolpe, 1973). This is typically used when the individual suffers from a simple phobia: an anxiety response to a specific stimulus that is out of proportion to the real risk (see Chapter 6 for a discussion of how phobias are learnt).

Common phobias include fear of spiders, flying, hypodermic needles and heights. A very common but seldom recognised phobia among students is examination anxiety. It is important to distinguish degrees of anxiety. A slight fear of spiders is probably a good idea as it sensitises us to a genuine environmental danger, and a slight fear of heights may keep us from doing dangerous things. A degree of anxiety about examinations motivates us to study and will stimulate our maximum level of performance. However, when a phobia prevents an individual from carrying out their normal activities, it needs attention. A severe phobia or a phobic reaction to a wide variety of stimuli (e.g. social situations) is a more serious psychological condition, which is best dealt with by seeking professional help.

Systematic desensitisation involves linking exposure to the stimulus that produces anxiety with the practice of relaxation. This begins with exposure to a very small dose of the stimulus and gradually works up to the desired level of desensitisation. The first step is to identify a hierarchy of exposure to the stimulus from a level that the individual can almost deal with now, up to the highest level of exposure that the individual feels is desirable (Rimm & Masters, 1979). For example, an individual with a fear of flying may wish to have no fear at all so they can fly in comfort, regardless of the length of the flight or size of the plane. For a fear of spiders, the individual would probably be wise to stop short of being comfortable picking up venomous varieties.

> **Systematic desensitisation**
> A cognitive behavioural strategy for dealing with phobic anxiety by linking increasing exposure to the stimulus that produces anxiety with the practice of relaxation.

> *Optimal level theories of motivation are discussed in Chapter 6.*

PAUSE & REFLECT

Abel has a phobia about flying. Thinking about flying makes him feel so anxious that he cannot get onto a plane.

How could systematic desensitisation be used to help him to overcome this phobia?

It is possible to imagine a stimulus hierarchy of events; for example, gradually increasing amounts of exposure to snakes. However, even thoughts about events are often enough to trigger anxiety. This means that steps in the hierarchy may include just thinking about events, such as thinking about snakes. To deal with a fear of examinations, the hierarchy might look something like this:

1   thinking about exams that are a long time away;

2   studying for exams that are a long time away;

3   thinking about exams that are closer in time;

4   studying for them;

5   doing practice exams;

6   thinking about exams immediately before they happen;

7   sitting minor exams;

8   sitting major exams.

At each level in the hierarchy, the individual would carry out the activity while practising relaxation. They might start by holding an exam paper and, if they felt anxious, meditating or relaxing until they felt comfortable. When they were able to hold the paper without anxiety, they could move to the next level in the hierarchy. If they were to experience anxiety while studying, they would practise relaxing until they were comfortable, then resume studying. Gradually, they would become more comfortable with studying and could move on to the next stage. If, at any time in the process, they felt anxiety at a lower level in the hierarchy, they could return to that level then resume progress to higher levels when ready to do so. Dropping down a level does not indicate failure; it shows only that that stage was not yet complete.

The most important aspect of this approach is that it is systematic: there is a defined progression of steps, and at each step the individual can gain a sense of self-efficacy with regard to their anxiety. Self-reinforcement should be given at every step. Whether a therapist is involved or not, positive reinforcement for progress is critical.

13.3 CASE STUDY

EDUARDO (CONT.)

There has been a serious deterioration in Eduardo's performance at work due to his substance abuse. His job is at risk, and his employer insists that he seek professional help. His wife threatens to throw him out of the house unless he gets help. Eduardo and the psychologist spend the first session talking about which elements of his life are most important to him. Eduardo realises that he is in danger of losing what he values most due to his use of alcohol and drugs as stress management tools.

It is decided that he needs strategies to help him deal with the unrealistic anxiety caused by his negative thinking about his work. This includes developing skills that enable him to think about work only when it is useful to do so (i.e. when he is preparing strategies for it) and not to think about it when he does not need to. He has to learn to focus his attention on positive thoughts. With ongoing practice of these techniques, Eduardo finds that many of the other issues simply go away when he is not worrying about work. Being able to focus on positive and realistic thoughts means that he is less tempted to drink, which means that he is more able to control his irritability and comfort eating. Spending more time at home repairing his relationships with his wife and children provides him with additional positive experiences.

Of course, all this takes time. Fear that he will lose the support of his wife and lose his children are powerful motivations for him to stick to his treatment. Support from his employer is also vital, as it makes work issues less negative and gives him a sense that his employer really wants him to succeed.

1   How important is unrealistic negative thinking to the experience of stress?

2   What techniques might be used to reduce unrealistic negative thoughts in your own experience?

Mental imagery

Mental imagery involves using positive images to counteract the negative thoughts that cause or accompany stress responses. Positive images are incompatible with feeling stressed; active images are incompatible with feelings of helplessness. One example from 'positive psychology' is for a person to look at themselves in a mirror and repeat positive slogans over and over. While this is somewhat simplistic, an extraordinary number of people benefit considerably from it.

Physiological or biochemical theories about the effects of positive imagery and related techniques suggest that they increase circulating endorphins, or interrupt positive feedback loops in adrenal functioning. Other theories have focused on psychological factors. Whatever the source of the effects, there is a considerable literature that mental imagery can produce genuine benefit (Tolgou et al., 2018). Mental imagery can help patients with chronic or serious pain to feel more comfortable, frequently in conjunction with drugs, but it can also reduce the need for those drugs. Imagery can help to improve immune function, speed healing and slow the progression of illness. It is often used in conjunction with relaxation techniques or meditation as a way of enhancing the effects of a relaxed state.

PAUSE & REFLECT

Think of a peaceful place that you have visited. Close your eyes and imagine that you are there again. Recall as much detail as you can about how it looked, felt and smelt, and how you felt while you were there.

How did this exercise make you feel?

How did it compare to the physical relaxation that you experienced after clenching your fist very hard?

The range of benefits reported for imagery is very similar to those for placebos, for relaxation in general, for meditation and for other mind–body techniques. It is likely that the mechanism for all of these relates to preventing the wastage of resources on unproductive, ineffective or untimely coping strategies. Instead, they allow the parasympathetic system to restore resources.

Placebo effects are discussed in Chapter 7.

Imagery is frequently combined with relaxation techniques—the individual is asked to focus on a specific mental image. As already mentioned, this is an integral part of some meditation techniques. It can also be used as an adjunct to physical relaxation. Many people find it useful to think of a specific image while they are relaxing to help block other thoughts that might interrupt relaxation. The image could be a place, person or object, and it becomes conditioned to relaxation. This means that the individual may later be able to induce relaxation by thinking about that image.

Covert self-control

Individuals who are feeling stressed frequently carry out internal discussions that are often dominated by negative thoughts or cognitive distortions. These might involve the person thinking that they are weak because of difficulty handling stressful situations, or thinking that terrible things will happen if they do not handle those situations.

Some cognitive distortions

1 *All-or-nothing thinking.* If your performance falls short of perfect, you see yourself as a total failure.

2 *Overgeneralisation.* You see a single negative event as a never-ending pattern of defeat.

3 *Mental filter.* You pick out a single negative detail and dwell exclusively on it.

4 *Disqualifying the positive.* You reject positive experiences by insisting that, for some reason, they don't count.

5 *Jumping to conclusions.* You make a negative interpretation even though there are no facts.

6 *Magnification (catastrophising) or minimisation.* You exaggerate the importance of things or dismiss things so they appear less significant.

7 *Emotional reasoning.* You assume your negative feelings reflect the way things really are.

8 *'Should' statements.* You try to motivate yourself with 'should' and 'shouldn't' statements.

9 *Labelling and mislabelling.* Instead of describing your error as an event that occurred, you attach a negative label to yourself.

10 *Personalisation.* You see yourself as the cause of some negative external event.

These thoughts serve as a form of punishment and share all the drawbacks of punishment. They cause the individual to avoid situations that cause them to have the distressing thoughts (avoidance learning) and produce negative emotions towards the punisher, in this case the self. And, most importantly, they give no information about the desired response.

Cognitive restructuring
A technique aimed at interrupting patterns of negative thinking by training the individual to recognise that they are occurring, and replace them with positive thoughts.

Cognitive restructuring (Lazarus, 1971; Clark & Beck, 2011) is a technique aimed at interrupting these patterns of negative thinking. It involves training the individual to recognise that these patterns are occurring, and replace them with positive thoughts. This positive self-talk is used to define and increase the probability of adaptive behaviour; it is a positive reinforcer. A therapist may model this kind of reinforcement by encouraging adaptive behaviour for a client, then hand the task of reinforcement to the client to carry out mentally (covertly) for themselves. There is ongoing research into the neurological bases of how CBT and cognitive restructuring work (Crum, 2021).

Negative cognitions often serve as antecedents for undesirable behaviour; for example, thinking "I'm a fat slob and I'll never lose weight" can trigger eating. Covert self-control—replacing these maladaptive thoughts with adaptive ones—attempts to trigger desirable behaviour instead. When a lapse occurs, it is then possible to minimise its importance and resume adaptive behaviours.

SOCIAL SUPPORT

Social support is an important resource that has far-ranging effects on stress and coping. Types of support include instrumental/tangible support (money, labour, time), informational support (advice, suggestions, evidence), emotional support (affirmation, affection, concern, listening) and social networking (building and maintaining a support network). Support may help individuals to deal with stress or illness when it occurs, and may also lessen the likelihood of occurrence by reducing the likelihood of adverse life events.

Social support has been linked to mental health among several populations, including university students (McKimmie et al., 2020). There are indications that women are more likely to have good social support than men, possibly because they are better at maintaining and using the relationships they have with others. It has been suggested that this may be one of the factors contributing to women's longer lifespan. Particularly in the later years of life, when more support is required, greater access to social support is a key resource. As with coping in general, the better the match between the types of social supports available and demands of the situation, the more effective the support will be. In severe and uncontrollable situations, emotional support is seen to be the most helpful; however, when events are controllable but overwhelming due to lack of time or money, instrumental support may be far more helpful. It is important to recognise that social support is not always helpful. It may in fact do more harm than good if the help offered does not fit the individual's perceptions of what is needed, if it reduces the individual's self-esteem by suggesting that they are incapable, if it isn't perceived as support but as interference or if it encourages damaging behaviours, such as smoking or drinking heavily to relax.

Managing COVID-19 stress

A great deal of attention has been devoted to the stress experienced by people worldwide during the COVID-19 pandemic, and the consequences for mental health (Salari et al., 2020). Multiple sources contributed to COVID-19 stress. They included concern about catching the virus, the potential severe short-term and long-term effects (long COVID) and the threat to life. There were also indirect stressors, such as lockdowns, effects on employment and education and the broader economic impact. Even the need to comply with simple public health measures such as hand-sanitisation and mask-wearing added stress to daily living. The loss of or severe restriction in normal social activity was probably the greatest stressor.

At the same time, access to health resources was widely affected. There were cutbacks in elective treatments, overload on health professionals—particularly as many became infected themselves and were not available to provide care for a period of time—and diversion of resources from general health care to management of the pandemic. Resources to help individuals cope with stress were also affected, with mental health services often conducted online or postponed. Many resources have been made available to guide people in dealing with COVID-19 stress (APA, 2021b). These are generally the same as those discussed in this chapter, but adapted for online presentation and use at home instead of a specialised setting.

13.4 CASE STUDY

MAHMOUD AND HIGH BLOOD PRESSURE

Mahmoud is a 53-year-old chef. He works evenings and weekends, which are the busiest times. He finds it quite exciting, as his restaurant is popular and there is a long rush hour at dinner. The kitchen is hectic and hot, with staff following his direction to ensure that all orders are dealt with promptly and correctly. Time pressure doesn't allow Mahmoud to take regular meal breaks so he tends to eat on the run—whatever looks good to him at the time. Because his customers prefer food to be fairly high in salt, he has grown used to his food tasting that way. He also likes fried foods. Although he enjoys the stress of his work, he does find that he gets very wound up and it takes a while to wind down when the restaurant closes. He has taken to having several glasses of wine with his staff to unwind, and later to help him sleep.

What he does find very stressful is the paperwork involved in running the restaurant. This involves everything from ordering supplies for the kitchen to organising workers' compensation for staff, paying taxes and getting insurance—the list seems endless to him.

Even though he has an office assistant who is good at processing the paperwork, Mahmoud has to make all the decisions. He frequently finds that his heart is beating rapidly and that he has tension headaches during the day. One day, Mahmoud had a terrible headache that kept getting worse. When he tried to stand, he collapsed. His office assistant, unable to get him to respond, called an ambulance and Mahmoud woke in hospital several hours later. He was told he had had a stroke—fortunately a minor one—and would need time off work to recover. He was also told that his blood pressure is disturbingly high; he has been given medication to bring it down to safe levels.

When Mahmoud visits his doctor after discharge from hospital, his blood pressure remains elevated. In spite of medication, his systolic pressure is still 140 mm/hg (the preferred level is around 120) and his diastolic pressure is 95 mm/hg (preferred level around 80). The doctor has Mahmoud lie down for 10 minutes before measuring his blood pressure again. Mahmoud spends the 10 minutes worrying about the possible result, thinking about having another stroke and not being able to work again. At the end of the 10 minutes, his blood pressure has gone up to 200/100. The doctor decides that Mahmoud's blood pressure responds quite quickly and strongly to stress, and that this needs to be part of his long-term management strategy.

A multifactor strategy involves continuing Mahmoud on medication, but also includes lifestyle changes. Mahmoud has to reduce the amount of salt in his diet and eat more fruit and vegetables. He is given an exercise program that he can fit around his work schedule.

Mahmoud and his doctor then tackle the problems created by stress. After trying several relaxation techniques, Mahmoud reads about mindfulness meditation. This approach appeals to him. He likes the idea of relaxing his muscle tension while also clearing his mind of worrying thoughts. He sets aside three regular times during the day to complete a 20 minute meditation exercise and finds the results so helpful that he adds another at the end of each night's work. This makes it much easier for him to wind down without alcohol. He also falls asleep more quickly and has more restful sleep.

As Mahmoud continues to practise his relaxation and meditation skills, he finds that he can use them for very short periods during stressful moments even while the restaurant is busy, without interfering with his efficiency. Eventually, the lifestyle changes combined with stress management allow Mahmoud to reduce his medication and maintain a normal blood pressure.

1   Which of Mahmoud's behaviours prior to his stroke could be classified as problem-focused or emotion-focused?

2   What changes have taken place in Mahmoud's cognitions about his health and lifestyle as a result of this experience?

3   Can you identify the impact of stress on medical conditions of people you know?

4   Do you use stress management techniques? Are these things that you do intentionally (e.g. yoga) or unintentionally (e.g. going to the movies to unwind)?

5   How common are inappropriate coping strategies among the people you know?

Points to consider

Hypertension (high blood pressure) is not the only medical condition that does not produce obvious symptoms in many sufferers, but it is the most common. Because of the lack of obvious symptoms, the psychophysiological impact of stress may go unnoticed or be attributed to other causes. In other conditions (e.g. asthma), the relationship between stress and symptoms may be immediately obvious, as the symptoms quickly worsen. The important issue is that all physical and psychological conditions are in fact psychophysiological to some degree. This indicates the importance of everyone—no matter how healthy—developing and practising some positive life skills. University students who suffer from examination anxiety (as almost all do) benefit most if they develop stress management skills early and practise them regularly, rather than delaying their use until exam time. As noted above, such skills can be as simple as regular exercise, getting enough sleep and improved time management. The key is that practice improves these skills, so that they become part of everyday life.

CHAPTER SUMMARY

- Coping strategies may be problem-focused (modifying the balance of demands and resources) or emotion-focused.

- Stress responses are emotional and, as a result, involve the interaction of physiological arousal and stress-related cognitive appraisals. Techniques aimed at stress management involve the modification of one or both of these components.

- Relaxation is central to stress management. Breathing, exercise and progressive muscle relaxation are techniques that are primarily effective in modifying the physiological arousal component of stress. To develop these skills, training and practice are required.

- Meditation is also targeted at reducing arousal. It includes techniques designed to affect cognitions.

- Cognitive behavioural techniques may be primarily aimed at changing cognitions (i.e. mental imagery and cognitive restructuring) but may incorporate relaxation as well, as in systematic desensitisation.

- Social support is an important resource for coping, and may work in a variety of ways.

Learn more
Access additional resources to broaden your understanding of this chapter. See the Guided Tour for access details.

FURTHER READING

Dolan N, Simmonds–Buckley M, Kellett S, Siddell E & Delgadillo J (2021) Effectiveness of stress control large group psychoeducation for anxiety and depression: Systematic review and meta-analysis. *British Journal of Clinical Psychology* 60(3), 375–99.

Folkman S & Lazarus RS (1985) If it changes it must be a process: Study of emotion and coping during three stages of a college examination. *Journal of Personality and Social Psychology* 48(1), 150–70.

Selhub E (2020) *The Stress Management Handbook: A Practical Guide to Staying Calm, Keeping Cool, and Avoiding Blow-Ups.* Skyhorse.

Toussaint L, Nguyen QA, Roettger C, Dixon K, Offenbächer M, Kohls N, Hirsch J & Sirois F (2021) Effectiveness of progressive muscle relaxation, deep breathing, and guided imagery in promoting psychological and physiological states of relaxation. *Evidence Based Complementary Alternative Medicine* July, 5924040. doi: 10.1155/2021/5924040

PART IV
FACTORS AFFECTING HEALTH AND BEHAVIOUR

» Chapter 14: Socio-cultural Influences and Inequalities 242

» Chapter 15: Health Literacy 258

» Chapter 16: Promoting Health and Preventing Illness............................ 275

DOES SOCIETY HAVE A ROLE IN HEALTH AND HEALTHY BEHAVIOUR?

This book has explored the nature of agency and health. Part I examined how health, illness and diseases are defined, and explored ways in which people react to illness across the lifespan. Reactions to illness can be explained by the capabilities and vulnerabilities that an individual (as an agent of their own health) brings to the experience of having an acute illness or living with a chronic condition. Part II explored the effects of beliefs and attitudes on behaviour in order to understand how health behaviours develop and are maintained. Part III investigated the links between mind and body in response to illness. Our appraisal of symptoms (e.g. pain) and our capacity to meet these demands can be experienced as stressful. Fortunately, stress can be managed and coping behaviours developed to enhance health and well-being. But an individual's cognitions alone cannot explain all that needs to be known about agency.

In this final Part, we explore agents of health and behaviour that exist outside the individual, in the form of social, cultural and even physical or environmental influences. Ignoring the importance of these factors can lead to placing too much responsibility on the individual (known as blaming the victim). Social agents include family, friends, communities, organisations, cultures, media, many levels of government, and so on. It is a very long list and health professionals have an important place in it. These agents can have an effect on the individual in numerous ways. An alcohol company, for example, might try to influence

OXFORD UNIVERSITY PRESS

individuals' thoughts about its products by depicting attractive and healthy sportspeople drinking alcohol in its advertisements. At the other end of the scale of influence, other agents (e.g. government) may require or ban certain actions by introducing a law; for example, people involved in car accidents while under the influence of drugs or alcohol can be sent to prison. Another influence on health is economic. Health insurance could be made more expensive for people who are obese. Although some agents would like people to eat healthy organic food, barriers exist because it is usually more expensive, either in terms of money or time (and time is money), than many unhealthy foods. Physical barriers can also serve as agents that affect the behaviour of people who live with a disability, or are outside the normal range of strength, agility and size. The variety of external agents is discussed in Chapter 14.

A person may not have the capabilities to be an agent of change. Recent studies suggest that limited health literacy in adults contributes to disparities in health, even though it is potentially modifiable. Chapter 15 defines health literacy, and explores possible ways to improve a person's capacity to obtain, process and understand information to assist them to make appropriate health decisions. The ultimate goal is to promote healthy behaviours and reduce the occurrence of harmful ones. Understanding how people learn and apply health messages to their lives can inform the development of communication strategies to promote healthy behaviour and better adherence to treatments for illness.

Chapter 16 examines some of the ways in which illness can be prevented and health promoted. Much of this is about empowering people to care for their own health, and about providing services to encourage that process to happen. The distribution of health care is not equal across any country or society in the world. There are many different systems for supplying health care, each of which produces different patterns of inequity in health. As a result, there are many different ways to promote health, and some of them will require exactly the skills you are developing through your studies to become a health professional. Individuals can be helped to change, as can families, social systems, the media, communities and governments.

14 Socio-cultural Influences and Inequalities

CHAPTER OBJECTIVES

By the end of this chapter, you should be able to:

» explore the agents of socialisation and their influence on health and health behaviour

» understand culture as a dynamic construct

» identify how culture is transmitted and influences an individual's fundamental values and health beliefs

» understand the socio-cultural factors that influence health and access to health services

» draw connections between socio-cultural influences, explanatory models of health and health behaviour on individuals and groups

» develop an awareness of stereotypes, misconceptions and attitudes relating to race, cultural practices and ethnicity on health inequality

» understand the impact of disability as a significant contributor to inequality

» understand cultural awareness as the first step towards cultural safety

KEYWORDS

» agents of socialisation
» anti-social influences
» communication disabilities
» culture
» ethnicity
» ethnocentrism
» evidence-based health care

» explanatory model
» First Peoples
» Indigenous
» inequality
» inequity
» intellectual disabilities
» nationality
» physical disabilities

» prosocial influences
» race
» sensory disabilities
» social capital
» socialisation

Introduction

There are many influences on health that arise outside the individual. One observation, known as the Inverse Care Law (Hart, 1971) suggests those who most need medical care are least likely to receive it. This observation is true across the world, whether the health system is organised on a publicly or privately funded basis, and whether the nation is poor or rich. This inequality indicates the presence and importance of social influences on health. These influences include culture, race, ethnicity, social class, gender and disability. Each of these factors can influence health by impacting an individual's understanding and experience of the world, their access to health care, health knowledge and healthy environments, and their treatment by others.

Culture

Health and illness are social concepts. What is regarded as illness or health by members of one group is not always regarded the same way by another group. Even families can differ from one another in their understanding of these concepts. A critical contributor to these understandings of health and illness is culture.

Culture refers to a way of life, or characteristics, shared by members of a group. According to Taylor, an anthropologist, culture refers to "the complex whole which includes knowledge, belief, art, morals, law, customs and any other capabilities acquired … as a member of society" (1871, p. 42). Members of a cultural group may be characterised by their shared language, beliefs and values, the way they dress and communicate and the food they eat. Culture is a significant contributor to identity by establishing "who we are", "where we belong" and "where we aspire to fit in". This notion of belonging is reflected in Maslow's hierarchy of needs model, which is discussed in Chapter 8.

> *Health, illness and disease as social constructs are discussed in Chapter 1.*

Culture
The way of life and beliefs shared by members of a group.

PAUSE & REFLECT

What do you consider to be your own cultural identity? Is it defined by where you or your ancestors were born, by what religious group you or your family belong to, or other factors?

How similar, or different, are your health beliefs to those of your grandparents?

It is worth emphasising that culture is learnt. We start learning about culture from birth and so our cultural understanding seems to be an ever-present part of our lives. Encountering an individual who does not share the same cultural assumptions can be quite disturbing. Unfortunately, all cultures seem prone to **ethnocentrism**: the belief that their own culture is the natural or best culture. Ethnocentrism is the conviction that others who do not share a particular culture are inferior in some way. Such views can contribute to arrogance, misunderstanding and conflict.

Some elements of culture are obvious and consciously recognised as cultural. Values associated with religion, ideology and morality are easily recognised as potentially different from one culture to another. Obvious differences are often tolerated well, and even those who dislike some elements of a culture may be fond of its food, music, religious ceremonies or dress styles. Other cultural elements are less obvious but perhaps more important in

Ethnocentrism
The belief that a person's own culture is the natural, or best, culture.

society. These subtle differences include preferences about personal space and acceptable level of touching, and small rituals such as taking off shoes before entering someone's house, or not speaking about or showing pictures of a deceased person. Because these differences may not be consciously recognised as cultural, individuals may feel uncomfortable or even irritated by them, without fully realising why.

PAUSE & REFLECT

Think about the language, customs and experiences of refugees in their home country.

What are some of the challenges experienced by refugees when seeking medical help in a different culture?

Race and ethnicity

Race
The biological (physical) characteristics of an individual's features.

Ethnicity
How people define themselves, and how they are defined by others.

Nationality
An acquired classification generally based on a person's country of birth or, in some instances, their parents' country of birth.

First Peoples
Australia's Aboriginal and Torres Strait Islander peoples.

Indigenous
A term used with respect when referring to First Peoples of all countries.

When we encounter the term culture, we tend to consider characteristics of race and ethnicity. **Race** is defined as the biological (physical) characteristics of an individual's features including eye colour and shape, bone structure, hair colour and texture and skin tone (Berman et al., 2020). Examples of race classification includes African, Latino, Pacific Islander and First Peoples. **Ethnicity** relates to shared traditions and behaviours such as language and customs. For example, Arab people as an ethnic group are linked by language as well as their history, nationality, geographic location and political views (often related to religion and cultural identity). Arab people often emanate from countries such as Saudi Arabia, United Arab Emirates, Egypt, Jordan, Iraq and Iran. While there are vast differences between individuals who consider themselves to be Arab, including customs, dress and foods (leading to classifications of subgroups), a common link is language.

Ethnicity and **nationality** are usually closely aligned. Nationality is an acquired classification generally based on a person's country of birth or, in some instances, their parents' country of birth. As a person can hold dual nationalities, the notion of nationality pertains to laws such as visas, freedom to enter certain countries, and social support entitlements such as medical access or unemployment benefits.

Many nationalities are prone to stereotyping. A 'true-blue Aussie' is a phrase generally understood as referring to a person who lives in Australia, is laid-back, loves sport and values friendships with 'mates'. The reality is, of course, more complex. Australia's Aboriginal and Torres Strait Islander peoples, referred to here as **First Peoples**, are the **indigenous** inhabitants of Australia with a history dating back 65 000 years (Clarkson et al., 2017). First Peoples should therefore feature prominently within Australia's national identity, but this is not the case. Adding to the complexity, there is no singular definition of First Peoples culture. Their cultural diversity includes more than 250 Indigenous languages including 800 dialects. Each language is specific to a particular place and people. So, what constitutes 'Australian' culture remains unclear and previous descriptors no longer apply to everyone living in Australia (Cultural Atlas, 2021).

We often think about ethnicity in terms of disadvantages. People from minority ethnic groups are often the victims of discrimination and stereotyping, and have poorer access to the resources of the dominant society. But being a member of a disadvantaged group may also carry benefits such as access to housing or education grants, land rights or job opportunities as part of an affirmative action strategy. Ethnicity is often statistically related to health but this relationship is, like that of race, related more to social factors or behaviour than anything else. Ethnicity may contribute to a person's access to healthy living conditions, or even their access to health services, which can have major consequences for health.

14.1 CASE STUDY

MRS MECIR AND UNDIAGNOSED ABDOMINAL PAIN

This case study considers how the identification, experience and treatment of health issues can be influenced by cultural, social, family and gender issues.

Mrs Mecir is a 65-year-old woman of Turkish ancestry. She moved to Australia from Albania to live with her recently widowed son in the small country town where he runs a mixed business. She cares for his children, aged four and 10, while he works long days in his shop. Mrs Mecir has been suffering abdominal pain for several weeks, and the pain is increasing.

In Albania, Mrs Mecir lived in a world of extreme hardship and deprivation. For decades, there was little food beyond the staples such as bread, rice, yogurt and beans. She was overjoyed when her son was able to arrange for her to migrate to Australia. Albanian cuisine is meat-oriented, and since arriving in Australia Mrs Mecir has eaten meat twice a day. Mrs Mecir also likes to makes a custard dish and a special *ashura* (pudding) made of cracked wheat, sugar, dried fruit, crushed nuts and cinnamon. Her diet is high in red meat and sugar with little fresh fruit or fibre.

1 How might culture contribute to Mrs Mecir's physical and psychological health?

2 How might culture affect Mrs Mecir's experience of illness?

Culture and health beliefs

The understanding of health and illness is part of an individual's culture. Not all cultures agree on what health is, and there are wide variations in beliefs about the causes and treatments for illness. All cultures provide an **explanatory model** about the cause of an illness, its course and treatment (Kleinman, 1988). Although the explanatory model needs to be logical within the context of a culture, different cultures may produce quite different kinds of logic.

Within Western cultures, explanatory models tend to be based largely on biomedical science. Typical causes of illness include infections, injuries and problems within the body's systems. Mechanisms are usually at a biological level, although more attention is being given to the role of lifestyle and psychological factors. Treatment tends to fall into the categories of medicine (drugs), manipulation (including surgery), diet and rest. When modern medicine fails, people often seek alternative models that may promise more positive outcomes.

Outside of Western cultures, explanatory models may be based on different philosophies. Traditional Chinese medicine bases much of its explanatory model on balance within the person; for example, between hot and cold, and motion and stability. In such a model, treatment aims to restore balance. However, a recent study with Chinese men with HIV reported that 42.5% expressed some endorsement of belief in a supernatural explanatory model (a higher power that influences their health and treatment outcomes) (Pan et al., 2020).

Explanatory model
Perceptions and expectations about health and illness, including causes and mechanisms, timing, future course and outcome, and appropriate treatment.

In some African cultures, illness may be viewed as the manifestation of witchcraft. In such a model, the first step in treatment is identification of the source of the curse, followed by intervention to remove it. It surprises some people to discover that models based on witchcraft can often easily accommodate modern medicine. Modern medicine may provide an explanation for the symptoms while witchcraft is still seen as providing the cause—the curse made the individual catch the infection. In this case, the treatment might be to placate the witch who applied the curse, and complete a course of antibiotics. As the recommendations provided by the two explanatory models do not actually contradict one another, both can be followed.

Closely linked to the biopsychosocial-spiritual model of health (discussed in Chapter 1) is the Indigenous world view of health. Elements that build on the biopsychosocial model include First Peoples' connection to Country as the basis of their understanding of health (Best & Fredericks, 2014). Country is not just a location and way of life, but an identity relationship for First Peoples that represents each moiety (group). Each group has different stories about the creation of elements in their landscapes, as well as a vast array of words (languages) used to describe these places and events. For First Peoples, health is tied to Country and to the social, emotional and cultural well-being of not only an individual but the whole community. First Peoples have a whole-of-life view that includes a cyclical concept of life-death-life (Commonwealth of Australia, 2013; Wettasinghe et al., 2020). First Peoples' ceremonies and the Dreaming establish behavioural standards and ideals as well as instructions on how to respect sacred places, and preserve the land and its inhabitants. Lessons taught through ceremonies have clear links to the concepts of communal well-being and environmental protection and connection. Traditional teaching by Elders includes understanding how to preserve land fertility, reduce fire hazards and maintain adequate numbers of animals, birds, insects and fish (as both food supplies for hunting and a way to achieve balanced ecosystems and health) (Australian Museum, 2021).

The biopsychosocial-spiritual model of health is discussed in Chapter 1.

It is important to understand that not all people share a common set of beliefs about health. This is particularly true within multicultural societies such as Australia, where there can be a significant potential for misunderstanding and conflict.

PAUSE & REFLECT

Think of some common symptoms, such as pain and tiredness.

How is the meaning of symptoms influenced by culture?

14.2 CASE STUDY

MRS MECIR (CONT.)

While it is extremely unlikely that ethnicity alone played a part in Mrs Mecir's health problem, gender and cultural factors may influence her condition in a variety of ways. For example, culture has a clear influence on her diet. The fact that Mrs Mecir is a recent immigrant and has significant household responsibilities will influence her stress levels, which may affect her condition directly or indirectly. Culture will also affect her sense of responsibility to her family, her view of appropriate roles for females within her community, and her beliefs about health. These are all important influences on her thinking about her abdominal pain.

She may see her pain as being within the acceptable range for health and simply tolerate it. Or she may treat herself using traditional methods, or seek medical help. She might even see her pain as a matter to be dealt with through faith, and use prayer. She may consider stomach and bowel problems as too intimate and embarrassing to discuss.

1   How might Mrs Mecir's perceptions of her abdominal pain affect her behaviour?
2   What factors might influence her ability to obtain care from a health professional?

Three-tier system of socialisation

Shared features of cultural behaviour form our core values and beliefs, but how do we come to 'know' these values and beliefs? **Socialisation** theory operates on the idea that adults want to pass their knowledge of traditional beliefs, values and ways of understanding to the next generation. Some researchers refer to a two-tiered system of socialisation—within the family (internal influences) and outside the family unit (external influences). Others pose a six-tier system that breaks down tertiary agents into subgroups. Here we consider the three-tiered system of primary, secondary and tertiary **agents of socialisation**.

PRIMARY AGENTS OF SOCIALISATION

The primary agent of socialisation is the family, where a child learns how to interact with their environment. From birth, a child learns about who provides care and they develop a sense of attachment with that person(s), who is usually a parent. Through family life, a child learns the fundamental rules of safety and danger (e.g. not touching the hot stove, safe storage of medications) and right and wrong. They model the behaviours they see in others. While most influences in these formative years are positive, having been generated by prosocial role models, adverse childhood experiences can contribute to a poor sense of safety and security and have life-long negative health consequences.

Prosocial influences (positive or protective factors) are those perceived to add value or create advantages that are beneficial to the individual and society overall. **Anti-social influences** (negative or risk factors) exert negative influences and increase the risk of disadvantage. Anti-social behaviours include illicit drug use and criminal activities (e.g. wilful damage with graffiti, underage drinking).

The family also educates members about a shared understanding of health and illness. Some families are relatively tolerant of complaints about feeling unwell, while others are intolerant. Most families have knowledge about health problems that have affected their members, and this may sensitise the family to certain symptoms. If a father suffered from asthma when he was a child, for example, he may be more watchful for signs of breathlessness and wheezing in his own children. If several members have had a particular kind of cancer, others in the family may watch for signs, or change their diet or behaviour to try to prevent its occurrence.

Most family explanatory models of health and illness work in much the same way as those of others in the broader culture (i.e. explaining cause, modes of treatment), but models

Socialisation
The process of learning the culture of a society or group, its language and customs.

Agents of socialisation
External influences that establish and reinforce norms of expected behaviour and therefore shape an individual's characteristics.

Prosocial influences
Positive or protective factors that add value or create advantage.

Anti-social influences
Negative influences on a person's well-being.

can also differ quite considerably. There may be family rituals based on habit or traditions passed down from earlier generations. Individual members may have had experiences of successful or unsuccessful treatments, which may add to a family's model.

Families regulate access of members to health care. Parents decide when children are sick, when they are sick enough to see a health professional, and which health professional will be seen. In most families in high-income countries, parents have responsibility for health matters. In other cultures, health may be a religious matter and regulated by the family's religious authority.

PAUSE & REFLECT

Think about some of the illness prevention strategies used in your family when you were a child.

Are there any identified events that confirmed or altered your approach to health, help-seeking and management of health conditions in adulthood?

SECONDARY AGENTS OF SOCIALISATION

The impact of developmental milestones and rites of passage are discussed in Chapter 2.

Secondary agents of socialisation involve the environment outside of family. Around the age of five, many children commence primary school. This environment brings new exposures such as rules that have not been encountered before; for example, raising a hand and waiting for permission to speak, or new eating routines. As the child socialises (interacts with others in ever-expanding environments) they are socialised (learn the rules and regulations) about the norms of behaviour in those circumstances. As the child progresses into high school, different factors pose an impact.

During adolescence, most teenagers take an interest in music and social media. In Australia, around 99% of teenagers aged 15 to 17 reported access to a smartphone and spending an average of 18 hours per week on the internet (ABS, 2018b). Interacting with technology and networking and socialising with peers are important agents of socialisation. Smart technologies are quickly shaping socio-cultural practices (Briziarelli, 2019). Social media platforms can be used to educate, promote and popularise health behaviours through peer influence. This is an example of a value-adding or prosocial consequence. However, Shin et al. (2020) found that adolescents were more susceptible than older adults to continuous advertising on social platforms because of their social media usage patterns, which could be seen as a negative consequence.

TERTIARY AGENTS OF SOCIALISATION

Tertiary agents of socialisation include environments such as university, work, sporting participation and other recreational and social activist groups (e.g. Greenpeace, environment protection, political groups), along with charity and welfare activities. Tertiary agents represent the wider world and contain the most diverse influences—both prosocial and anti-social.

Events that occurred during the COVID-19 pandemic provide salient examples of tertiary agents of socialisation. Our socialisation practices were negatively impacted by lockdown requirements, social distancing and the wearing of personal protective equipment such as masks. The concept of personal space changed. Whereas once we smiled, hugged or shook hands as a greeting, this changed to masking our face and drastically minimising our physical contact.

Maintenance of these new behaviours was reinforced not only by family influences (e.g. parents restricting children's activities, and reminders to wash hands frequently) but also by society—people reminded others to maintain social distancing and avoid physical contact. Even after restrictions were lifted, many of the legal enforcements remained in place, such as the requirement to prove full vaccination against COVID-19 before accessing community places.

Health care as a culture

As most countries become progressively multicultural, health care must account for a variety of explanatory models and value systems. However, health care providers form subcultures within the larger community with their own values and beliefs. Conflicts over what is acceptable health care practice inevitably arise between health professionals and other groups within society.

Some conflicts involve the beliefs or behaviours of some groups that are seen as medically unjustifiable by most health professionals. A dramatic example includes female genital mutilation. Other conflicts involve practices that are seen as acceptable or best practice by health professionals but are opposed by small or large groups within society. These include autopsies, abortion, blood transfusions, birth control, organ transplants, in vitro fertilisation, inoculation programs and fluoridation of the water supply.

In Western societies, health professionals accept scientific evaluation as the dominant model for determining standards of good practice (**evidence-based health care**), and follow laws and regulations for the provision of safe care. Complementary treatments—whether they involve herbal medications, acupuncture or physical therapies—are required to meet the same tests of validity and efficacy as new medical treatments. As evidence-based health care becomes the standard for evaluating treatments, some traditional procedures have been banned or regulated, while many others have been accepted and incorporated into best practice.

Evidence-based health care
The view that all clinical practice should be based on evidence from randomised controlled trials to ensure treatments are effective and better than a placebo.

PAUSE & REFLECT

Behaviours associated with the COVID-19 pandemic have become commonplace and therefore shape our daily lives.

To what extent has a contemporary pandemic culture resulted?

CULTURAL SAFETY IN HEALTH CARE

In addition to providing evidence-based health care, all registered health professionals in Australia are required to practise in ways that are culturally safe (AHPRA, 2018). Cultural safety involves non-Indigenous health professionals working in partnership with First Peoples to help address significant health disparities (AHPRA, 2018). Practice standards for cultural safety are critical to eliminating institutional racism in health care. A recent review of 16 discipline-specific Codes of Conduct found that most health disciplines combined cultural safety practices for First Peoples with the needs of culturally and linguistically diverse communities (Milligan et al., 2021). The exceptions were nursing and midwifery. This catch-all approach to cultural safety is inappropriate.

Cultural safety is underpinned by a social justice framework. To become culturally safe, every health professional needs to undertake personal reflection to examine how race, whiteness and privilege contribute to First Peoples' health disadvantage, understand the effects of colonial ideology on the health care system, and identify how they can stop racism (Mills & Creedy, 2019). Cultural awareness (the first step in the process towards becoming culturally safe) acknowledges difference and contributes to cultural sensitivity (building on the awareness of difference through cultural acceptance, respect and understanding) (Mills et al., 2021). Cultural safety is therefore a holistic and shared approach to health care, where First Peoples feel safe and are treated with dignity.

Inequalities and inequities

The range of social factors discussed in this chapter often create challenges or barriers to a person's well-being and participation in society. The terms **inequity** and **inequality** are often used interchangeably, but they are distinct from one another. Inequity refers to "unfair, avoidable differences arising from poor governance, corruption or cultural exclusion" (Global Health Europe, cited by Goh, 2017, p. 356). This means that an action has purposely created difference. Inequality refers to the "uneven distribution of health or health resources as a result of genetic or other factors or the lack of resources" (Global Health Europe, cited by Goh, 2017, p. 356). This means there is an unequal distribution, which disadvantages one or more groups. A pictorial example on how to address differences in terms of inequality and inequity is provided in Figure 14.1.

Inequity
Unfair, avoidable differences arising from poor governance, corruption or cultural exclusion.

Inequality
The uneven distribution of health or health resources as a result of genetic or other factors or the lack of resources.

FIGURE 14.1 Equality vs equity

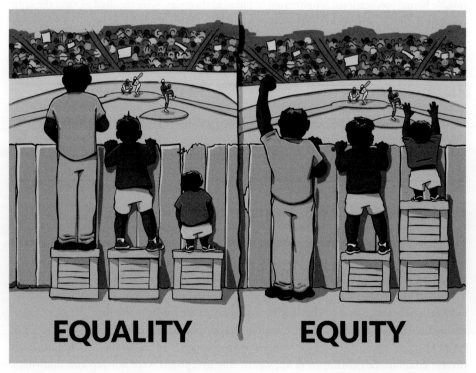

EQUALITY   EQUITY

IISC (n.d.)

Social determinants of health

Inequity and inequality in health outcomes and care access are influenced by a range of factors. Social determinants of health include socio-economic differences, behaviour, geography, social selection, race, disability and gender.

SOCIO-ECONOMIC

Socio-economic status (SES) is one of the strongest predictors of health in industrial nations (Wouk et al., 2021). Across many countries, and racial and cultural groups, it has been observed that the higher an individual's income, the better their health. This includes outcomes related to infant mortality, heart disease, infections, cancer and respiratory problems.

Although the work activities of poorer-paid jobs may involve more physical effort, this is usually not the healthier aerobic kind of exercise that produces the most health benefit. The work in poorer-paid positions tends to be less interesting and more repetitive. People on low incomes also tend to drive older, less maintained cars, resulting in an increased risk of accidents and injuries in getting to and from work.

BEHAVIOUR

For whatever reason, health-related behaviours of individuals from different socio-economic classes can, and do, differ. Diet, for example, can be dictated by social class, with individuals on lower incomes eating less fruit and fibre and more fried food. Inexpensive ways of making uninteresting but cheap food more palatable include frying it and adding salt but this increases dietary fat and sodium intake (McKay et al., 2019). Poor nutrition or overreliance on fat-laden and nutrient-poor fast foods contribute to obesity (Ridoutt et al., 2019).

While we think of Australia as a high-income (developed) nation, it may be confronting to realise that some people experience food insecurity (O'Kane, 2020). Food insecurity occurs when individuals cannot access either the quantity or quality of food necessary for a healthy and active life (Bowden, 2020). Food insecurity is clearly linked to reduced health outcomes. For example, poorly nourished children have impaired development and poorer educational achievement than well-nourished children.

GEOGRAPHY AND LIVING CONDITIONS

Australia may be considered a land of extremes, with a geographically diverse population ranging from high-density metropolitan, through regional to rural, remote and very remote areas (ABS, 2021b). Globally, while Australia is seen as having a world-class health system, there is a clear divide in the provision of basic health care to city-based and remote area populations (Bourke et al., 2021). Cardiovascular disease, for example, is higher among Australians with low socio-economic status and in regional areas (Jacobs et al., 2018). Families and individuals with less income tend to have poorer physical and social living conditions (Markham & Biddle, 2018). Old or damp buildings, high population density, urban fringe location and environmental pollution all tend to make housing cheaper, but also less healthy. There are fewer educational, recreational and work choices in areas where people on restricted incomes live (Frier & Devine, 2020).

SOCIAL SELECTION

Social selection is based on the assumption that society filters people according to a variety of characteristics. The fittest, tallest, strongest individuals are more likely to experience better life circumstances, including health care. Access to education by means of a scholarship or sponsorship also produces access to better health. Conversely, disadvantaged groups—such as those who face discrimination based on race or ethnicity, those living with a disability, or those with a mental health condition—tend to be 'selectively' downwardly mobile.

RACE: FIRST PEOPLES

Australia's First Peoples continue to experience significant adverse health outcomes. The latest Australian Burden of Disease study (2018–19) (AIHW, 2018c) reported that Indigenous health and well-being remains lower than the national average. Male First Peoples have a life expectancy of 71.6 years compared with 80.2 for non-Indigenous Australian males, and females have a life expectancy of 75.6 years compared with 83.4 (AIHW, 2021b). While there are many causal factors, the gap is influenced by behaviour, geography, living conditions and resource access and allocation. The leading illnesses and diseases among First Peoples are mental health and substance disorders, injuries and suicide, cardiovascular disease, cancer and respiratory disease (AIHW, 2021c). While the *Closing the Gap* report in 2021 identified some improvements through Indigenous-led policy developments and service delivery, the prevalence of complex issues such as suicide continues to be high (AHRC, 2021). An example of a successful Indigenous-led health service is the Deadly Ears program in Queensland, that aims to reduce hearing loss in children. Hearing impairment is frequently associated with difficulties in speaking, delayed learning, poor academic achievement and subsequent unemployment as an adult. Without intervention, a ripple effect has an exponential impact that maintains a state of disadvantage throughout the lifespan (Guenther, 2021).

The challenges faced by people with a disability are discussed in Chapter 5.

DISABILITY

In the last decade, greater recognition has been given to supporting people living with disability and the need for inclusive practices facilitated by legislation. In Australia, around 4.4 million people live with some form of disability; that is, a chronic impairment that restricts everyday living (ABS, 2018a). People living with disability continue to experience lower community participation, reduced education and employment opportunities, and ultimately reduced health outcomes (AIHW, 2019).

Disability is an overarching term for a variety of conditions, each impacting on individuals in different ways. Disabilities are categorised according to communication, physical, sensory and intellectual impairments. People living with disability may have challenges with visible and less obvious health conditions, as discussed in Chapter 5. An invisible disability such as intellectual impairment may not always receive the acceptance or allowances made for the rights and obligations of the sick role (Howie et al., 2021). **Communication disabilities** occur when a person is not able to speak or has difficulty speaking or sequencing thoughts or is non-verbal. **Physical disabilities** are conditions that reduce a person's mobility, stamina and agility; they include neurological conditions (e.g. cerebral palsy and post-stroke syndrome), missing or deformed limbs and reduced

Communication disabilities
Inability to or difficulty with speaking or sequencing thoughts, or being non-verbal.

Physical disabilities
Reduced mobility, stamina and agility; neurological conditions; missing or deformed limbs; and reduced muscle mass or bone strength.

muscle mass or bone strength. **Sensory disabilities** affect vision, hearing, tactile, olfactory and taste responses. **Intellectual disabilities** can affect learning, problem-solving, logic, impulse control and reasoning.

In addition to legislative efforts such as the *Disability Discrimination Act 1992* and provision of funding for additional support through the National Disability Insurance Scheme (NDIS), simply increasing public awareness will increase the health literacy of the general public and facilitate greater understanding of the contributions of people living with disability.

GENDER

Gender has a complex effect on health and the equity of care. In this section we use 'female' and 'male' as biological classifications, unrelated to gender identity which may change over a person's life. At any age of life, females are more likely to be sick, but males are more likely to die. Several factors contribute to this imbalance, partially related to the age of the individuals as well as their gender. Early in life, male babies are very slightly more prone than female babies to a variety of genetic and biological problems. At this stage, the male death rate is only very slightly higher than the female death rate.

During childhood and into adulthood, gender differences tend to relate more to differences in behaviour than to biology. Male children are more prone to accidents than female children because of different preferences for activities or differences in physical development. Later, males are more likely than females to be involved in risky behaviours, including working in riskier environments (e.g mining or construction) and playing dangerous sports. They are also more likely to have a poorer diet, become overweight, and have riskier drinking and smoking behaviours than females (AIHW, 2019).

As a generalisation, females appear to take better care of their health and are more likely to seek professional help when ill. This may be because females are more likely to be responsible for taking children or elderly relatives to the doctor, which could lead to feeling comfortable in that setting. Pregnancy and childbirth can expose females to some health risks (e.g. high blood pressure, gestational diabetes, surgery); however, their more frequent interactions with health care professionals may lead to a better level of lifestyle advice than males receive during the equivalent adult years of life.

Sensory disabilities
Impaired vision, hearing, tactile, olfactory and taste responses.

Intellectual disabilities
Difficulties with learning, problem-solving, logic, impulse control and reasoning.

PAUSE & REFLECT

Consider the major factors that influence differences in health and death rates between females and males.

What can be done to change them?

Should they be changed, or are there actually advantages to society in allowing some of these differences to exist?

Differences in male and female death rates lead to an increasing predominance of females over males as people get older. In middle age, there are slightly more females than males (ABS, 2019b). Among the very old—say, greater than 100 years of age—the proportion of males is only about 10%. This longer survival for females means that they need a different kind and level of care than males. Hip fractures provide a good case. Most hip fractures occur among the elderly; since most of the elderly are female, they would benefit from calcium supplements, regular weight-bearing exercise and screening for bone density.

Lifespan development is addressed in Chapters 2 and 3.

Differences in treatment can also arise from a variety of factors. Health professionals may treat females and males differently, even when the problem is the same. Also, males may be less likely than females to seek and to accept social support, thereby missing out on an important contributor to health and well-being. Within some cultural groups, women's access to health care is controlled by fathers, husbands or brothers; women in those groups may be denied needed care for reasons of modesty, because they are considered not worthy of the expenditure, or from fear that they may lose their value as workers.

14.3 CASE STUDY

BELINDA AND SOCIAL DETERMINANTS OF WELL-BEING DURING PREGNANCY

This case study explores the social determinants that increase the likelihood of poor health outcomes for First Peoples. With a focus on maternal mental health during childbearing, it aims to identify how this mother's experience differs from the experiences of non-Indigenous mothers.

Belinda is a 17-year-old woman of the Kalkadoon people who live in the area around Mt Isa in the Gulf region of Queensland. Officially she has completed Year 10, but her reading and numeracy skills are poor due to absenteeism from school. She has never been in paid employment. She is one of 10 people who live in the house. Most of the adult members of the family receive Centrelink payments. Her parents are heavy drinkers and two years ago her father was involved in a fight. He caused grievous bodily harm to a hotel owner and is currently serving three years in prison. Belinda had a boyfriend, but they broke up when she became pregnant. He left the community and she has not heard from him since. Belinda drinks every day and smokes around 10 cigarettes, but she has been trying to cut down since she became pregnant. There is a health service near where Belinda lives. Belinda went to the clinic when she thought she was pregnant but has not been back. She said, "That nurse there, she was rude and told me I was stupid to get pregnant. She told me to stop smoking and don't come back until I do." Belinda's grandmother talks to her about the baby, and one day they walked into the bush to find some bush bananas which are good for mothers and babies.

At 32 weeks, Belinda was not feeling well. Investigations at the clinic identified that Belinda had a urinary tract infection, was anaemic (low red blood cell count) and had high blood pressure, all of which could threaten the safety of her baby. The Flying Doctor Service was available that day to take Belinda to Mt Isa and then to Townsville (the closest tertiary health provider) for care during her pregnancy. Belinda had never been away from her family and wanted the baby to be born on Country. But she was told that if she did not go, the baby would not survive.

1   What are some of the immediate and long-term medical and psychosocial implications of Belinda's decision? Should she have choices about where and how she gives birth? If not, why not?

2   What are the social, psychological and spiritual factors contributing to the health and well-being of Belinda and her baby?

Implications of inequalities for health care: Challenges for the individual

Most societies regard health as something to which everyone has an equal entitlement. The World Health Organization has long had a policy of 'Health for All'. Ensuring equity in health, however, may be very difficult to achieve. The health of most people living in Australia has improved due to better control of infectious diseases, increasing life expectancy from birth and decreasing death rates from coronary heart disease and stroke as well as downward trends in deaths from lung, colorectal and breast cancer (AIHW, 2021d). However, health gains have not been shared equally between population subgroups. Each kind of disadvantage discussed in the previous section contributes to the likelihood of others also occurring. For example, no single factor explains all health disadvantages faced by the world's Indigenous peoples. However, many of these disadvantages directly affect an individual's ability to access important resources related to health.

PAUSE & REFLECT

Many Indigenous peoples, including First Peoples, Māori in New Zealand, First Nations in Canada and Native Americans in the US have poorer health than non-Indigenous people in those countries.

What are some of the common factors that all Indigenous peoples share that may help to explain this observation?

If we allocate resources in the same way across all individuals and groups, there are vast differences in outcomes. Allocating scarce resources, where, when and to who they are needed most, facilitates more advantageous, cooperative and negotiated outcomes. In this way, equal outcomes should eventuate. Changing health systems to create cultural inclusion and acceptance can be achieved by individuals gaining a greater voice and implementing a coordinated group-action approach. For example, adjustments by health services could accommodate First Peoples' sense of community and cultural practices. Grief customs within First Peoples communities indicate that when one member is nearing the time of death, as many people from that community as possible will visit that person in their final days (Best & Fredericks, 2014; Berman et al., 2021). Rather than limiting the number of visitors (which is usual hospital policy), arrangements could be made for care to be offered in the home and for support to be encouraged.

This kind of intervention builds **social capital** within society. Working in a respectful partnership with recipients of health care services increases the trust that people have in one another, in government institutions within their society and in the health professions. This increase in trust is associated with a willingness to cooperate for the mutual benefit of all. Where social capital is low, cooperation is less likely; individuals will tend to fight for their own interests and hoard their own resources rather than work for the interests of the whole social group.

Social capital
The level of trust people have in one another, government institutions and the health professions.

Could differences in social capital help in understanding the different reactions of people living in areas that suffered disasters?

Health professionals encounter a wide cross-section of people when providing care, and these interactions require insight into the person's life. To develop therapeutic relationships with users of health services, is it necessary for health professionals to understand a person's capabilities, vulnerabilities, motivators, strengths and challenges. Equally important is for the health professional to be aware of their own potential bias and prejudice. All individuals function within complex social environments, and our interactions with others impact on our own sense of who we are and our well-being to varying degrees.

Professional development and education enable us to gain an understanding of diverse and often contrasting cultural perspectives to which we may not have been previously exposed. This learning and understanding can be translated across different practice environments. As discussed in Chapter 1, a contemporary care framework (i.e. client-centred care within a biopsychosocial model) involves the consumer/client as the focus and most important contributor, as well as input from significant others in their life such as family carers and support workers. Understanding a client's needs and providing interventions that align with their goals, beliefs and values as well as their capacities, facilitates optimal health outcomes and promotes equity and equality.

The biopsychosocial model of care is discussed in Chapter 1.

14.4 CASE STUDY

JING AND YAN

Jing is 15 and his older brother Yan is 18. Both attend the local high school, and work in the family business each evening and on weekends. Jing and Yan were born in Australia. Their parents, along with their paternal grandmother, immigrated from China 20 years ago. The youths are accomplished musicians and have played the piano and violin from an early age. The parents hope their sons will enter university and study medicine. Jing and Yan achieve very high grades at school and excel in mathematics, physics and chemistry.

Apart from working in their restaurant, the parents do not have much outside social contact. At home, the family speaks Mandarin as the mother has struggled to speak English fluently. Recently, the mother developed a gynaecological condition and she now attends frequent medical appointments. The grandmother, who lives with the family, is elderly and has multiple health issues. Both women rely on Yan or Jing to accompany them to medical appointments and act as the translator. The boys are frustrated with their mother and grandmother who, despite being prescribed medication, often do not follow the doctors' advice. Instead, they use traditional Chinese medicines and acupuncture to address their health concerns.

Yan recently gained his driver's licence and bought a late model sports car from his savings. He and Jing are enjoying the newfound freedom that the car offers. Lately, both Jing and Yan have changed their style of dress from their usual black trousers and white shirts; they now tend to wear designer jeans with distressed contemporary styling, and t-shirts depicting popular music and social logos. Yan is planning to get a tattoo soon. He also has a girlfriend who, until recently, he had been seeing without his family's knowledge. The discovery that he is dating has caused problems in the family as his mother does not want Yan to be distracted from his studies. Further, Yan's mother does not approve of his girlfriend as she is from a different ethnicity.

1   What stereotypes of cultural indicators are depicted here?

2   There are indicators of a generational or cultural clash. What contributed to these differences?

3   What challenges are faced by the youths, the parents and the grandmother?

CHAPTER SUMMARY

Learn more
Access additional resources to broaden your understanding of this chapter. See the Guided Tour for access details.

- Culture is a dynamic concept. It reflects shared behaviours and characteristics exhibited by individuals to then form a group.

- Agents of socialisation are commonly termed primary, secondary and tertiary.

- Through self-reflection and critical analysis, we shape our own values and beliefs. We may reaffirm core values and beliefs, consider challenges to our understanding and shape new practices.

- Our self-esteem and concept of who we are is shaped from a range of social influences.

- The family serves as the main transmitter of cultural beliefs and values regarding health.

- Medicine needs to be understood as a culture with its own values and standards.

- Socio-cultural factors affect if, when, how, where and who we interact with to address our health needs.

- Socio-economic status has a strong impact on health, through behaviour, living standards and social selections, which interact with one another.

- The process of ensuring equity in health involves more than ensuring equity in health care. It may include steps to increase the total pool of health resources available or to ensure there is equal access to resources. Several factors—including location, travel, time and isolation—may have significant impacts on access.

FURTHER READING

Closing the Gap (2021) https://www.pc.gov.au/closing-the-gap-data/annual-data-report/2021

Godding R (2014) The persistent challenge of inequality in Australia's health. *Medical Journal of Australia* 201(8), 432. doi: 10.5694/mja14.c1020

Mills K & Creedy DK (2019) The 'pedagogy of discomfort': A qualitative exploration of student learning in a First Peoples health course. *Australian Journal of Indigenous Education* [online] 1–8. doi.org/10.1017/jie.2019.16

15 Health Literacy

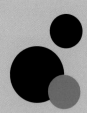

OXFORD UNIVERSITY PRESS

What is health literacy?

Health literacy is the ability to read, comprehend and use medical information to make health decisions and effectively use health care services (WHO, 2016). Health literacy affects the ways in which health information is accessed, understood and shared with others. It also affects the health and well-being of individuals and the delivery of health care services. While low health literacy is often linked with low education levels, along with ethnicity, age and ability to understand and communicate in English, it must not be seen as a reflection of an individual's intellectual ability or motivation to learn. Chapter 14 addressed similar factors that may act as barriers to health care; however, this chapter draws on cognitive psychology and learning theories to explain why some people may have difficulty learning, remembering and applying health information in their lives to make good decisions about their health.

There are over 20 different forms of literacy. Each of these types of literacy contributes to health. Fundamental skills in reading, numeracy, scientific, technological (e-Health) and cultural literacy are particularly important. Some forms of written and spoken medical/health information can be complex and not easily understood. Individuals with low literacy often have a reading ability equivalent to a 10-year-old child in Year 5. An individual who has limited reading ability may find it difficult to understand more complex words or phrases, and as a result they may take a long time to read a short passage or may misunderstand the meaning.

Scientific literacy refers to the ability to understand scientific (including medical) concepts. It would be difficult for a person to understand their cardiac condition, for example, if they have no or limited understanding of what the heart looks like, how it functions and how fat can build up in the blood vessels feeding the heart muscle, resulting in impaired blood flow and subsequent heart attacks.

Increasingly, various forms of information technology (e.g. the internet and mobile devices) are used to communicate health messages. Individuals who do not have the necessary skills to access, understand and critically review electronic sources of information are disadvantaged compared with those who do.

Electronic health (e-Health) literacy allows individuals to navigate through the vast (and sometimes misleading) web-based world. People increasingly use online health communities to learn about and manage their health, but there have been warnings about the quality and relevance of some shared information. One study of registered users of a popular online health site that used the e-Health-E scale (Neter et al., 2015) measured the extent to which respondents were aware of sources, recognised quality and meaning, understood information, perceived efficiency, validated information and "being smart on the Net" (Petric et al., 2017).

Based on e-Health-E scores and reported behaviour, participants were categorised as active help-seekers (49%), lurkers (31%), core relational users (17%) and low-engaged users (3%) (Petric et al., 2017). Active help-seekers had the highest scores in all areas. Core relational users performed worse on validating information and being smart on the Net but were more likely to post information than any other group. These findings highlight the need for health professionals to ask patients about their engagement with online sites and encourage them to check and be critical of posted information.

e-Health literacy can inform a person about health issues, community services in their area, and changes in government health policy that might affect the care or support they

Health literacy
The ability to read, comprehend and use medical information to make health decisions, and effectively interact with the health care system and health professionals.

Scientific literacy
The ability to understand scientific (including medical) concepts.

Electronic health (e-Health) literacy
The ability to navigate through the vast (and sometimes misleading) online world.

receive. Online information and e-Health communities can influence personal behaviours and choices and be far-reaching as they are not limited by geographic boundaries. Examples include choices about cigarette smoking and vaping in public places, or voluntarily being vaccinated against a range of diseases such as measles, influenza and coronavirus (COVID) strains.

While the scientific and medical consensus on the benefits of vaccination is clear and unambiguous, some people perceive vaccines as unsafe and unnecessary. The World Health Organization identified people's reluctance or refusal to vaccinate despite the availability of vaccines as one of the 10 top threats to global health in 2019. The negative influence of anti-vaccination movements is believed to increase vaccine resistance in the public. Two factors related to vaccine resistance are low health literacy levels and widespread misinformation (mostly designed to generate fear) through electronic (social media) channels. Health professionals must be aware of these influences in their practice, while respecting the rights of the individual to choose what they believe is best for themselves. Health professionals can attempt to shift a patient's beliefs and behaviours towards healthier options in a safe and culturally appropriate way.

Cultural literacy
The ability to identify, understand and respect the collective beliefs and customs of diverse groups in the community.

Cultural literacy refers to individuals' abilities to identify, understand and respect the collective beliefs and customs of diverse groups in the community (Zarcadoolas et al., 2006). For example, childbearing women of Chinese ethnicity commonly 'do the month' or *zuo yuezi* after giving birth. During this time, new mothers receive considerable social support from family such as the woman's mother, mother-in-law or other female relative. The woman is encouraged to rest, feed the baby and restore the lost *yang* (heat) to her body. All health professionals have a responsibility to practise cultural safety and must understand the influences of culture on patients' health beliefs and behaviours.

The role of culture in defining illness and reactions to illness is discussed in Chapters 1 and 4.

As outlined in Chapter 14, Australia's First Peoples continue to have poorer health outcomes than non-Indigenous Australians. A systematic review on the effectiveness of health literacy interventions with First Peoples (Nash & Arora, 2021) included only five studies, suggesting a lack of quality research in this area. Interventions included exercise classes, more affordable fruit and vegetables in order to improve nutrition, and raising awareness about oral health. All included studies reported some improvement; however, there was limited involvement of First Peoples in designing the interventions, participation rates were low, and few participants actually completed an intervention. New collaborative and co-designed interventions are needed to improve the health literacy of Australia's First Peoples and culturally and linguistically diverse groups.

Prevalence of poor health literacy in the community

Governments must have a vested interest in determining and improving health literacy in the community. Adequate levels of health literacy in the population reduce health care costs, prevent illness and chronic disease, and can reduce rates of accidents and death (AIHW, 2020c). The Adult Literacy and Life Skills Survey (ABS, 2009) measures the literacy of adults aged 15 to 74 and the results can be compared against those of the seven collaborating countries, which include Canada, Hungary and the US.

Skill levels are categorised from Level 1 (lowest) to Level 5 (highest). Skill Level 3 is regarded as the minimum required for individuals to meet the demands of everyday life. The 2009 survey found that 19% of adults had Level 1 health literacy skills and 40% had Level 2. These people had difficulty reading information on a medicine bottle to find out the maximum number of days the medicine should be taken, or drawing a line on a container to indicate where one-third would be. Only 41% of adults had adequate or better health literacy skills (Level 3 or above). At this level a person can combine written and numerical information (e.g. understanding data on a graph) to correctly assess the safety of a product for them (e.g. the recommended dose of a drug for their weight).

These disturbing results prompted the Australian Bureau of Statistics to conduct the **Health Literacy Questionnaire** in 2018. The Health Literacy Questionnaire reports a larger range of health literacy characteristics than the Adult Literacy and Life Skills Survey and is useful for individuals, practitioners/clinicians and policy-makers. There are 44 questions across nine domains of health literacy, with responses according to level of agreement ('Strongly agree' to 'Strongly disagree') or perceived difficulty ('Always easy' to 'Always difficult'). Each domain covers different aspects of individual, environmental and/or institutional health literacy. The questionnaire provides a broad picture of the functional, social and systemic factors that influence the health literacy of the population, rather than a level of health literacy (e.g. 'Adequate' or 'Low') (ABS, 2018c, ABS, 2019a; Osborne, 2013). The nine domains are:

Health Literacy Questionnaire
A national survey in Australia that measures the health literacy of adults aged 18 and older across nine different domains.

1 feeling understood and supported by health care providers;
2 having sufficient information to manage my health;
3 actively managing my health;
4 social support for health;
5 appraisal of health information;
6 ability to actively engage with health care providers;
7 navigating the health care system;
8 ability to find good health information;
9 understand health information well enough to know what to do.

A sample of 5790 adults (aged 18 and older) completed the Health Literacy Questionnaire. Overall, 91% of people strongly agreed or agreed that they could actively manage their health (Domain 3). Those who disagreed were more likely to be in poorer health, have less education, live alone and smoke cigarettes (ABS, 2019a). In regard to actively engaging with health care providers (Domain 6), 89% of people 'always found it easy or usually easy'. Those who disagreed were more likely to be older, have fair or poorer health, or a disability.

Around a quarter (26%) of people found it 'always easy' to navigate the health care system (Domain 7), but this was harder for people who were older or reported very high levels of psychological distress. While younger people predominantly had positive responses on the questionnaire, other research with younger people aged 13–25 identified that although they regularly sought online information, they reported it could be confusing and difficult to access (QFCC, 2019). They valued clear 'how to' instructions from sources such as YouTube. Formats such as podcasts and simple infographics could be viable solutions for future effective interventions.

15.1 CASE STUDY

ANNE AND UNDERSTANDING HEALTH RESEARCH ON HORMONE REPLACE-MENT THERAPY

Anne is 52 and experiencing symptoms associated with menopause. Her doctor prescribed hormone replacement therapy (HRT) three years ago. At the time, Anne recalled that the doctor told her the tablets were to reduce symptoms such as hot flushes and improve her mood so she would be less prone to tears and irritability. While driving to work one morning, she heard a radio news segment: "Researchers from the University of Queensland released a report that links HRT to ovarian cancer. Furthermore, recent trials that randomly assigned women to HRT or a placebo found that women on HRT were at increased risk for heart attack or stroke."

To better understand this information, Anne drew on her scientific and health knowledge from reading about health topics in magazines and online. Let us consider possible outcomes for Anne, depending on her health literacy level.

Limited health literacy. Anne decides she is satisfied with her tablets. Her symptoms reduced in frequency and intensity, although they did not disappear. Her mother never had HRT but nevertheless passed away from ovarian cancer. The news report annoys Anne, who thinks how scientists are always finding out that they did not know what they thought they knew. Consequently, she chooses to ignore the report. She does not discuss her risk of ovarian cancer during her next medical appointment for a new prescription for HRT.

Adequate health literacy. Anne knows that she has been on HRT for three years. Because her mother passed away from ovarian cancer, she knows that she has a higher risk of cancer herself. She is not sure what a placebo is, but decides to talk with her doctor about the news report during her scheduled appointment next month.

Good health literacy. Anne knows that long-term HRT may have associated health risks. She recognises that the news report discussed the findings of a well-conducted study by reputable researchers. Given that the report linked HRT and ovarian cancer, and that her mother died from ovarian cancer, Anne believes that she may be at increased risk (susceptibility) for this type of cancer. She does an online search for more information about HRT and ovarian cancer. She also makes an appointment to discuss her HRT protocol with her doctor in the next day or so, with a view to discussing her risk/s and possibly stopping the medication.

We can foresee different health outcomes for Anne, based on her level of health literacy. In the third scenario, as an informed consumer of health care services, Anne proactively looks after her health, seeks to keep informed about medical research and has a 'partnership' relationship with her GP. Her health outcomes are likely to be significantly better than if she had limited health literacy.

1   How could researchers and health professionals better convey important findings in the media?

2   From your reading about social inequalities and health in Chapter 14, what socio-cultural factors might positively influence Anne's level of health literacy?

3   What are the advantages for health professionals if they work with people (like Anne) who have good health literacy?

Socio-cultural factors associated with low health literacy

There are several social and cultural factors associated with health literacy. These factors include age, education, income, self-assessed health status, employment status, occupation, being born overseas, and birth language. Unfortunately, relatively few health professionals are aware that rates of health literacy vary with age, or they may assume that young or old adults are well informed about health matters. However, a study showed that around two-thirds of males and females aged 15–19 had inadequate or low health literacy (ABS, 2009). The proportion of people with low health literacy decreased to around half of all people aged 20–49, before increasing again in older age groups. Low health literacy in younger people may occur because they are still completing their education and have fewer health-related experiences to draw upon. Low health literacy levels in older age groups may be associated with the effects of age on information-processing skills, or fewer years of formal education.

Social and cultural factors in defining and reacting to illness are discussed in Chapters 1 and 4.

The relationship between education and health is well documented. People who complete higher levels of education are more likely to have higher rates of adequate health literacy (ABS, 2009). Around 75% of people with a bachelor's degree or higher have adequate to good health literacy compared with only 16% of people who finished their education at Year 10 (ABS, 2009). Generally, people with higher incomes have higher levels of education, as well as better health literacy skills. Like income, workforce status is influenced by educational attainment. Consequently, people employed in occupations requiring a high level of education and skill are more likely to have higher levels of health literacy.

People born overseas or whose first language is not English may have more difficulty understanding health information. In 2016, nearly 5 million Australians aged 15–74 spoke English as a second language (ABS, 2019a). Based on previous surveys, only 25% of this group will have adequate health literacy.

PAUSE & REFLECT

Think about when you began your program of study to become a health professional.

What terms were new to you? How did your classes help you to better understand and remember these medical/scientific terms or concepts?

What learning strategies have you employed to increase your health literacy levels?

Implications of low health literacy

There are several implications of low health literacy. Individuals with low health literacy may experience difficulty understanding what doctors, nurses, pharmacists and other health professionals tell them, as well as difficulty understanding written medical instructions. Even when individuals can access good health services, a lack of understanding of relevant information can make it challenging for them and their families to manage illness or a condition and to make informed decisions (UNESCO, 2016). Individuals with low health literacy are more likely to be hospitalised (Bourne et al., 2018). Importantly, people with low health literacy access less preventive health care (e.g. screening for cancer and cardiovascular disease) and are likely to attend emergency departments more often.

On a day-to-day basis, people with low health literacy may have trouble with a range of tasks that health professionals consider routine. Challenges can include getting a prescription filled, understanding information about how to take medication and its possible side effects, understanding appointment slips and reading a health promotion brochure. These routine skills are essential for a person to better understand and manage a health condition and be able to act on health-promoting information. According to the Australian Institute of Health and Welfare (AIHW 2020c), a person's health literacy influences behaviours such as:

- adopting healthier habits in their daily lives;
- responding appropriately to health-related information;
- sharing relevant information with health care providers;
- managing their own health;
- accessing available health and well-being services.

People with limited health literacy may feel ashamed about their lack of knowledge and skills and may not voluntarily speak up if they do not understand information provided to them (Wolfe et al., 2007). Unfortunately, many health professionals seriously underestimate or ignore patients' health literacy levels. To investigate health professionals' estimation of health literacy, researchers asked new parents with an infant about to be discharged from intensive care to complete a brief health literacy measure (Mackley et al., 2016). Attending nurses also rated parents' understanding about the discharge instructions. The study found that there was no relationship between parents' health literacy scores and nurses' perception of parental understanding, with nurses erroneously perceiving adequate comprehension in 83% of parents who scored low on the health literacy scale (Mackley et al., 2016).

Similarly, in an online survey of Australian midwives, most of them (77.1%, n = 221) gave little consideration to women's health literacy (Creedy et al., 2020a). This suggests that health literacy was deemed to be a low priority in the provision of care. Around 60% of respondents never or only sometimes used specific techniques to promote maternal health literacy. Importantly, 75% of the surveyed midwives had not received any prior education about health literacy.

The role of health professionals in promoting health and health literacy is discussed further in Chapter 16.

15.2 CASE STUDY

KAMALA AND DIABETES SELF-MANAGEMENT

Kamala was born in Singapore to Indian parents. At the age of 32 she migrated to Australia to take up a senior position with a multinational accounting firm. She is married and has two adult children. Due to her long hours at work and sedentary lifestyle, Kamala has noticed an incremental weight gain. Now aged 58, she weighs 86 kg and has a BMI (body mass index) of 30. Recently she has felt very thirsty throughout the day and night, urinated frequently and had extreme unexplained fatigue.

At the doctor's office, Kamala was given a brochure that contained information about diabetes: "According to the Australian Diabetes Association, diabetes is a disease in which the body does not produce or properly use insulin. Insulin is a hormone that is needed to convert sugar, starches and other food into energy needed for life. The cause of diabetes is a mystery, although both genetics and environmental factors appear to play important roles."

Kamala did not understand some of the terminology or scientific concepts in the brochure but agreed with her doctor's suggestion to have tests to confirm the provisional diagnosis of diabetes. She was referred to a diabetes clinic at the local hospital and had an appointment for the following day. That night Kamala searched online for more information. She learnt that some of her symptoms indicate diabetes, but she didn't understand what caused them. She decided to write down each symptom and learn about the related physiology, such as how the body produces insulin and the role of insulin in regulating the amount of sugar in the blood. Kamala accessed a medical dictionary online and looked up words that were unfamiliar to her. She found that type 2 diabetes is a chronic disease associated with physical inactivity, poor diet and excess body weight. She was shocked to see that she had all the risk factors.

The next day at the hospital clinic, Kamala had more tests and spoke with the endocrinologist about her condition. She was prescribed medication and told to change her diet and exercise regularly. She was also told to have her eyes checked and to take good care of her feet by going to a podiatrist; she was not told why. She then had a session with the clinic nurse who showed her how to measure her blood sugar (glucose) levels by pricking her finger (which hurt more than she thought it would) and testing the blood in a small device. Based on the reading, she then had to calculate how much insulin to inject. She was taught how to give herself an injection, which she found difficult. Five hours later, Kamala left the clinic and went to a chemist to purchase the blood glucose machine and have her prescription filled. By the end of the day she was exhausted and overwhelmed. She burst into tears when her husband asked how the day went.

1   After initially reading the passage on diabetes, Kamala didn't understand several words (e.g. 'insulin', 'hormone', 'properly convert'). Indeed, there are several key scientific concepts embedded in the case study. Identify these scientific concepts.

2   What could Kamala do to reduce the high level of stress she is experiencing?

3   What strategies could Kamala have used to remember all the information she was given throughout the day?

4   How could the clinic change its process to reduce stress and information overload for patients?

Points to consider

Kamala, like many others in similar circumstances, has a great deal to learn about her condition. Although patient education is considered a key component of diabetes care, studies show that many patients who have attended a diabetes education program, especially those with low health literacy, do not know the basis of their disease or essential self-management skills (Rafferty et al., 2021). For example, 50% of people with low health literacy did not know that all people have some glucose (sugar) in their blood. One reason may be that most diabetes self-management education programs introduce too much information in a complex manner. Often that information is not relevant to what a person needs to do on a day-to-day basis. Therefore, a person receiving this education will not retain essential information because it's not seen as useful to them.

Theoretical considerations to enhance health literacy

MEMORY AND COGNITIVE LOAD

Several steps must occur for learning to take place. According to Wolfe et al. (2011), a person must go through five steps (see Figure 15.1).

FIGURE 15.1 Five steps necessary for learning to take place

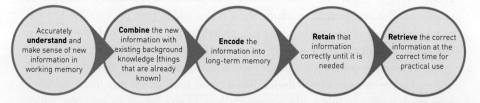

Learning
A change in understanding and/or behaviour that results from experience with the environment.

Schema
A mental map of ideas about a topic that is stored in long-term memory.

Learning can be defined as a change in long-term memory. When a person with a health condition successfully learns new information, this information is processed in working memory, combined with pre-existing knowledge, and placed into long-term memory as part of a connected system of ideas. The act of combining new and existing knowledge helps a person build mental **schemas** (Wolfe et al., 2011). A schema is a mental map of ideas about a topic or issue (e.g. the five steps presented in Figure 15.1). As a person encounters new information, they revise and update their existing schema. A new pattern of ideas is then encoded (stored) into long-term memory for retrieval at a later time when needed.

From cognitive psychology research, we know that **working memory** allows us to temporarily store and use information in short-term memory (Van Dyke et al., 2019). Working memory is critical in almost all complex cognitive tasks (e.g. reading, reasoning and problem-solving). These tasks require us to hold information in memory while doing something else or while being distracted by other stimuli.

For example, working memory helps a reader to focus on certain elements of what they are reading, as well as keeping track of and monitoring their understanding of information in the text. So, when you are reading a novel, you use your working memory to understand what you are reading in the third paragraph on the current page, but you also remember the key ideas in the previous paragraphs and previous pages and thus form a schema of the overall plot.

Working memory also allows individuals to ignore non-essential information and thus avoid cognitive overload. **Cognitive load** is how much information a person can keep in their working memory. Kamala, for example, complained of information overload when she was confronted with a lot of new information in a short space of time.

The capacity of the working memory is relatively fixed. Miller (1956) first reported that the maximum number of elements that a person could remember and manipulate was seven (plus or minus two). It is important to remember that the more a person has to learn in a short amount of time, the more difficult it is to process that information in working memory. Thus, communicating health information may need to be spaced out according to individual capabilities, including the level of health literacy. Ideally, a health professional would objectively assess the health literacy of a person, using relevant existing measures (Mackley et al. 2016), before providing complex health information.

The amount of information that can be stored in memory is much greater if the individual is familiar with the content being presented. This is because related information is already available in long-term memory. This stored information can be retrieved and placed into the working memory, allowing the individual to focus on making links between the new information and what they already know. People who have limited knowledge of a health topic will experience greater cognitive load when learning about the topic because all the information is new to them.

Although Kamala spent time researching her diabetic condition, most concepts would still be new to her. Looking up the information on the internet then discussing this newly acquired information at the diabetes clinic would have assisted her understanding and retention of key points. However, it would not guarantee full understanding and recall in one visit. Key ideas or concepts may need to be discussed with Kamala several times before she has adequate learning about her health condition.

Working memory can be expanded if the information is stored in schemas that can be recalled from the long-term memory (Simon et al., 2016). New health education should be presented in smaller blocks of information so that individuals can build comprehensive schemas of information that can be recalled and used later. People with low health literacy are less likely to use long-term memory because they have less background knowledge and no relevant schemas to draw on, compared with individuals who have higher literacy (Wolfe et al., 2011). This does not mean that they are less intelligent; rather, they may have had limited prior exposure to ideas about health, physiology and blood chemistry that are relevant to their health condition.

New basic concepts need to be learnt and understood by an individual before they can process further new knowledge and apply it when managing their health condition.

Working memory
Information that is stored temporarily for short-term use.

Memory and learning are discussed in detail in Chapters 6 and 7.

Cognitive load
The amount of information kept in the working memory.

Teaching strategies to help Kamala form appropriate mental schemas could include having a plan or an overview of key topics to be learnt, using diagrams to explain key concepts, encouraging her to take notes and ask questions, and the health professional checking understanding before communicating more detailed information. Kamala could have been given printed materials to take home, information about useful online sites and a written summary of key points. There are different types of learning preferences: read/write, visual, auditory, kinesthetic or multimodal. It is important to determine which type of learning preference best suits each individual. Tools such as the VARK questionnaire (https://vark-learn.com/the-vark-questionnaire/) may be helpful.

MASTERY LEARNING

Mastery learning theory (Bloom, 1968) proposes that people learn at different rates but can master material if given multiple opportunities to process and practise information. Although the amount an individual can learn in a given time is relatively fixed, with repetition, most people can achieve mastery. It is essential to go through four key steps in a cyclical manner, as demonstrated in Figure 15.2.

Mastery influences self-efficacy beliefs and behaviour, as discussed in Chapter 7.

FIGURE 15.2 Mastery learning

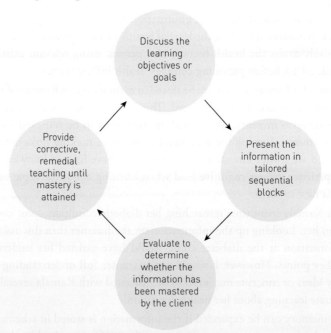

Mastery learning
The repetition of a task until learning occurs.

The importance of **mastery learning** was demonstrated in a study that examined the number of times patients needed information to be repeated in order to understand informed consent (Sudore et al., 2006). Informed consent must always be obtained by a health professional before conducting an invasive procedure on a patient. The individual indicates in writing that they have been informed about what the procedure involves and of the risks involved. All participants in the study mastered the material: 28% achieved mastery on their first attempt, 52% after two attempts and 20% required three or more repetitions. Importantly, people with adequate health literacy were more likely to achieve mastery on the first attempt.

INTERVENTIONS TO ENHANCE HEALTH LITERACY

Sheridan et al. (2011) undertook a systematic review of 38 published studies that tested the effectiveness of interventions for people with low health literacy. They concluded that four specific design features of an intervention improved comprehension:

1 presenting essential information either by itself or first in a list;

2 presenting information so that the higher numbers represent better outcomes;

3 adding graphics to numerical information (e.g. a cartoon figure of a person where one figure represents 100 people);

4 adding visual resources (e.g. media clips, YouTube segments) to verbal discussions of topics.

The review also identified that interventions about self-care and disease management delivered in a shorter timeframe (intensive mode, e.g. four sessions in a week rather than one session a week) reduced the likelihood of the disease getting worse. People who received health education in an intensive way also had fewer emergency department visits and hospitalisations. However, the extent to which the interventions were effective in changing other health outcomes (e.g. adherence to health screening follow-ups) was not clear. The review concluded that interventions with multiple components showed most promise for addressing low health literacy in clinical practice. Multiple components include discussions, media clips, pictures, diagrams and practice sessions for skill development.

Self-care is discussed in Chapter 5.

Common features of effective interventions that are likely to increase understanding of health information are frequent sessions within a shorter timeframe, using a framework (from learning theories) to inform the design of the intervention, doing a pilot test to identify any problems early on, an emphasis on skill-building, and delivery by an expert health professional such as a pharmacist or a health educator.

The results also indicated the importance of first assessing a person's level of literacy and then discussing the best approach for them, rather than offering universal interventions (Sheridan et al., 2011). This means tailoring each health education session to the needs of the individual, rather than offering the same information and strategies to everyone in the same way. Other successful features included using simplified text and teach-back approaches.

Teach-back is a useful strategy for improving the understanding and recall of health information among people with low literacy (Dinh et al., 2016). It is a learning cycle, as demonstrated in Figure 15.3.

Teach-back
A learning cycle involving repetition and reinforcement of new learning.

Teach-back is an effective way to support long-term learning because it slows down the learning process and allows for repetition and reinforcement of new information. Cognitive experiments have shown that repeating short sequences of information helps to activate the memory dedicated to storage and recall of information.

FIGURE 15.3 Teach-back learning cycle

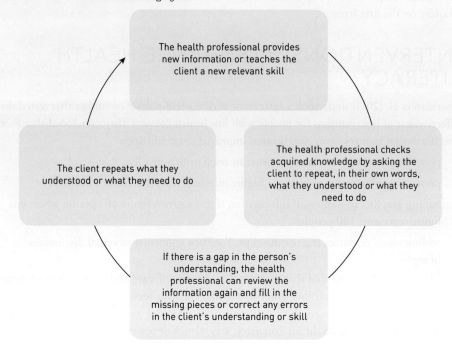

GUIDING PRINCIPLES FOR INTERVENTIONS TO ENHANCE HEALTH LITERACY

Some guiding principles for effective interventions were proposed by Baker and colleagues (2011).

1   *Establish a defined set of learning goals and develop the learning program.* There needs to be a limited set of learning goals for any educational program or set of materials. There is often a tendency to try to cover too much information. All information in a health education program should explain a behaviour, provide background information to understand a recommended behaviour (i.e. explain the underlying scientific concept) or promote attitude change about the behaviour (e.g. explain how the behaviour helps the person). It may be helpful to work backwards in order to identify what information is necessary so that the individual can understand the concept and change their behaviour.

2   *Present information in discrete units.* A health education program should be divided into simple units of learning. The plan needs to be logical, easily understood and memorable. The program should start with behaviours that could prevent deterioration in the condition (what the person needs to do to stay well) and finish with the most crucial behaviours for monitoring their condition and maintaining their well-being. People are more likely to remember information if they are presented with only a few key points rather than a lot of content. This approach reduces information overload.

3   *Determine the optimal order for each topic.* The order of content needs to prepare learners for what is to follow.

4   *Use simple language.* Using simple language to explain essential concepts is important, but there are other considerations as well. The information needs to be presented in an

organised way (see point 1). Consideration needs to be given to the amount of information presented (point 2) and background information needs to be provided first (point 3).

5   *Use pictorial aids*. Different forms of graphics (e.g. diagrams, media and animations) can be used to increase understanding and recall. Individuals with low health literacy may have limited reading fluency. They typically read slowly, struggle with individual words and phrases and may not grasp the meaning of a sentence or paragraph. Graphics can assist understanding by presenting complex concepts in a visual format. The saying 'A picture paints a thousand words' is useful—in health education, a picture can be far easier to understand and remember than words.

6   *Confirm mastery of learning goals*. Health professionals should confirm the person's understanding after each session, perform corrective or remedial instruction until mastery is attained, and review learnt concepts until the person consistently masters the task. Learning could be checked through teach-back methods.

7   *Link information to behaviour change*. Knowledge, skills and behaviours need to be closely linked. This approach, known as **teach to goal**, involves the clear identification of information and skills that an individual needs to learn in order to change their behaviour. All too often, health education interventions deliver information but do not teach the associated behaviour at the same time. Goals for specific behaviours should be established immediately after a person has understood the reasons for it and mastered the skills for performing it. The approach of linking education immediately to personal action plans has been used successfully in programs addressing chronic conditions such as diabetes (Rafferty et al., 2021). It can also be applied to other chronic conditions.

Teach to goal
Information and skills that need to be learnt in order to change understanding and behaviours.

Getting the most from existing health services

In Australia, primary health care is most often provided through general practices. General practitioners (GPs), nurses, allied health professionals, health educators and other health professionals are a valuable resource for information and health promotion. However, opportunities to enhance an individual's health literacy during a routine consultation are limited because of time constraints and a lack of evidence-based health materials available as hand-outs.

Many people find health information difficult to understand. This includes advice from doctors, nurses, pharmacists and other health professionals, along with written medical instructions and medical forms. Research is continuing to determine the best way to improve health literacy. The internet is a good source of health information if reliable sites are accessed. Government websites (e.g. Australian Institute of Health & Welfare, National Health & Medical Research Council) and many not-for-profit organisations (e.g. Cancer Council, Heart Foundation) are trustworthy sources and offer regularly updated information. Increasing knowledge and empowering individuals to make informed decisions improves not only their health status, but also that of their family and community.

PAUSE & REFLECT

What advice would you give to a family member with a chronic condition so they can make the most of a visit to their GP?

According to Health Direct (2019) (a government-sponsored website), when visiting a GP, individuals could consider the following six actions:

1 write down their questions and concerns prior to the visit so they don't forget anything;

2 take a trusted person, such as a family member or close friend, with them;

3 always ask questions if they don't understand something. The health professional wants to make sure the patient knows about their condition and understands how to follow their medical instructions;

4 always bring an up-to-date list of all medications, including over-the-counter drugs and any natural or herbal preparations;

5 ask the health professional to write down the information and instructions that were discussed during the visit;

6 if they have hearing or sight difficulties, ask the doctor to provide information in large print or use other resources.

15.3 CASE STUDY

PETER AND CARDIAC FAILURE

This case study explores how the learning principles for effective health education can be applied to assist a person who has heart failure.

Peter was born in 1958 and migrated to Australia from Italy in 1971 with his parents, three younger brothers and sister. He attended high school but struggled with English as a second language. At 15, he left school and commenced a carpentry apprenticeship with his uncle. Peter eventually established his own business. He married in 1984 and had three children. Because he did a lot of physical work, he was able to eat and drink what he wanted without gaining a lot of weight. He smoked a pack of cigarettes a day and had beer in the afternoon after work and a glass of wine nearly every night.

Two years ago, he suffered shortness of breath and, after urging from his wife, went to see his GP. He was diagnosed with mild emphysema and hypertension (high blood pressure); he also had high cholesterol readings. Medication was prescribed, but Peter took it only when he experienced some symptoms. He subsequently suffered heart failure and, after recovery in hospital, was discharged home and referred to a cardiac rehabilitation clinic.

When Peter attended the cardiac rehabilitation clinic, he was asked to complete a short questionnaire to assess his level of health literacy. Peter read slowly and struggled with some words and phrases. He had relatively good numeracy skills due to his work as a carpenter.

The cardiac rehabilitation program was run by a team of nurses in consultation with specialist doctors, a pharmacist, physiotherapist, occupational therapist and exercise physiologist. As the program aimed to meet individual needs, the nurse educator met with Peter to discuss his learning goals. For Peter to manage his condition, he needed to learn how to monitor his physical symptoms every day, take his medications as prescribed, have a low-salt diet, exercise regularly and adjust the dose of his diuretic medication if there were signs of fluid build-up in his body.

In line with the learning goals, Peter was given information about five topics: the nature of heart failure, medication, lowering his salt intake, exercise and daily check-ups. Peter found this approach easy to understand and could remember the four things he needed to do. He needed to learn how to prevent deterioration of his heart condition (medication adherence and low-salt diet) and maintain health (daily check-up and exercise).

When he was discharged from hospital, Peter was told to weigh himself daily and was given an action plan to be implemented if his weight changed by a certain amount (e.g. take two diuretic pills instead of one if his weight increased by more than 2 kg).

To maintain a low-salt diet (the goal), Peter was taught that salt is the same as sodium, that some foods are high in sodium even if salt is not added, and that foods labelled as low sodium have 140 mg or less of sodium. Peter acknowledged that because his wife does all the shopping, he had little knowledge about the information on food labels. He needed this skill to calculate his daily sodium intake and therefore maintain a low-salt diet.

Addressing this learning goal highlighted to the team that not everyone possessed certain skills (e.g. reading a food label) that they had thought were well understood by the general public. The team thought it might be useful to include Peter's wife in the education sessions.

For every topic there was an immediate behaviour that Peter had to practise. He learnt how heart failure occurs and so he understood the importance of his daily weight check-up. He also knew why he had to change existing behaviours (e.g. stopping smoking, consuming less salt). Six months later, Peter had lost 8 kg, stopped smoking and was taking his medication regularly. He and his wife were looking forward to a more active and enjoyable life.

1　Based on his case history, what do you think Peter's level of health literacy would be? Why?

2　What are Peter's likely strengths and challenges in learning new health information?

3　Peter struggled to understand the need to weigh himself daily and vary his intake of diuretic pills accordingly. What could be the reasons for this?

4　What could be the benefits of including Peter's wife in his rehabilitation?

Points to consider

Cardiovascular disease (CVD) is the largest cause of premature death in Australia. CVD relates to the health of the heart, blood vessels and organs that depend on a strong blood supply (AIHW, 2020d). The major CVDs are coronary heart disease, stroke, heart failure and peripheral vascular disease. CVD is usually due to a build-up of fat, cholesterol and other substances in the inner lining of arteries (atherosclerosis). Atherosclerosis accounted for one in four of all deaths in 2018. Around 1.2 million Australians have one or more long-term diseases of the circulatory system (AIHW, 2020d). Around one in four people with CVD also report having a disability that restricts their self-care, mobility or communication. People with CVD are more likely to report medium to high levels of psychological distress, fair or poor mental and physical health, and depression (AIHW, 2020d).

Learn more
Access additional
resources to broaden
your understanding
of this chapter. See
the Guided Tour for
access details.

CHAPTER SUMMARY

- Health literacy is the ability of individuals to understand health information, to make healthy decisions and to access the care needed to stay well.

- Individuals with low literacy have difficulty reading and understanding written information, comprehending numerical information, performing calculations, and understanding ranges of normal values (e.g. the normal range for blood pressure). They tend to have poorer baseline knowledge, short-term memory and working memory than individuals with higher literacy.

- Inadequate health literacy is common among the young, the elderly, individuals with chronic conditions or disability, individuals who do not speak English as a first language and people with a mental health condition.

- Many health professionals underestimate the prevalence of low health literacy, and often fail to identify individuals with low health literacy. Understanding health literacy and its importance is critical for effective provision of health care and health education.

- Improving health literacy through targeted education programs that provide information and motivate individuals to adopt healthy behaviours is important for illness prevention, reducing hospitalisations, improving quality of life and reducing health care costs.

- Communication plays an important role in care. The health professional's knowledge of characteristics associated with low health literacy influences interactions between the health care provider and the patient.

FURTHER READING

ABS [Australian Bureau of Statistics] (2018) *National Health Survey: Health Literacy, 2018*. Cat. no. 4364.0.55.014. Australian Bureau of Statistics.

Health Literacy Questionnaire. https://bmcpublichealth.biomedcentral.com/articles/10.1186/1471-2458-13-658

Liu C, Wang D, Liu C, Jiang J, Wang X, Chen H et al. (2020) What is the meaning of health literacy? A systematic review and qualitative synthesis. *Family Medicine and Community Health* 8(2), e000351. https://doi.org/10.1136/fmch-2020-000351

Nutbeam D & Lloyd JE (2021) Understanding and responding to health literacy as a social determinant of health. *Annual Review of Public Health* 42, 159–73. https://doi.org/10.1146/annurev-publhealth-090419-102529

Osborne RH, Batterham RW, Elsworth GR, Hawkins M & Buchbinder R (2013) The grounded psychometric development and initial validation of the health literacy questionnaire (HLQ). *BMC Public Health* 13, 658. https://doi.org/10.1186/1471-2458-13-658

Weiss BD, Mantz W, De Walt DA, Pignone MP, Mockbee J & Hale FA (2005) Quick assessment of literacy in primary care: The newest vital sign. *Annals of Family Medicine* 3, 514–22.

Wolfe MS, Williams MV, Parker RM, Parikh NS, Nowlan AW & Baker DW (2007) Patients' shame and attitudes towards discussing the result of literacy screening. *Journal of Health Communication: International Perspectives* 12(8), 721–32.

16 Promoting Health and Preventing Illness

Introduction

Much can be done to decrease the occurrence of illness and increase levels of health and well-being. This is a highly desirable outcome because of the reduction in suffering and improvement in quality and quantity of life that would follow. It would also be likely to result in reduced costs of treatment. Illness prevention and health promotion are key considerations for health professionals working with individuals, organisations, communities and governments.

Illness prevention involves interventions by health care professionals or institutions to prevent the occurrence of illness. Two examples—smoking and injury prevention—have been selected for discussion as they represent important areas for illness prevention and health promotion.

Strategies to prevent serious illness and death due to smoking

Consider the advantages that would result for a community if health professionals across all disciplines could manage to discourage young people from becoming smokers. The amount of day-to-day ill health that results from smoking—including reduced fitness, breathing difficulties and high health care costs—would be drastically reduced. In the longer term, less damage would be done to lung tissues, decreasing the occurrence of emphysema and lung cancer. The largest gain would be in cardiovascular health indicators, as smoking is a major risk factor for heart disease and stroke.

Mortality and morbidity are discussed in Chapter 1.

What does smoking cost the Australian community? A report from the National Drug Research Institute (NDRI, 2019) estimated the social cost of smoking across the whole of Australia to be $137 billion annually, of which $118 billion was due to premature death and loss of quality of life due to illness.

Smoking cessation interventions should try to reach populations, communities and individuals. At a population level, many governments have launched campaigns to reduce the likelihood of someone starting or continuing to smoke using a variety of means such as higher taxes on tobacco products, elimination of subsidies to tobacco growers (to encourage them to change crops), bans on advertising and sponsorships, and health warnings and graphic pictures of the physical damage related to smoking. At a community level, smoking cessation interventions can be co-designed to be culturally responsive and locally tailored (Bovill et al., 2021). Importantly, intensive smoking cessation interventions at an individual level can also reduce other risky behaviours such as heavy alcohol use (Philibert et al., 2022).

Strategies to prevent and address injury

The costs associated with preventable injuries are massive for both taxpayers and the individuals directly impacted. This includes road accidents (estimated cost of $30 billion), workplace accidents (estimated cost $28 billion), sporting injuries (60 000 Australians hospitalised in 2016–17), injuries to children, and even injuries in the home. Many of these injuries are not only preventable but also have easily identifiable causes.

According to insurance claims data, two out of three Australians have been in a car accident (including minor ones). Although car accidents are one of the leading causes of death for Australians aged one to 24 (child deaths included) (AIHW, 2021d), an informal survey discovered that one in five Australians is more afraid of vaccine side effects than of a car accident (BudgetDirect, 2021). As knowledge is power, be aware that the top causes of car accidents are speeding, distracted driving (phone calls, changing music, eating/ drinking, applying makeup while driving, smoking, other activities that take the driver's focus away from the road), fatigued driving, and driving under influence of alcohol or other drugs. While you cannot control the behaviour of other drivers, you can control your own behaviour if you choose to and not partake in risky behaviours. Additionally, you can encourage your peers to do the same. While driving, you can choose to respect road rules, drive under the speed limit, stay alert and maintain a safe distance from other drivers as they may put you at risk.

Workplace accidents leading to injury and death are also a significant cost to the community. Safe Work Australia (SWA, 2015) estimated the total cost of work-related injuries at $28 billion based on 2012–13 data. Many accidents are preventable by improving workplaces, using safety equipment, changing work practices or educating workers.

Sporting injuries may seem random, but they result from the combination of a predisposed athlete (i.e. limited neuromuscular control, limited muscle strength, weak ligaments, previous injury), external factors (equipment, facilities, weather) and a particular inciting event (e.g. contact with another player). Over the course of a sport season, there is increasing likelihood that all these factors will occur together. However, each of the factors can be changed. Prevention could include testing athletes for potential vulnerabilities and counselling them about risks, improving equipment and venues, avoiding dangerous conditions, and perhaps changing the rules of a sport to reduce the occurrence of inciting events. The Australian Football League and National Rugby League, for example, have modified their rules regarding players tackling late or high (above the shoulders). From a health promotion perspective, availability of social support after an injury has been shown to reduce the recovery period of both members of the general population and elite athletes.

In young children, after the first year of life, accidents become the major cause of illness and death (AIHW, 2021d). Based on 2017–19 data, the top two leading causes of death for children aged one to 14 were car accidents, followed by perinatal and congenital health conditions. The third cause of mortality in this age group was brain cancer, the fourth was accidental drowning (unintentional injury), and the fifth was suicide (intentional injury). In the 15–24 age group the top three causes of mortality were either intentional or unintentional injuries: suicide was the number one cause of death, followed by car accidents then accidental poisoning (including alcohol-related events).

Adults need to be involved in risk-reduction strategies that address injuries in children. For example, to reduce the number of car accidents that claim young lives, parents need to not only drive safely, but educate their children about not distracting them while driving. Similarly, greater attention needs to be given to improving parenting skills so that parents are better able to provide safe home environments for their children. Other interventions performed by parents can involve screening their children for health conditions (e.g. hearing and vision checks, monitoring for mental health conditions that can lead to suicide) and involving their children in swimming lessons. Some health promotion programs work directly with children (e.g. SeeMore Safety), start early in life (ages four to six) and aim to build children's capacity to stay safe and identify safety hazards for themselves and others from an early age (Peck & Terry, 2021).

For young people aged 14–24, school-based interventions and availability of social support from peers as well as the entire community are critical for early identification of individuals at risk and reduction of risk factors. Using a health promotion approach, programs focused on building protective factors such as resilience can improve quality of life among people at risk and create conditions that encourage individuals to want to live a fulfilling life (Shahram et al., 2021). Injury prevention and health promotion initiatives can be delivered through local and digital solutions developed in collaboration with potential beneficiaries, including First Peoples (Toombs et al., 2021). Electronic health technologies have been used for substance use treatment or prevention, suicide prevention, parenting support, goal-setting and behaviour change. Since smoking prevalence among Australia's First Peoples is nearly three times higher than in non-Indigenous Australians, innovative solutions are needed. For example, locally designed programs to reduce smoking have effectively used Facebook.

About one-third of all injuries happen at home and there is a higher incidence in children and those over 75 years of age. This indicates that much of the risk is related to individual vulnerabilities, such as vision and balance problems in the elderly, and lack of understanding of risks among children. Another important cause of in-home injuries is burns, including hot beverage scalds to children which can be addressed through better environmental controls (don't leave cups of coffee within a child's reach, angle saucepan handles away from edge of stove) and improving parents' knowledge.

PAUSE & REFLECT

What are some other major health issues that would make a positive difference in society if people changed their risky behaviours to healthier ones?

16.1 CASE STUDY

JULIE AND A YOUNG MOTHERS' PROGRAM

This case study examines the role of illness prevention and health promotion in advancing the health of a group with special needs.

Julie is a midwife who works with mothers and babies in the maternity unit of a general hospital. She believes that many of the youngest mothers, who are often in their early to mid-teens, do not have enough knowledge and skills to successfully mother their babies during the first weeks at home. Along with other midwives in the unit, Julie would like to improve the health of babies and their mothers during this critical time.

Young mothers are usually at high risk for parenting stress. Many will have dropped out of school, be unemployed and in an unstable relationship with poor social support, meaning they are unlikely to receive the support they need to mother their baby successfully. Young mothers can potentially experience a great deal of difficulty if the baby cries for prolonged periods or cannot settle at night. Crying is a common trigger for child abuse. All infants cry; crying generally begins in the first month of life, and its duration increases and peaks between two and four months of age. Understanding why the baby is crying and learning how to soothe the baby are important mothering skills.

1   What approaches could Julie and her colleagues use to prevent illness or promote health for young mothers and their babies?

2   Some young mothers may have unrealistic expectations of motherhood and of their baby. What might be some common misconceptions held by young mothers?

3   How can Julie and her team engage with young mothers to provide information and support?

Illness prevention

Although it may appear that prevention of illness and promotion of health are the same thing, there are significant differences in the approaches that these two terms describe. The key element of **illness prevention** is interventions by health care professionals or institutions to prevent the occurrence of illness. This generally describes things that are done for people (actions that may be carried out by health professionals). It includes actions by governments, companies, charities and other groups in society.

There are as many ways to prevent illness as there are illnesses. Prevention could include preventing individuals from injuring and killing one another during attacks of road rage, decreasing the occurrence of dental caries by fluoridation of the water supply, draining pools of water where mosquitoes breed, and making it less likely that individuals confined to bed by disability will develop bed sores. Epidemiology provides necessary data about the nature, distribution and determinants of health issues so that interventions can be developed and implemented.

> **Illness prevention**
> Interventions by health care professionals or institutions to prevent the occurrence or lessen the severity of illness.

> *Epidemiology is discussed in Chapter 1.*

Types of prevention

It is helpful to look at two dimensions of prevention: type and level. Types of prevention are primary, secondary and tertiary, depending on who the intervention is intended to reach (Calvet et al., 2021). Level refers to the agent involved, which may be government, community or health professionals.

PRIMARY PREVENTION

Primary prevention describes interventions that are aimed at healthy (well) individuals or groups with the intention of keeping them in that state. Examples are interventions aimed at stopping people from being injured or killed in car accidents or reducing the number of young people who take up smoking. The first could be accomplished by legal requirements for fitting cars with seatbelts (made compulsory for the first time anywhere in the world in Victoria in 1971) and airbags, which prevent injury once an accident has occurred. It could also be accomplished by improving roads or brakes so that accidents are less likely to occur. In either case, the behaviour of the individual is not the target.

> **Primary prevention**
> Interventions by health professionals and institutions that are aimed at (healthy) well individuals or groups, with the intention of keeping them in that state.

The number of young people who smoke could be reduced by decreasing the availability of cigarettes and tobacco products, and perhaps by eliminating cigarette vending machines. Smoking could also be reduced by decreasing its desirability. Increasing the cost of cigarettes by raising taxes is a common approach.

Perhaps the most familiar example of primary prevention is immunisation. Immunising children against poliomyelitis has nearly eliminated risk of a disease that most older people remember very well. The sight of friends in iron lungs or wearing leg braces occupies a place in the memories of people aged over 60 that is not shared to the same extent by the under-60s. Smallpox vaccinations are no longer required for most of the world's children because most of the world's adults were vaccinated in the past. The discovery of a vaccine for human papilloma virus (HPV) is expected to result in a massive reduction in the risk of genital warts and cervical cancer for girls who have not been exposed to HPV, and may even help those who have already been exposed.

Health education has an important role in primary prevention, but because the agent is different it is best considered as a separate area of action for creating health.

PAUSE & REFLECT

Consider a particular problem associated with primary prevention in which the individuals being targeted are not ill, and therefore may not be motivated to do anything.

What would be the major difficulties in implementing a primary prevention program for reducing sexually transmitted diseases?

SECONDARY PREVENTION

Secondary prevention
Interventions by health professionals and institutions that are aimed at reducing the prevalence of illness at a particular point in time by targeting at-risk individuals.

Secondary prevention aims to reduce the prevalence of illness at a particular point in time by targeting at-risk individuals. Examples of secondary prevention include screening for signs of the early development of cancers, getting those who already smoke to quit before they develop significant disease, or reducing high blood pressure and cholesterol levels in individuals so that the pathological changes that result in heart disease do not occur. Screening for cancer includes a range of techniques; for example, blood tests that may indicate the presence of prostate cancer, mammograms that look for early signs of breast cancer, taking tissue samples or inspecting the body to detect skin cancers. These are aimed at case finding, so that treatment can begin when it is most effective.

Smoking cessation programs are based on the prevention of damage to cells and tissues, or reversing these effects. After an individual quits smoking, some of their risks decrease rapidly, and others more slowly. Where pathological cell changes have already taken place, some risks may not decrease at all.

Limiting the amount of disability that the individual experiences from disease is also an element of secondary prevention. Such limiting may involve treatment that arrests the effects of a condition (e.g. the surgical removal of a tumour) or provision of facilities that limit the disability experienced (e.g. exercise and lifestyle change programs for victims of a heart attack in order to prevent the occurrence of another).

An example is minimising the risk of premature illness and death from heart disease and stroke through reduction in blood pressure. The essential first step is identification; blood pressure testing in at-risk groups, such as people over the age of 40, has become a routine part of medical appointments. Intervention to reduce blood pressure is increasingly common, but because this includes daily medication for most people, there are some problems with compliance. The same is true for high cholesterol. Compliance problems can arise with any secondary intervention because the process may involve inconvenience, cost, discomfort or side effects for an individual who does not experience any of those from the condition that puts them at risk. Healthy lifestyle programs for high blood pressure often combine medication with healthy diet (including losing weight and reducing salt, caffeine and alcohol intake), exercise and stress management.

TERTIARY PREVENTION

Tertiary prevention aims to decrease the adverse consequences experienced by people who already have a disease or condition. This can involve rehabilitation, or the provision of treatment to manage disability arising from disease. Reducing the disability experienced by children with asthma could involve identifying appropriate medications to prevent asthma attacks occurring or treat breathlessness when such attacks occur. It can also involve identifying situations that increase the risk of an attack, so that they can be avoided.

Tertiary prevention
Interventions by health professionals and institutions that are aimed at decreasing the adverse consequences experienced by people who already have a disease or condition.

16.2 CASE STUDY

JULIE (CONT.)

Julie has decided that teenage mothers are an at-risk group, so secondary prevention activities will aim to reduce the likelihood of this risk resulting in actual disease. One target may be to encourage breastfeeding among this group, as this has advantages in terms of encouraging bonding between the mother and baby, and ensuring that the baby gets adequate nourishment, which helps with the development of their immune systems. Another may be to ensure that the mothers keep in touch with their midwife or attend health centres to get expert help with any problems that arise.

A common perception is that formula feeding is perfectly adequate, and breastfeeding is 'a little bit better'. However, there is a great deal of scientific evidence about the benefits of breastfeeding and the potential health hazards of formula feeding (e.g. infections and higher level of fat intake). Successful breastfeeding is best fostered when mothers and babies are kept in close proximity (including uninterrupted skin to skin contact immediately after birth) and when infants are allowed to suckle from the breast whenever needed. However, in our fast-paced, highly mobile society, many new mothers expect their babies to conveniently fit into a structured routine. They may be unprepared for the high frequency and unpredictability of breastfeeding and the fact that breastfeeding cannot be delegated to anyone else.

Julie and her team decide that mother-to-mother support groups may be a good way to support young mothers. They can observe other breastfeeding mothers and learn how they accommodate breastfeeding within their busy schedule. The group may also help the young mothers to view their breasts as a source of infant nutrition rather than as a sensual organ—thinking of breasts as sex-related causes many nursing mothers to feel self-conscious when they need to breastfeed in public and makes some people feel uncomfortable in the presence of a breastfeeding woman. Breastfeeding mothers can learn how to nurse discreetly in public and receive frequent reassurance that breastfeeding babies is supported.

Another important issue is that teenage mothers may be less confident about what services are available to them and how to obtain those services. In addition to health education, personal development programs offering assertiveness skills could be offered to young mothers to encourage them to take control of their own and their baby's health. Another approach might involve encouragement to share knowledge and skills, and develop social networks through the creation of a mothers' social group.

1   What strategies could be used to attract young mothers to the social group?
2   What approaches could Julie and her colleagues use to promote health for babies and mothers?
3   What factors could affect access of these mothers and babies to health and health care?

Levels of prevention

Regardless of whether they are primary, secondary or tertiary, preventive interventions can occur at various levels within society. Some highly effective primary preventive measures have been brought about by action at a government or legislative level. These include changes to laws or regulations aimed at protecting health. For example, seatbelt laws have decreased injuries and deaths resulting from car crashes and gun-control laws have reduced gunshot wounds.

Governments may provide funding or other resources for a preventive program. Changing the funding patterns for doctors so that they receive money for health promotion activities and prevention of illness activities as well as clinical treatments is an important example of such an intervention. In Australia, a great deal of attention is being paid to encouraging health professionals to practise in rural areas and, once there, to stay. These programs involve providing better support for rural practitioners, and encouraging more applicants from rural areas to apply for undergraduate and postgraduate health professional programs.

Government programs can also be aimed at secondary prevention. Mandatory identification by health professionals of child abuse is aimed at preventing long-term consequences of such abuse. Regulatory change to prevent the consequences of behaviour for at-risk individuals—such as placing clocks on gambling devices so that gamblers do not lose track of time, or placing limits on alcohol consumption—are often controversial. Many people feel that it is not the role of government to protect individuals from the consequences of their own decisions. Considering the compliance problems that have been noted in secondary prevention, this should not be surprising. Tertiary government programs can include things as varied as regulation of the quality of care provided by nursing homes and fortifying beer with vitamins to prevent dietary deficiencies among problem drinkers.

There are also changes that take place at a societal level. Such changes are not legal or regulatory, but often arise out of grassroots demand for change. If enough people demand foods with lower levels of salt, sugar or animal fats, that demand will eventually be met by the market. The mechanism for much of the change that takes place at the societal level is political advocacy.

Individual-level interventions play an important part in illness prevention, most often through the influence of health professionals. Identification of health needs for the individual health consumer (client) is increasingly seen as part of the role of all health professionals. Some individuals—both consumers and professionals—see this as an unwarranted interference with the rights of the consumers, but that attitude is rapidly changing. It is much more common now for a client to be disappointed if their health professional sees a risk and does nothing about it; there may even be legal action against the health professional.

The most basic barrier to individual-level prevention is that the professional may not be aware of the risk that the individual client faces. It is still common for doctors and nurses not to know that particular clients smoke, or that they have undesirable levels of alcohol consumption. Other health professionals may also not have information that bears on their professional activities. Consider the importance of a nurse or physiotherapist, for example, knowing whether a client experiences dizzy spells or has brittle bones because of osteoporosis. Similarly, it is vital for a radiographer to know if a woman is pregnant before risking exposure of the foetus to radiation.

PAUSE & REFLECT

Parents often bring teenage children to see health professionals and stay with them during examinations. Imagine the situation in which a 15-year-old girl is pregnant but has not told her parents. Because she has abdominal pain, she is sent for X-rays. Her mother insists on staying with her daughter while the X-rays are taken. The radiographer asks the girl if she is pregnant, because the X-rays could potentially harm a foetus.

What medical and privacy issues are involved, from the viewpoint of the girl and the radiographer?

Behaviour change for the individual is discussed in Chapter 8.

Once the professional has knowledge about the health needs of the client, modifications can be made to the behaviour of either. Sometimes illness prevention is the responsibility of the professional (e.g. providing shielding material during radiation, or support during a period of bereavement) and sometimes it is the responsibility of the client. Responsibility usually involves changes in the client's behaviour. Achieving this change generally involves health promotion as distinct from illness prevention.

Health promotion

This book has discussed the influence of genetics and biological, psychological and environmental factors on health. **Health promotion** involves changing some of these factors. Health professionals, even governments, cannot always enforce such changes, but they can help by providing the information, skills, resources, environments, policies and legislation to support healthy changes.

The World Health Organization's **Ottawa Charter for Health Promotion** signified the official introduction of health promotion as a field of practice and research. It defines health promotion as the process of enabling people to increase control over, and to improve, their health. Importantly, health promotion involves activities carried out by any person for their own benefit, rather than activities done for them by experts or governments. These activities may involve individuals, groups, communities or entire societies, and comprise a number of action areas: build healthy policies, create supportive environments, strengthen community action, develop personal skills (a major focus of this book) and reorient health services (WHO, 2022).

Health promotion
The process of enabling people to increase their control over, and to improve, their health.

Ottawa Charter for Health Promotion
An international agreement that identifies five areas for health promotion action (Building healthy public policy, Creating supportive environments, Strengthening community action, Developing personal skills, Re-orienting health care services towards prevention of illness and promotion of health) and three strategies for health promotion action (Advocate, Enable, Mediate).

Primary health promotion
Enabling people in a healthy population to promote health.

Secondary health promotion
Enabling people in an at-risk population to promote health.

Tertiary health promotion
Enabling people who already have a disease or condition to promote health.

As with illness prevention, health promotion can be primary, secondary or tertiary. **Primary health promotion** involves enabling people in a healthy population to promote health. **Secondary health promotion** involves enabling people in an at-risk population to promote health. **Tertiary health promotion** involves enabling those who already have a disease or condition to promote health. Table 16.1 gives some examples.

TABLE 16.1 Examples of health promotion interventions

LEVEL/S	INDIVIDUAL	GROUP	SOCIETY
Primary	Teaching a child how to brush their teeth regularly and thoroughly	Stress management workshop for university students	Mass media campaign to encourage seatbelt use
Secondary	Individual coping skills training for siblings of a person with an addiction	Weight loss group for sedentary office workers	Meals on Wheels program to improve nutrition for the elderly
Tertiary	Developing a diabetes management plan for a client	Self-help group for consumers with schizophrenia	Lobbying for public transport with easy access for people with a disability

Health promotion can be carried out in a variety of settings, such as schools, workplaces, health care settings or in the community. It may be more accurate to say 'communities' in the latter case, as there are often advantages in targeting specific groups within the larger society, such as people with a disability, the elderly, rural residents or First Peoples (Baxter et al., 2021; Seaman, 2021).

The potential scope of health promotion is enormous, and there are many groups in society involved in activities that could be seen as health promotion. One of the largest groups is health professionals.

HEALTH PROFESSIONALS AND HEALTH PROMOTION

Health professionals are ideally placed to assist their clients with health promotion as they are seen as having expertise, access to knowledge and resources, and prestige. Helping clients to gain control over their health outcomes is more effective than trying to exert that control for them. Techniques for encouraging behaviour change have been discussed at length in this book. Importantly, by educating themselves and empowering their clients, health professionals can be active in tailored health promotion and illness prevention while delivering clinical treatments (see Figure 16.1).

An emerging concept is that of precision health promotion, where health promotion and disease prevention programs are tailored to a new level through the availability of digital health data. The benefits could be both immediate, such as informing health decisions related to HPV vaccinations and safe sexual practices, and long-term, such as prevention or immediate identification of HPV-associated cancers (Olusanya et al., 2021). Another emerging concept is the combination of clinical treatment with health promotion in psychotherapy, where sessions are provided by a trained therapist to a client while walking together whenever the weather permits (Koziel et al., 2022). In addition to improvements in mental health, participants reported increases in non-sedentary behaviour outside therapeutic sessions (Koziel et al., 2022).

FIGURE 16.1 Health as the focus of three complementary areas of action for health professionals: health promotion, illness prevention and clinical treatment

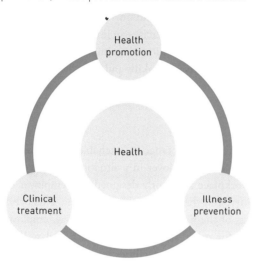

Some health professionals become so focused on changing the behaviours of their clients that they overlook the gains that can be made by changing their own behaviours or changing their practice procedures or settings. The environments in which health care is provided need to be supportive, in the terms of the Ottawa Charter. The easiest way to prevent falls for clients who are having X-rays (a not uncommon problem) is not to warn them to avoid falling but to make falls less likely to occur, or the consequences less serious, by changing the environment. This could involve taking X-rays of frail or physically unstable clients while they are seated, designing tables that are hard to roll off (or providing pads that prevent rolling) or carpeting floors so that slips are less likely and falls will be less damaging.

None of this should minimise the high level of impact that professionals can have in promoting health. Clients are generally keen to have information about what can be done to improve their health and well-being and are often willing to devote large amounts of time and energy to the process. Well-designed and readable information pamphlets, contact information and plans that have reasonable and achievable goals are well received by most consumers.

SUPPORTIVE ENVIRONMENTS

Schools, workplaces, clinical environments and communities provide considerable opportunity for health promotion via **teachable moments** (Wortley & Hagell, 2021).

Schools and universities

Teachable moments are particularly effective times for concepts to be learnt or behaviours to be developed. As an example, schools are able to require healthy behaviours on the part of students, such as wearing sunscreen and hats during outdoor activities. As a result, these behaviours can become habits that are carried over into life outside school. Provision of safe play areas and healthy food, health screening and inoculations, and education about hygiene and risky behaviours have long been seen as responsibilities of schools. Sex education, coping skills and conflict resolution are other areas in which schools have become involved.

Teachable moments
Particularly effective times for concepts to be learnt or behaviours to be developed.

Well-being is covered in Chapter 1.

It would be ideal if universities and their students were aware of, and focused on, creating health promotion settings that reduce stress and improve well-being. One of the simplest forms of health promotion at individual and university level is short-term exercise. Evidence suggests that even a single episode of exercise can improve mood states in stressful situations (Pascoe et al., 2021). For such interventions, it is important to address multiple behavioural health determinants such as motivation, skills and self-efficacy while clarifying for students the benefits of short-term exercise on stress and anxiety (Pascoe et al., 2021).

Workplaces

Stress and coping are covered in Chapters 12 and 13.

Workplaces, like schools, provide a range of teachable moments. Health risks within the workplace frequently place the employer in a situation of legal liability. If equipment or environments in the workplace are poorly designed, the employer is likely to be found at fault in the case of injury, and the costs can be significant. This liability can be avoided by improving these aspects of the workplace. In a similar way, employers can be encouraged to accept responsibility for other aspects of the health and well-being of workers. This could include the provision of exercise facilities for workers with sedentary jobs, childcare facilities to reduce worry about the well-being of children and the stress of meeting pick-up times, stress and conflict management courses, and a large variety of educational programs. Employers are recognising that provision of health promotion programs pays off in the form of reduced health costs and less absenteeism, and contributes to improved morale, with a resulting positive effect on productivity and profits.

Clinical environments

In clinical environments such as nursing homes, health promotion can take the form of health education based on social cognitive theory, with a focus on improving the mental health of residents (Abusalehi et al., 2021). In any type of setting, it is important to consider the potential contributions of peers in the delivery and success of health promotion programs (Wehner et al., 2021) with a particular emphasis on teachable moments for health professionals and their clients. Examples of behaviours relevant to teachable moments are self-care behaviours such as mindfulness, focus on recognising, understanding and managing emotions (link to emotional intelligence) and opportunities for incidental exercise during daily activities.

PAUSE & REFLECT

For health professionals, what might be a teachable moment related to personal safety in a clinical setting?

Workplaces would greatly benefit from illness prevention and health promotion initiatives that are provided either by an external entity or by internal working groups. As discussed previously, injuries greatly impact workplaces and people working in clinical environments have a higher exposure to infection risks that can be reduced through primary, secondary and tertiary illness prevention. Complementing these, primary, secondary and tertiary health promotion programs can be implemented in clinical environments for the benefits of health professionals working in such settings (e.g. mental health programs) and consumers using services in clinical environments (e.g. health literacy assessment and education on multiple topics during a clinical visit or stay).

Communities

Communities have a major role to play in promoting health. They can serve as focal points for education programs, provide access to facilities at low or no cost, help to define an agenda for health promotion that fits community needs and co-design locally relevant interventions. Local communities often carry out this role on a geographical basis. Some activities, such as those requiring regulation or accreditation, can only realistically be carried out at local community level.

Schools and universities are examples of communities that can greatly benefit from health promotion initiatives. First, they already have a way to reach a large population of students. Second, there are formal structures in place with a focus on health and safety that can be further enhanced by health promotion initiatives. Third, the students themselves can be prepared and supported to be agents of change (a central tenet of health promotion) in initiatives that support their own health and the health of their peers and teachers.

The health needs of rural communities, and even of outer suburban ones, are different from those of urban communities, and the appropriate programs need to be tailored to those needs. Tailored interventions are more likely to result in positive health outcomes, particularly when health literacy is accounted for and measured in the process (Kinsman et al., 2021). New models of engaging with the community for health promotion purposes are being developed and tested in the field. An example is the Optimising Health Literacy and Access (OPHELIA) process, which has been successfully used in Tasmania to engage with underrepresented groups and encourage them to have input in health promotion processes focused on reducing organisational barriers and health inequities (Kinsman et al., 2021).

Health literacy is covered in Chapter 15.

ACCESS AND EQUITY

It is easy enough to see that health promotion and illness prevention produce win–win situations. The individual wins by having better health, and the community or society wins by having to devote less of its resources to the treatment of illness. Within the health promotion planning, it is important to consider the structural or societal causes of ill health. Those who have the most to gain by avoiding illness and maximising their health are often those who are least able to do so. This may be because services are unevenly available within the community. For example, if most programs were run in populated urban centres, rural dwellers would miss out. Some programs are dependent on access to facilities such as gyms, sports grounds, community centres or large medical practices, and access to these facilities is unequally distributed in the community.

Programs that are provided only through health professionals in private practice are going to miss the individuals who do not use those practices as their source of primary health care. The homeless, the very poor and others on the margins of society are likely to spend larger proportions of whatever resources they have on cheap but unhealthy food and accommodation, or to self-medicate in unhealthy ways, such as with alcohol and tobacco use. They are less likely to have resources that can be invested in potential future benefits, as all their resources need to be used for survival today.

Access to health will probably be affected by financial issues (e.g. teenage mothers are unlikely to have the education or training to be in well-paid employment), by lack of education about health, by problems of transportation and frequently by isolation. A variety of programs at all levels is needed to ensure the maximum level of health. These include not only health care programs but also financial aid, support and development programs.

Access and equity issues are discussed in Chapter 14.

What are some of the costs to individuals when a society adopts a strongly preventive model of health?

ENVIRONMENTS

Environments are also inequitably distributed. Those who live in polluted areas or work in unhealthy workplaces are more likely to be financially vulnerable. High crime rates, community unrest and war are all relevant to health, and again it is the poor who are most vulnerable as they are least able to move from riskier environments.

It is imperative for societies to ensure that health is distributed equitably. This means more than just throwing money at health problems. In many cases, health resources are adequate, but the approach taken is not appropriate or is unacceptable to some communities. Many charitable schemes fail because the recipients do not wish to accept charity, particularly when the distributors of that charity sometimes restrict or deny what is provided if the recipients do not seem to be adequately grateful for it.

Health promotion programs may be rejected if they are seen as labelling people as unhealthy or if they have a moralistic tone; for example, laying the blame for being sick or at risk on the individual. Management of relapse is a particularly important consideration. Relapse must not be seen as a moral failure for the individual (e.g. a lack of willpower) as this is likely to lower self-efficacy and drive participants out of health promotion activities. Setting unrealistic goals for participants can lead to failure and the abandonment of a perfectly viable program.

Use of symbols must also be considered. Some women with breast cancer object to the use of symbols such as pink ribbons and teddy bears because they are seen as infantilising their experience. Many people with chronic health problems feel that too much emphasis on positive outcomes, regardless of how unlikely they may be, diminishes the seriousness of their situation. They may feel closed out, as if their failure to gain benefit from a program is somehow a personal flaw. Involvement of the individual, the family and the community in controlling health programs is one way of avoiding these negative consequences.

The importance of cognitions about the illness and the self is discussed in Chapter 7.

Health and human behaviour

Health promotion can be seen as the logical end point of the study of health and human behaviour. Because health relates in so many ways to behaviour, promotion of better health essentially means promotion of healthier behaviours. This might involve modifying habits, such as new approaches to diet, exercise or the use of substances such as alcohol and tobacco. It might involve changing emotional responses, such as coping with stress or reducing levels of arousal. It may involve shifting broad societal approaches to health and illness, such as community development and support of the disadvantaged. Ultimately, it may involve changing our shared beliefs about what health is and how it can be created and maintained. Beliefs about the responsibility for health have been changing over recent decades and will continue to change in response to new knowledge and technology. This book has aimed to increase understanding of some of these issues and provide information about possible directions and methods to create healthy changes within and around us.

16.3 CASE STUDY

ALFIE AND HIS FALL INJURY

This case study considers how an accident may occur, and what factors may influence the timing, nature and consequences of that accident.

Alfie is an 82-year-old Navy veteran. The local town hall is having a display of old photos of the history of the Navy—several of them contributed by Alfie—so he has walked down to see the exhibition. Although he wears glasses with bifocal lenses and finds walking easier with the aid of a cane due to arthritis in one hip, Alfie does not think of himself as being disabled. He is proud of his general health and well-being. On arrival at the town hall, Alfie enters the dark lobby from the sunshine outside, and finds it hard to see. As a result, he walks over the edge of a ramp installed for wheelchair access, and falls sideways, breaking the flimsy handrail in the process. He attempts to regain his balance with his cane, but the cane tip slips on the highly polished wooden floor of the lobby—a heritage feature of the century-old hall—and Alfie falls. He braces his arm to prevent his head hitting the floor. On landing, he feels something break in his forearm, and his hip begins to hurt badly. Several people in the lobby rush to help him, and one of them attempts to lift him into a seated position. This causes intense pain in his hip, and Alfie begs his helpers to let him lie flat.

An ambulance arrives within minutes. On reaching hospital, medical imaging shows that Alfie has broken a bone in his arm and aggravated the existing arthritic damage to his hip joint. At his age, healing is slow, so Alfie becomes an invalid for an extended period while healing takes place. Eventually, it is determined that he will require a hip replacement to recover his mobility. Until that occurs, he largely relies on using a wheelchair and generally stays inside his flat. As his flat is on the second floor and the lift in the building is often out of order, his ability to participate in his usual activities is severely limited. As a result, Alfie becomes somewhat socially isolated, unhappy and less physically fit than before.

1 What environmental factors contributed to Alfie's injuries?

2 Are there individual characteristics of Alfie himself that contributed to this injury?

3 What prevention and promotion strategies in relation to the floor surface could be applied by the council to reduce the risk of injuries?

4 What are the financial, social and other costs associated with this accident? To what extent could they have been prevented or lessened?

Points to consider

The council staff member who is responsible for health and safety received the incident report about Alfie's fall. The next day he interviewed Alfie at home and did an inspection of the town hall area. The staff member noted that the ramp, although designed to help one group of disabled people, was a significant health risk due to the absence of an adequate handrail. A high-visibility strip marking the edge of the ramp might have prevented Alfie walking over the edge, as might have better lighting. Although the wooden floor is an attractive heritage feature of the hall, it was a significant contributor to Alfie's injuries in this case. The slippery surface of the polished wood floor made his cane useless as a balance aid in this situation, and the hard surface worsened the impact of his fall. The separation of the ramp, with its non-slip surface, and the floor might have been adequate in this case if the handrail had been adequate. Other people entering the lobby might also have problems with the floor's slickness; for example, women in high heels, people with ordinary plastic soles on wet days, or people with minor balance or mobility problems.

It would probably be unviable, and undesirable, to change the surface by coating it or covering the floor (primary prevention). The heritage value would be reduced or destroyed by too much change. However, at the simplest level, warning signs to let people know about the risks could be a help, or perhaps alternative access points could be provided for those at risk (secondary prevention).

Learn more
Access additional resources to broaden your understanding of this chapter. See the Guided Tour for access details.

CHAPTER SUMMARY

- Illness prevention and health promotion are major growing areas of health care.

- Illness prevention principally concerns programs that are done for people by health professionals, governments or other institutions.

- Primary prevention refers to programs aimed at keeping well individuals well. Secondary prevention is aimed at decreasing the prevalence of disease in at-risk groups. Tertiary prevention's goal is to reduce the negative consequences for those who already have an illness or disease.

- Prevention can take place at the legislative level by constraining behaviour, both at the societal level by changing policy or procedures, and at the individual level.

- Health promotion enables people to exert more control over their own health. Health promotion may be primary, secondary or tertiary.

- Health professionals can play a key role in health promotion and illness prevention.

- Schools, workplaces, clinical environments and communities can provide additional teachable moments for influencing and encouraging change.

- Local communities and local groups can co-design and provide support for health promotion programs.

- Equity in the provision of health promotion is vitally important. It may involve helping disadvantaged groups to develop the necessary skills to take control of their own health.

- Health promotion is a logical endpoint for the consideration of the interactions between health and human behaviour that have been the focus of this book.

FURTHER READING

Bowden J & Manning V (2017) *Health Promotion in Midwifery: Principles and Practice.* Taylor & Francis.

Fleming M & Parker E (2020) *Health Promotion: Principles and Practice in the Australian Context.* Taylor & Francis.

Fleming M-L & Baldwin L (Eds) (2020) *Health Promotion in the 21st Century: New Approaches to Achieving Health for All.* Routledge.

McKinnon M (Ed.) (2021) *Health Promotion: A Practical Guide to Effective Communication.* Cambridge University Press.

Naidoo J & Wills J (2016) *Foundations for Health Promotion.* Elsevier Health Sciences.

GLOSSARY

Abnormal illness behaviour

The persistence of inappropriate or maladaptive modes of perceiving, evaluating or acting in relation to health after the person has received an appropriate explanation of the nature and management of the illness from a professional.

Acceptance

A more neutral or middle-of-the-road reaction to a condition that diminishes the negative meaning of the condition and thus represents a decrease in negative thinking.

Accommodation

The modification of existing behaviours or the development of entirely new behaviours to enable an individual to deal with a new experience.

Acute illness

A single episode of illness or disease, generally severe and over a limited period of time.

Acute pain

Pain that is intense and gains the individual's immediate attention, but usually disappears within hours, days or weeks.

Advance health care directive (living will)

A statement signed by an individual about the treatment they will accept when they are dying.

Affective support

The act of communicating feelings and providing constructive feedback and advice.

Agent

The person who has control over the stimuli and/or reinforcements for change.

Agents of socialisation

External influences that establish and reinforce norms of expected behaviour and therefore shape an individual's characteristics.

Algorithm

A mechanical routine or simple set of rules that can be used to solve all problems of a particular kind.

Allostasis

The process of maintaining balance in bodily systems, through physiological or behavioural means, in the face of a demand.

Allostatic load

The cumulative cost to the body of allostasis.

Alzheimer's disease

A significant impairment of cognitive ability, memory or problem-solving ability resulting from abnormalities of cells in the cerebral cortex.

Antecedents

Stimuli that precede and lead to the occurrence of a behaviour.

Anticipatory decision-making

Advance planning by an individual regarding a significant future event. Directives provide guidance for family members and others regarding the decision-maker's preferences and wishes.

Anticipatory grieving

Grieving that takes place before an expected loss has occurred.

Anti-social influences

Negative influences on a person's well-being.

Appraisal

Cognitions that an individual holds about the situation they are in at a given time.

Arousal

Activation of the sympathetic nervous system, which produces visceral changes and provides energy for behaviour.

Assimilation

The use of existing knowledge or habits to enable the individual to deal with a new experience.

Attitudes

An individual's thoughts, feelings and readiness to act in relation to any object, person or event.

Attribution theory of emotion

The idea that emotion results when physiological arousal and emotion-related cognitions about that arousal exist at the same time.

Automatisation

The carrying out of patterns of behaviour or thinking that are so well learnt that they require no apparent thought.

Aversive conditioning

The use of punishment to decrease the occurrence of unwanted behaviour.

Avoidance learning

The learning of a response, such as fear, that will allow the individual to escape punishment. It is reinforced by a reduction in the level of fear experienced.

Balance theory

An approach that suggests consistency is the organising principle of an individual's cognitions.

Bariatric surgery

Surgery aimed at weight loss in the obese that works by reducing the size of the stomach, either by insertion of a mechanical device (e.g. lap-band) or removal of part of the stomach.

Behavioural predispositions

Actions that have been learnt by the individual as a response to situations.

Biofeedback

Control of internal processes through conditioning, using mechanical devices to make those internal processes perceptible.

Biopsychosocial model

A model of health that considers the individual as a whole person in a social setting, who may or may not be ill at any given moment.

Biopsychosocial-spiritual model
A humanistic and holistic view of a person and their environment.

Body mass index (BMI)
An approximate measure of an individual's amount of body fat, frequently used by health professionals because it is easy to calculate.

Capability
A characteristic or behaviour of the individual that protects against a negative event.

Catastrophising
The appraisal by an individual that a situation is impossible for them to cope with when in fact it is not.

Chronic condition
A medical condition that is permanent, incurable and irreversible.

Chronic strain
Repeated or constant occurrence of a minor physical stressor.

Chronological age
The number of years that have passed sequentially since a person was born.

Classical conditioning
A learning process through experience where an already existing response to the presentation of food (e.g. salivating) becomes connected to a previously irrelevant stimulus (e.g. bell ringing).

Cognition
A general concept embracing all types of knowing, judging, thinking, reasoning and so on.

Cognitive behavioural therapy
Counselling therapies in which an individual can learn to control or modify worrying or intrusive thoughts, thereby improving their mental health.

Cognitive load
The amount of information kept in the working memory.

Cognitive responses
How a person views their condition.

Cognitive restructuring
A technique aimed at interrupting patterns of negative thinking by training the individual to recognise that they are

occurring, and replace them with positive thoughts.

Collaborative model
A model in which patients are active participants, in partnership with health care providers, in regulating and managing their chronic condition.

Comfort food
Food, often with traditional or nostalgic connections, that is eaten primarily for positive emotional reasons rather than because of hunger.

Communication disabilities
Inability to or difficulty with speaking or sequencing thoughts, or being non-verbal.

Compassion fatigue
A deep physical, emotional and spiritual exhaustion related to repeated exposure to another's suffering.

Compliance
Obeying another person's instruction, or acting as they would like. It does not necessarily mean agreeing with the reasons behind the instructions.

Complicated or chronic grief
Unresolved grief characterised by an impaired ability to recall personal life details, as well as imagine and plan for the future.

Confabulation
The addition of plausible detail to a memory to make it seem more complete. This process takes place without the individual being aware of it.

Conservation withdrawal
An extreme pattern of withdrawal from interaction with a neglectful or abusive environment by an individual in order to preserve life.

Controllability
The level of control over a condition. It can be both actual and perceived.

Coping
Any strategy by which an individual attempts to manage the perceived discrepancy between demands and resources.

Crystallised intelligence
Accumulation of knowledge that comes with life experience and education.

Cultural literacy
Ability to identify, understand and respect the collective beliefs and customs of diverse groups in the community.

Culture
The way of life and beliefs shared by members of a group.

Cytokines
A group of proteins and peptides that work as signalling compounds, enabling cells to communicate with each other; they regulate the body's response to infection, inflammation and trauma.

Disability
A chronic condition of the body, mind or senses that results in a limitation, restriction or impairment in performing activities of daily living.

Disease
An abnormal state of a person's body or mind, as identified by a qualified observer.

Disengagement theory
The idea that ageing individuals tend to modify their amount of interaction with society to suit their capabilities.

Dysregulation of emotions
Poor understanding or insight, negative reactivity and ineffective or maladaptive coping intelligence.

Ecological model
A model which proposes that overweight and obesity include biological, behavioural and environmental factors in addition to food intake.

Efficacy beliefs
A person's belief that they can carry out required treatments and that the treatments will be effective.

Electronic health (e-Health) literacy
Ability to navigate through the vast (and sometimes misleading) online world.

Emotional intelligence
Ability to perceive, use, understand and regulate emotion.

Emotion-focused coping
Behaviour, such as relaxation, distraction or prayer, aimed not at dealing with situational demands but with the way the demands make an individual feel.

Emotions

Positive or negative responses to external stimuli (situations, events, things and people) and/or internal mental representations (thoughts, dreams and ideas).

Endogenous opioid peptides

Opiate-like neurochemical substances, produced in the body, that act as an internal pain regulation system.

Endorphins

Endogenous substances that are considered to be the body's own pain relievers, binding to the same receptor sites on neurons as morphine.

Epidemiology

The science of measuring the health status of a community.

Ethnicity

How people define themselves, and how they are defined by others.

Ethnocentrism

The belief that a person's own culture is the natural, or best, culture.

Evidence-based health care

The view that all clinical practice should be based on evidence from randomised controlled trials to ensure treatments are effective and better than a placebo.

Expectancy–value theory

A model that suggests that rational choices between alternatives are based on the perceived probability of occurrence of each option and its value to the individual.

Expectations

Cognitions held by an individual about what is likely to happen in a given situation.

Explanatory model

Perceptions and expectations about health and illness, including causes and mechanisms, timing, future course and outcome, and appropriate treatment.

Extinction

The gradual lessening of a conditioned response when reinforcement is removed.

Fight or flight response

The release of catecholamines, which prepare the body for action.

First Peoples

Australia's Aboriginal and Torres Strait Islander peoples.

Fitness

A condition of health or physical soundness, which may be general or related to the ability to meet a specific demand ('fit for purpose').

FITT principle

Four conditions that determine the appropriateness of an exercise program for an individual at a specific time: frequency, intensity, time and type.

Fluid intelligence

The use of flexible reasoning to draw inferences, solve problems and understand the relationships between concepts.

Food pyramid

A triangular figure divided into segments to indicate what proportion of the diet each food group should comprise.

Gate-control theory

The idea that that the brain controls the experience of pain by influencing the amount of pain stimulation that is allowed to pass a sensory gate at the level of the spinal cord.

Good behaviour bond

A sum of money (or equivalent goods or services) that is set aside to be returned only if a behaviour change program is successfully completed.

Goodness of fit

Appropriateness of the individual's resources to the specific demands that they face.

Habit

An activity that has become automatic through prolonged practice.

Habituation

Adaptation to a stimulus so that it no longer arouses the level of response that it originally aroused.

Hardiness

A behaviour pattern of commitment, a belief in the individual's ability to control events and a willingness to tackle challenges in the face of high levels of stress.

Hassles

Apparently minor events that can cause irritation, aggravate existing health problems or (in large numbers or over a prolonged period of time) affect an individual's health.

Health

A dynamic concept that varies over time and is influenced by social situations, cultures, ethnicities, families and individuals.

Health behaviours

Behaviours that are carried out specifically to promote the health of the individual.

Health literacy

Ability to read, comprehend and use medical information to make health decisions, and effectively interact with the health care system and health professionals.

Health Literacy Questionnaire

A national survey that measures the health literacy of adults aged 18 and older across nine different domains.

Health promotion

The process of enabling people to increase their control over, and to improve, their health.

Helplessness

A negative and maladaptive response to a condition that has long-term adverse implications for psychological and physical health.

Heuristics

Problem-solving strategies based on general rules that usually or often work.

Holism

A word derived from Greek, meaning entire or total.

Homeostasis

Tendency of the body to maintain internal constancy, and to try to restore equilibrium when that constancy is disturbed.

Hypnosis

A deep, trance-like state of relaxation.

Hypothalamus

A small structure in the midbrain that regulates behaviour to maintain homeostasis.

Illness

A subjective experience on the part of an individual that something is not quite right with their health.

Illness behaviour

The process by which an individual transitions from being a well person to an unwell person.

Illness perceptions

An individual's views or theories about their illness, based on bodily experiences such as symptoms, information from the external environment and previous experience with illness.

Illness prevention

Interventions by health care professionals or institutions to prevent the occurrence or lessen the severity of illness.

Incentive

An external object or stimulus that draws out behaviour or creates motivation in the absence of a need.

Incidence

The rate at which new cases of a specific disease occur in a particular population during a specified period.

Indigenous

A term used with respect when referring to First Peoples of all countries.

Inequality

Uneven distribution of health or health resources as a result of genetic or other factors or the lack of resources.

Inequity

Unfair, avoidable differences arising from poor governance, corruption or cultural exclusion.

Instincts

Patterns of behaviour that are genetically programmed to occur in response to internal or external events.

Instrumental support

The act of giving tangible assistance and practical aid.

Intellectual disabilities

Difficulties with learning, problem-solving, logic, impulse control and reasoning.

Learning

A change in understanding and/or behaviour that results from experience with the environment.

Learned helplessness

Distress to the point where behaviour is impaired or the individual gives up in the face of punishment that cannot be controlled.

Lifestyle diseases

Diseases in which behaviours of the individual over a prolonged period influence the development or course of disease, such as heart disease, many cancers and stroke.

Locus of control

Degree to which an individual attributes the cause of events to internal factors or external forces.

Low-awareness habits

Habitual behaviours that the individual carries out without being particularly aware that they are doing so (e.g. nail-biting).

Mastery learning

Repetition of a task until learning occurs.

Medical model

A model of health that considers the individual as a case or patient, primarily the host for some sort of disease or malfunctioning organ. The model is prescriptive and focused on patients' compliance with or adherence to medical management instructions.

Memory

Processes (including sensory, short-term and long-term memory) by which experience is retained within the organism.

Middle adulthood

A general classification of adulthood where social and personal role expectations and goals are achieved, re-evaluated, challenged or forfeited; the major timespan of the adult lifespan.

Morbid grief

Grieving that is too intense or inappropriate to the loss.

Morbidity

Amount of disease observed within a group.

Mortality

Number of deaths observed within a group.

Motivation

Factors that arouse, sustain and direct behaviour.

Multimorbidity

Presence of two or more chronic conditions in a person at the same time.

Myelination

Development of a fatty insulation on nerve cells that accelerates their development and efficiency in electrical transmission.

Nationality

An acquired classification generally based on a person's country of birth or, in some instances, their parents' country of birth.

Negative definition of health

The absence of disease equates with being healthy.

Neuroplasticity

The brain's ability to reorganise itself by forming new neural connections throughout life.

Nocebo effects

Negative experiences which follow a treatment, such as side effects or failure to work, that result from patient expectations and not from the treatment itself.

Nociceptors

Nerve endings in the peripheral nerves that identify injury and release chemical messengers that pass to the spinal cord and into the cerebral cortex.

Obesity

The label for a range of weight that is significantly above what is considered to be healthy, and documented as presenting a serious risk to health.

Obesogenic environment

An environment (including culture, physical structures and other elements) that encourages overeating and/or inadequate physical activity.

Older adulthood

Subjective classification of adulthood generally coinciding with retirement from the workforce and more focus on leisure activities; the latter stage of the lifespan.

Opponent–process theory

The idea that there are always two processes in motivation: the primary motivation or process, and a secondary and opposite process set up within the nervous system.

Optimal level theory

The idea that organisms have a preferred range of environmental stimulation, and that they will work to maintain themselves in that range.

Optimism

A tendency to expect that outcomes will generally be good.

Ottawa Charter for Health Promotion

An international agreement that identifies five areas for health promotion action (Building healthy public policy, Creating supportive environments, Strengthening community action, Developing personal skills, Re-orienting health care services towards prevention of illness and promotion of health) and three strategies for health promotion action (Advocate, Enable, Mediate).

Overweight

The label for a range of weight that is above what is considered to be healthy.

Pain control

Ability to reduce the experience of pain, report of pain, emotional concern about pain, inability to tolerate pain or presence of pain-related behaviours.

Pain management programs

Programs that address concerns associated with chronic pain, with strong emphasis on patient education, cognitive components and a physical therapy component.

Perceived benefit

A positive response to a condition that adds optimistic meaning through increased positive thinking.

Perception explanation

The idea that placebos affect the perception of the symptom rather than the symptom itself.

Perceptual constancy

The tendency to see objects as unchanged in spite of changes in sensory input.

Persistent (chronic) pain syndrome

A subtype of abnormal illness behaviour that can occur if an individual experiences pain over a lengthy period of time.

Personal fable

A person's belief that the world revolves around them.

Phobia

A strong, persistent and irrational fear of some object, person or event.

Physical activity

Bodily movement produced by skeletal muscles that requires energy expenditure.

Physical age

The state of a person's biological machine.

Physical disabilities

Reduced mobility, stamina and agility; neurological conditions; missing or deformed limbs; and reduced muscle mass or bone strength.

Placebo effects

Non-specific effects that any treatment produces.

Post-traumatic stress disorder

A persistent pattern of symptoms, including preoccupation, nightmares and flashbacks, that some individuals experience after a major stressful event.

Practical intelligence

Common-sense thinking that enables a person to successfully negotiate their daily activities.

Prepubertal growth spurt

A period of rapid and dramatic physical growth that occurs just before puberty.

Prevalence

Number of existing and new cases of a specific disease present in a particular population at a certain time.

Primary appraisal

The idea that, in the presence of an environmental demand, individuals first assess or appraise the severity of the demand.

Primary drive

An unlearnt drive, for which there is an organic or physiological basis.

Primary health promotion

Enabling people in a healthy population to promote health.

Primary prevention

Interventions by health professionals and institutions that are aimed at (healthy) well individuals or groups, with the intention of keeping them in that state.

Problem-focused coping

Behaviour, such as problem-solving or increased effort, aimed at modifying the balance between demands and resources in a particular situation by reducing the demand or increasing resources.

Progressive relaxation

A stress management strategy that involves relaxation of muscle groups one at a time so that the individual learns and remembers what relaxation feels like.

Prosocial influences

Positive or protective factors that add value or create advantage.

Psychological traits

Thought patterns such as feelings and emotions that produce a behaviour (action). They are uniquely formed by each individual.

Psychoneuroimmunology

The study of communications between the brain and the immune system.

Psychophysiology

The study of interactions between the physiological and psychological aspects of a situation as experienced by an individual.

Psychosocial interventions

Psychological, social and educational strategies that aim to minimise the adverse emotional and social impact of a condition on an individual and their family.

Psychosomatic illness

An outdated term reserved for a few specific conditions (e.g. bronchial asthma, neurodermatitis and gastric ulcers) that were incorrectly regarded as being caused by worry.

Puberty

A developmental stage defined by the appearance of secondary sexual characteristics, such as body hair and deepening of the voice in males, and menstruation and breast development in females.

Punishment

A consequence or outcome that, in conjunction with a behaviour, makes that behaviour less likely in future.

Race

Biological (physical) characteristics of an individual's features.

Reaction range

Total range of outcomes that are possible for a particular individual as a result of their genetic potential.

Reflex

An unlearnt response to stimulus.

Reinforcement

A consequence or outcome that, in conjunction with a behaviour, makes that behaviour more likely in future. Reinforcement can be positive or negative.

Relaxation

Placing the body into a low state of arousal by progressively relaxing sections of the body and taking deeper and longer breaths.

Religion

An organised system of beliefs and practices associated with a divine or sacred entity, often displayed by ceremony.

Risk-reduction behaviours

Avoidance of unhealthy behaviours specifically to protect the health of the individual.

Risky behaviours

Behaviours that increase the individual's chance of ill health.

Rooting reflex

An automatic reaction in newborns, where stimulation of the lips and tongue leads the newborn to turn towards the stimulus and initiate sucking activity.

Schedule of reinforcement

The pattern on which reinforcement is given. It may be continuous (every behaviour) or intermittent (less than every behaviour).

Schema

A mental map of ideas about a topic that is stored in long-term memory.

Scientific literacy

Ability to understand scientific (including medical) concepts.

Secondary appraisal

The appraisal that individuals make about their own resources.

Secondary gain

A gain or advantage received by an individual as a result of being ill.

Secondary health promotion

Enabling people in an at-risk population to promote health.

Secondary prevention

Interventions by health professionals and institutions that are aimed at reducing the prevalence of illness at a particular point in time by targeting at-risk individuals.

Self-agency model

A model in which individuals take charge of their condition, identify their responses and manage their lives accordingly.

Self-care

A person's capacity, disposition and activity when managing their multiple chronic conditions; taking time out from the usual business of life to care and nurture yourself through relaxing and restorative pleasurable activities.

Self-efficacy

The perception held by an individual that they can influence and control their own outcomes.

Self-esteem

An individual's perception that they are a good and worthy person.

Sensory disabilities

Impaired vision, hearing, tactile, olfactory and taste responses.

Set point theory

A theory that suggests that the body 'defends' a certain set weight against changes.

Settling point theory

A theory that changes in energy balance become habitual and remain at the new level.

Shaping

Teaching a complex behaviour by reinforcing, one at a time, the series of steps that make up the behaviour.

Sick role

A social agreement involving a balance of rights and obligations granted to an individual who is regarded by others as sick.

Social age

Points at which an individual has reached socially anticipated milestones in their life.

Social capital

Level of trust people have in one another, government institutions and the health professions.

Socialisation

Process of learning the culture of a society or group, its language and customs.

Socio-cultural indicators

Factors that shape or guide an individual's characteristics due to exposure to social and cultural norms within various environments.

Spirituality

A person's practice of creating meaning in their life, existence and purpose.

Stereotyping

Assuming that a member of a category of people will share all of the characteristics attributed to that category.

Stigma

A mark of disapproval that may be attached to an individual who differs from social or cultural norms.

Stimulus

Any change in physical energy that activates a receptor and activates or alerts an organism.

Stimulus control

Changing a behaviour by changing its antecedents.

Stimulus generalisation

The principle that a conditioned response will tend to occur in the presence of stimuli similar to the original conditioned stimulus.

Stress

A perceived imbalance between demands and resources.

Stress response

A pattern of physiological and cognitive reactions experienced by an individual in relation to a situation.

Stressor

An event that appears likely to an observer to produce stress.

Synaptic cleft

The tiny space between two nerve cells, across which they communicate using neurotransmitters.

Systematic desensitisation

A cognitive behavioural strategy for dealing with phobic anxiety by linking increasing exposure to the stimulus that produces anxiety with the practice of relaxation.

Teach to goal

Information and skills that need to be learnt in order to change understanding and behaviours.

Teachable moments

Particularly effective times for concepts to be learnt or behaviours to be developed.

Teach-back

A learning cycle involving repetition and reinforcement of new learning.

Tend and befriend

The idea that women, when stressed, look after their children or seek out social support in order to deal with their stress.

Tertiary health promotion

Enabling people who already have a disease or condition to promote health.

Tertiary prevention

Interventions by health professionals and institutions aimed at decreasing the adverse consequences experienced by people who already have a disease or condition.

Theories of ageing

Varying approaches to explaining the causal impacts of ageing within the human body.

Type A (coronary prone) behaviour pattern

The idea that individuals who show a pattern of competitive achievement, an exaggerated sense of time urgency, and aggressiveness and hostility are at greatly increased risk of heart attack.

Type C (cancer prone) behaviour pattern

The idea that a passive and emotionally repressed personality style is associated with higher rates of cancer occurrence and death from cancer.

Type D (distressed) personality

A tendency to feel negative emotions combined with a reluctance to discuss those feelings with others, that increases the probability of disease.

Unsafe sex

Having sex without using devices such as condoms to protect against pregnancy and STIs, and/or not finding out about a partner's sexual history.

Validation

The idea that patients assume that a health professional will not give them a diagnosis or treatment unless they have valid reasons for seeking a diagnosis or treatment.

Vulnerability

A characteristic or behaviour of the individual that increases the impact of a negative event.

Well-being

A state of complete physical, social and mental health that is consistent with living a full and satisfying life.

Wonder drug effect

Observed tendency for a new treatment to work better while it is new to the market.

Working memory

Information that is stored temporarily for short-term use.

Young adulthood

Arbitrary classification of the transition time from adolescent to an independent adult; the earliest phase of adulthood.

REFERENCES

Abbott R & Lavretsky L (2013) Tai chi and qigong for the treatment and prevention of mental disorders. *Psychiatric Clinics of North America* 36(1), 109–19. https://doi.org/10.1016/j.psc.2013.01.01

ABS [Australian Bureau of Statistics] (2009) *Australian Social Trends.* Cat. no. 4102.0. Australian Bureau of Statistics.

ABS [Australian Bureau of Statistics] (2018a) *National Health Survey: First Results, 2017–18.* ABS Cat. no. 4364.0.55.001. Australian Bureau of Statistics. http://www.abs.gov.au/ausstats/abs@.nsf/mf/4364.0.55.001

ABS [Australian Bureau of Statistics] (2018b) *Household Use of Information Technology, Australia, 2014-2015.* Cat. no. 8146.0. Australian Bureau of Statistics.

ABS [Australian Bureau of Statistics] (2018c) *National Health Survey: Health Literacy.* https://www.abs.gov.au/statistics/health/health-conditions-and-risks/national-health-survey-health-literacy/latest-release

ABS [Australian Bureau of Statistics] (2019a) *Census 2016.* Australian Bureau of Statistics.

ABS [Australian Bureau of Statistics] (2019b) *Disability, Aging and Carers, Australia: Summary of Findings, 2018.* Cat. no. 4403. https://www.abs.gov.au/statistics/health/disability/disability-ageing-and-carers-australia-summary-findings

ABS [Australian Bureau of Statistics] (2020a) *Births Australia.* https://www.abs.gov.au/statistics/people/population/births-australia/latest-release

ABS [Australian Bureau of Statistics] (2020b) *Labour Force Status of Families.* https://www.abs.gov.au/statistics/labour/employment-and-unemployment/labour-force-status-families/latest-release

ABS [Australian Bureau of Statistics] (2020c) *Marriages and Divorces in Australia.* https://www.abs.gov.au/statistics/people/people-and-communities/marriages-and-divorces-australia/latest-release#:~:text=Media%20releases-,Key%20statistics,a%2031.9%25%20decrease%20in%20marriages

ABS [Australian Bureau of Statistics] (2021a) *Causes of Death: Australia.* https://www.abs.gov.au/statistics/health/causes-death/causes-death-australia/latest-release

ABS [Australian Bureau of Statistics] (2021b) *Population.* https://www.abs.gov.au/statistics/people/population

Abusalehi A, Vahedian-Shahroodi M, Esmaily H, Jafari A & Tehrani H (2021) Mental health promotion of the elderly in nursing homes: A social-cognitive intervention. *International Journal of Gerontology* 15(3), 221–7.

Access Economics (2008) *The Growing Costs of Obesity in 2008: Three Years On.* Diabetes Australia.

Addison RG (1984) Chronic pain syndrome. *American Journal of Medicine* 77(3A), 54–8.

AHPRA [Australian Health Practitioner Regulation Agency] (2018) *Aboriginal and Torres Strait Islander Health Strategy: Strategic Plan 2018.* https://www.ahpra.gov.au/About-AHPRA/Aboriginal-andTorres-Strait-Islander-Health-Strategy.aspx.

AHRC [Australian Human Rights Commission] (2021) *Close the Gap.* https://humanrights.gov.au/our-work/aboriginal-and-torres-strait-islander-social-justice/publications/close-gap-2021

Ai A & Carretta H (2021) Depression in patients with heart diseases: Gender differences and association of comorbidities, optimism, and spiritual struggle. *International Journal of Behavioral Medicine* 28(3), 382–92.

AIHIN [Australian Indigenous Health InfoNet] (2018) *Summary of Indigenous Health 2018.* https://healthinfonnet.ecu.edu.au

AIHIN [Australian Indigenous Health InfoNet] (2021) *Social and Cultural Determinants.* https://healthinfonet.ecu.edu.au/learn/determinants-of-health/social-cultural-determinants/

AIHW [Australian Institute of Health and Welfare] (2017) *A Picture of Overweight and Obesity in Australia 2017.* Cat. no. PHE 216. Australian Institute of Health and Welfare.

AIHW [Australian Institute of Health and Welfare] (2018a) *Australia's Health 2018: In Brief.* www.aihw.gov.au/reports/australias-health/australias-health-2018-in-brief/contents/how-healthy-are-we

AIHW [Australian Institute of Health and Welfare] (2018b) *Older Australia at a Glance.* https://www.aihw.gov.au/reports/older-people/older-australia-at-a-glance/contents/healthy-ageing

AIHW [Australian Institute of Health and Welfare] (2018c) *Improving Australia's Burden of Disease.* https://www.aihw.gov.au/getmedia/28c917f3-cb00-44dd-ba86-c13e764dea6b/Improving-Australia-s-burden-of-disease-9-01-2019.pdf.aspx

AIHW [Australian Institute of Health and Welfare] (2019) *People with Disability in Australia.* https://www.aihw.gov.au/reports/disability/people-with-disability-in-australia/contents/summary

AIHW [Australian Institute of Health and Welfare] (2020a) *Australia's Children: In Brief.* https://www.aihw.gov.au/reports/children-youth/australias-children/contents/executive- summary

AIHW [Australian Institute of Health and Welfare] (2020b) *Australia's Health: Chronic Conditions and Multimorbidity.* https://www.aihw.gov.au/reports/australias-health/chronic-conditions-and-multimorbidity

AIHW [Australian Institute of Health and Welfare] (2020c) *Australia's Health: Social Determinants.* https://www.aihw.gov.au/reports-data/australias-health

AIHW [Australian Institute of Health and Welfare] (2020d) *Australia's Health.* https://www.aihw.gov.au/reports-data/health-conditions-disability-deaths/heart-stroke-vascular-diseases

AIHW [Australian Institute of Health and Welfare] (2020e) *National Drug Strategy Household Survey 2019.* Drug Statistics Series no. 32. Cat. no. PHE 270. Australian Institute of Health and Welfare.

AIHW [Australian Institute of Health and Welfare] (2021a) *Children and Youth.* https://www.aihw.gov.au/reports-data/population-groups/children-youth/overview

AIHW [Australian Institute of Health and Welfare] (2021b) *Deaths in Australia: Life Expectancy.* https://www.aihw.gov.au/reports/life-expectancy-death/deaths-in-australia/contents/life-expectancy

AIHW [Australian Institute of Health and Welfare] (2021c) *Indigenous Health and Wellbeing.* https://www.aihw.gov.au/reports/australias-health/indigenous-health-and-wellbeing

AIHW [Australian Institute of Health and Welfare] (2021d) *Life Expectancy and Death: Deaths in Australia.* https://www.aihw.gov.

au/reports/life-expectancy-death/deaths-in-australia/contents/leading-causes-of-death

AIHW [Australian Institute of Health and Welfare] (2021e) *Overweight and Obesity*. https://www.aihw.gov.au/reports/australias-health/overweight-and-obesity

Ajibewa T, Adams T, Gill A, Mazin L, Gerras J & Hasson R (2021) Stress coping strategies and stress reactivity in adolescents with overweight/obesity. *Stress & Health* 37(2), 243–54.

Ajzen I & Madden T (1986) Prediction of goal-directed behavior: Attitudes, intentions, and perceived behavioral control. *Journal of Experimental Social Psychology* 22, 453–74.

Akil H, Watson SJ, Young E, Lewis ME, Khachaturian H & Walker JM (1984) Endogenous opioids: Biology and function. *Annual Review of Neuroscience* 7, 223–55.

Alexander F (1943) Fundamental concepts of psychosomatic research: Psychogenesis, conversion, specificity. *Psychosomatic Medicine* 5, 205–10.

Allen F (1998) *Health Psychology: Theory and Practice*. Allen & Unwin.

Andreassi JL (2006) *Psychophysiology: Human Behaviour and Physiological Response* (5th edn). Lawrence Erlbaum.

APA [American Psychiatric Association] (2013) *Diagnostic and Statistical Manual of Mental Disorders: DSM-5*. American Psychiatric Association DSM-5 Task Force. American Psychiatric Association.

APA [American Psychological Association] (2021a) *APA Dictionary of Psychology*. https://dictionary.apa.org

APA [American Psychological Association] (2021b) *COVID-19 Stress Management Tools*. https://www.apa.org/topics/covid-19/stress-management-tools

Aparicio-Martinez P, Perea-Moreno AJ, Martinez-Jimenez MP, Redel-Macías MD, Pagliari C & Vaquero-Abellan M (2019) Social media, thin-ideal, body dissatisfaction and disordered eating attitudes: An exploratory analysis. *International Journal of Environmental Research and Public Health* 16(21), 4177. https://doi.org/10.3390/ijerph16214177

APBPA [Australian Preterm Birth Prevention Alliance] (2015) *Preterm Facts and Figures*. https://www.pretermalliance.com.au/About-Preterm-Birth/Preterm-Facts-and-Figures

Araja D, Berkis U, Lunga, A & Murovska M (2021) PMU29 burden of COVID-19 consequences: An example of post-viral chronic fatigue syndrome. *Value in Health* 24, S149–50.

Argyridis S (2019) Folic acid in pregnancy. *Obstetrics, Gynaecology and Reproductive Medicine* 29(4), 118–20.

Armstrong D (1980) *An Outline of Sociology as Applied to Medicine*. John Wright & Sons.

Arnold M (1960) *Emotion and Personality*. Columbia University Press.

Aschwanden C (2021) How COVID is changing the study of human behavior. *Nature* [online]. https://www.nature.com/articles/d41586-021-01317-z

Aschwanden D, Gerend M, Luchetti M, Stephan Y, Sutin A & Terracciano A (2019) Personality traits and preventive cancer screenings in the Health Retirement Study. *Preventive Medicine* 126, 105763. doi.org/10.1016/j.ypmed.2019.105763

Australian Government (2020) *National Agreement on Closing the Gap*. https://www.closingthegap.gov.au/national-agreement/national-agreement-closing-the-gap

Australian Museum (2021) *The Dreaming*. https://australian.museum/about/history/exhibitions/indigenous-australians/

Bailey RR (2017) Goal setting and action planning for health behavior change. *American Journal of Lifestyle Medicine* 13(6), 615–18. https://doi.org/10.1177/1559827617729634

Baker DW, DeWalt DA, Schillinger D, Hawk V, Ruo B, Bibbins-Dimingo K, Weinberger M, Macabasco-O'Connell A & Pignone M (2011) 'Teach to goal': Theory and design principles of an intervention to improve heart failure self-management skills of patients with low health literacy. *Journal of Health Communication* 16, 73–88.

Balis G (1978) Psychogenic aspects of the doctor–patient relationship. In G Balis, L Wurmser, E McDaniel & R Grenell (Eds) *The Behavioral and Social Sciences and the Practice of Medicine*. Butterworth.

Bandura A (1977a) Self-efficacy: Toward a unifying theory of behavioral change. *Psychological Review* 84(2), 191–215.

Bandura A (1977b) *Social Learning Theory*. Prentice-Hall.

Bandura A (1986) *Social Foundations of Thought and Action: A Social Cognitive Theory*. Prentice-Hall.

Bandura A (1998) Health promotion from the perspective of social cognitive theory. *Psychology and Health* 13, 623–49.

Bandura A, Ross S & Ross D (1963) Imitation of film-mediated aggressive models. *Journal of Abnormal and Social Psychology* 66, 3–11.

Banks E, Byles JE, Gibson RE, Rodgers B, Latz IK, Robinson IA, Williamson AB & Jorm LR (2010) Is psychological distress in people living with cancer related to the fact of diagnosis, current treatment or level of disability? Findings from a large Australian study. *Medical Journal of Australia* 193(5 Suppl.), S62–7.

Barlow DH (2000) Unraveling the mysteries of anxiety and its disorders from the perspective of emotion theory. *American Psychologist* 55(11), 1247–63.

Barlow F (2019) Nature vs nurture is nonsense: On the necessity of an integrated genetic, social, developmental, and personality psychology. *Australian Journal of Psychology* 71(1), 68–79.

Bavel JJV, Baicker K, Boggio PS et al. (2020) Using social and behavioural science to support COVID-19 pandemic response. *Nature: Human Behaviour* 4, 460–71. https://www.nature.com/articles/s41562-020-0884-z

Baxter R, Corneliusson L, Björk S, Kloos N & Edvardsson D (2021) A recipe for thriving in nursing homes: A meta-ethnography. *Journal of Advanced Nursing* 77(6), 2680–8.

Behan C (2020) The benefits of meditation and mindfulness practices during times of crisis such as COVID-19. *Irish Journal of Psychological Medicine* 37(4), 256–8. https://doi.org/10.1017/ipm.2020.38

Benjamin R, Haliburn J & King S (2019) *Humanising Mental Health Care in Australia*. Routledge.

Berkman ET (2018) The neuroscience of goals and behavior change. *Consulting Psychology Journal* 70(1), 28–44. https://doi.org/10.1037/cpb0000094

Berman A, Frandsen G, Snyder S, Levett-Jones T, Burston A & Dwyer T (2020) *Kozier and Erb's Fundamentals of Nursing*. Vols 1–3. Pearson Education Australia.

Berman A, Frandsen G, Snyder S, Levett-Jones T, Burston A, Dwyer T, Hales M, Harvey N, Langtree T, Reid-Searl K, Rolf F & Stanley D (Eds) (2021) *Kozier and Erb's Fundamentals of Nursing: Concepts, Processes and Practice* (5th Australian edn). Pearson.

Bernard W, Lambert C, Henrard S & Hermans C (2018) Screening of haemophilia carriers in moderate and severe haemophilia

A and B: Prevalence and determinants. *Haemophilia* 24(3), E142–4.

Best O & Fredericks B (2014) *Yatdjuligin: Aboriginal and Torres Strait Islander Nursing and Midwifery Care*. Cambridge University Press.

Bissell K & Mocarski R (2016) Edutainment's impact on health promotion: Viewing the biggest loser through the social cognitive theory. *Health Promotion Practice* 17(1), 107–15.

Bloom BS (1968) Learning for mastery. *Evaluation Comment* 1(2), 1–12.

Bontempo A (2021) The need for a standardized conceptual term to describe invalidation of patient symptoms. *Journal of Health Psychology* [online], 135910532110247–13591053211024718.

Boring B, Walsh K, Nanavaty N, Ng B & Mathur V (2021) How and why patient concerns influence pain reporting: A qualitative analysis of personal accounts and perceptions of others' use of numerical pain scales. *Frontiers in Psychology* 12, 2232. https://www.frontiersin.org/article/10.3389/fpsyg.2021.663890. DOI=10.3389/fpsyg.2021.663890

Bourke S, Harper C, Johnson E, Green J, Anish L, Muduwa M & Jones L (2021) Health care experiences in rural, remote, and metropolitan areas of Australia. *Online Journal of Rural Nursing and Health Care* 21(1), 67–84.

Bourne A, Peerbux S, Jessup R et al. (2018) Health literacy profile of recently hospitalised patients in the private hospital setting: A cross-sectional survey using the Health Literacy Questionnaire (HLQ). *BMC Health Services Research* 18, 877. https://doi.org/10.1186/s12913-018-3697-2

Bovill M, Chamberlain C, Bennett J, Longbottom H, Bacon S, Field B, Hussein P, Berwick R, Gould G & O'Mara P (2021) Building an Indigenous-led evidence base for smoking cessation care among Aboriginal and Torres Strait Islander women during pregnancy and beyond: Research protocol for the Which Way? project. *International Journal of Environmental Research and Public Health* 18(3), 1342.

Bowden M (2020) *Understanding Food Insecurity in Australia*. https://aifs.gov.au/cfca/publications/undehttps://aifs.gov.au/cfca/publications/understanding-food-insecurity-australiarstanding-food-insecurity-australia

BreastScreen Victoria (2021) *Your Breast Cancer Risk*. https://www.breastscreen.org.au/breast-cancer-and-screening/your-breast-cancer-risk/

Brewer NT, Chapman GB, Rothman AJ, Leask J & Kempe A (2017) Increasing vaccination: Putting psychological science into action. *Psychological Science in the Public Interest* 18(3),149–207. doi:10.1177/1529100618760521

Briziarelli M (2019) Snapchat's dialectics of socialization: Revisiting the theory of the spectacle for a critical political economy of social media. *Communication, Culture & Critique* 12(18), 590. doi:10.1093/ccc/tcz029

Brown WJ, Mummery K, Eakin E & Schofield G (2006) '10,000 Steps Rockhampton': Evaluation of a whole-community approach to improving population levels of physical activity. *Journal of Physical Activity and Health* 3(1), 1–14.

Brytek-Matera A & Czepczor K (2017) Models of eating disorders: A theoretical investigation of abnormal eating patterns and body image disturbance. *Archives of Psychiatry and Psychotherapy* 1, 16–26. doi: 10.12740/APP/68422

Buckinx F, Carvalho LP, Marcangeli V, Dulac M, Boutros GH, Gouspillou G et al. (2020) High intensity interval training combined with L-citrulline supplementation: Effects on physical performance in healthy older adults. *Experimental Gerontology* 140, 111036.

BudgetDirect (2021) *Almost One-fifth of Aussies Surveyed are More Scared of Vaccine Side Effects than Being Involved in a Car Accident*. https://www.budgetdirect.com.au/about-us/media-releases/2021/car-accident-risks.html

Bueter A (2019) On illness, disease, and priority: A framework for more fruitful debates. *Medicine, Health Care, and Philosophy*, 22(3), 463–74.

Burian H, Böge K, Burian R, Burns A, Nguyen M, Ohse L et al. (2021) Acceptance and commitment-based therapy for patients with psychiatric and physical health conditions in routine general hospital care: Development, implementation and outcomes. *Journal of Psychosomatic Research* 143, 1–9.

Calvet B, Vézina N, Laberge M, Nastasia I, Sultan-Taïeb H, Toulouse G, Rubiano P & Durand MJ (2021) Integrative prevention and coordinated action toward primary, secondary and tertiary prevention in workplaces: A scoping review. *Work* 70(24), 1–16.

Can Y, Iles-Smith H, Chalabianloo N, Ekiz D, Fernández-Alvarez J, Repetto C, Riva G & Ersoy C (2020) How to relax in stressful situations: A smart stress reduction system. *Healthcare* 8(2), 100. https://doi.org/10.3390/healthcare8020100

Cannon W (1932) *The Wisdom of the Body*. Norton.

CDCP [Centers for Disease Control and Prevention] (2011) *Health Weight: Assessing your Weight—BMI*. www.cdc.gov/healthyweight/assessing/bmi/adult_bmi/index.html

CDGN [Communicable Diseases Genomics Network] (2020) *Variants of Concern*. https://www.cdgn.org.au/variants-of-concern

Chabert J-L (2012) *A History of Algorithms: From the Pebble to the Microchip*. Springer Science & Business Media.

Chaput JP, Dutil C & Sampasa-Kanyinga H (2018) Sleeping hours: What is the ideal number and how does age impact this? *Nature and Science of Sleep* 10, 421–30. https://doi.org/10.2147/NSS.S163071

Charles ST, Piazza JR, Mogle J, Sliwinski MJ & Almeida DM (2013) The wear and tear of daily stressors on mental health. *Psychological Science* 24(5), 733–41. https://doi.org/10.1177/0956797612462222

Cheshire A, Ridge D, Clark L & White P (2021) Sick of the sick role: Narratives of what 'recovery' means to people with CFS/ME. *Qualitative Health Research* 31(2), 298–308.

Chida Y & Steptoe A (2009) The association of anger and hostility with future coronary heart disease. *Journal of the American College of Cardiology* 53(11), 936–46.

Chuang I, Shyu Y, Weng L & Huang H (2020) Consistency in end-of-life care preferences between hospitalized elderly patients and their primary family caregivers. *Patient Preference and Adherence* 14, 2377–87.

Clark DA & Beck AT (2011) *The Anxiety and Worry Workbook: The Cognitive Behavioral Solution*. Guilford Press.

Clarkson C, Jacobs Z, Marwick B et al. (2017) Human occupation of northern Australia by 65,000 years ago. *Nature* 547(7663), 306–10.

Clemmensen C, Petersen MB & Sørensen TI (2020) Will the COVID-19 pandemic worsen the obesity epidemic? *Nature Reviews Endocrinology* 16(9), 469–70.

Clucas C, Sibley E, Harding R, Liu L, Catalan J & Sherr L (2011) A systematic review of interventions for anxiety in people with HIV. *Psychology, Health and Medicine* 16(5), 528–47.

Coates J & Jha A (2019) A comparison between phantom breast syndrome and phantom limb: A systematic review. *Journal of the Neurological Sciences* 405, 107–8.

Cohen S, Kessler R & Gordon L (1995) Conceptualising stress and its relation to disease. In Cohen S, Kessler R & Gordon L (Eds) *Measuring Stress: A Guide for Health and Social Scientists* (pp. 3–26). Oxford University Press.

Colloca L (Ed.) (2018a) *The Neurobiology of the Placebo Effect*. Elsevier.

Colloca L (2018b) Preface: The fascinating mechanisms and implications of the placebo effect. *International Review of Neurobiology* 138, xv–xx. https://doi.org/10.1016/S0074-7742(18)30027-8

Commonwealth of Australia (2013) *National Aboriginal and Torres Strait Islander Health Plan 2013–2023*. https://www.health.gov.au/resources/publications/national-aboriginal-and-torres-strait-islander-health-plan-2013-2023

Corn B, Feldman D & Wexler I (2020) The science of hope. *Lancet Oncology* 21(9), e452–9.

Cox CE (2017) Role of physical activity for weight loss and weight maintenance. *Diabetes Spectrum* 30(3), 157–60. https://doi.org/10.2337/ds17-0013

Coyne E, Wollin J & Creedy D (2012) Exploration of the family's role and strengths after a young woman is diagnosed with breast cancer: Views of the women and their families. *European Journal of Oncology Nursing* 16(2), 124–30.

CPA [Cerebral Palsy Alliance] (2018) *What is Cerebral Palsy?* https://cerebralpalsy.org.au/our-research/about-cerebral-palsy/what-is-cerebral-palsy/

CPPSCG [Cochrane Pain, Palliative and Supportive Care Group] (2021) https://papas.cochrane.org/about-us

Crawley R, Wilkie S, Gamble J, Creedy DK, Fenwick J, Cockburn N & Ayers S (2018) Characteristics of memories for traumatic and non-traumatic birth. *Applied Cognitive Psychology* 32(5), 584–91. doi:10.1002/acp.3438

Creedy DK, Gamble J, Boorman R & Allen J (2020a) Midwives' knowledge and reported practices to assess and address maternal health literacy: A cross-sectional survey. *Women & Birth* 34(2), e188–95. https://doi.org/10.1016/j.wombi.2020.02.018

Creedy DK, Baird K & Gillespie K (2020b) A cross-sectional survey of pregnant women's perceptions of routine domestic and family violence screening and responses by midwives: Testing of three new tools. *Women & Birth* 33(4), 393–400. doi.org/10.1016/j.wombi.2019.06.018

Creedy D, Collis D, Ludlow T, Cosgrove S, Houston K, Irvine D, Fraser J & Maloney S (2005) The impact of a support program for children with a chronic condition on psychosocial indicators. *Contemporary Nurse* 18(1), 46–56.

Crielaard L, Nicolaou M, Sawyer A, Quax R & Stronks K (2021) Understanding the impact of exposure to adverse socioeconomic conditions on chronic stress from a complexity science perspective. *BMC Medicine* 19(1), 1–20.

Crum J (2021) Understanding mental health and cognitive restructuring with ecological neuroscience. *Frontiers in Psychiatry* 12, 697095. https://doi.org/10.3389/fpsyt.2021.697095

Cultural Atlas (2021) Australian Culture. https://culturalatlas.sbs.com.au/australian-culture/australian-culture-core

Cumming E & Henry W (1961) *Growing Old*. Basic Books.

Dadras O, Alinaghi SAS, Karimi A et al. (2021) Effects of COVID-19 prevention procedures on other common infections: A systematic review. *European Journal of Medical Research* 26, 67.

Dai M, Wombacher K, Matig J & Harrington M (2017) Using the integrative model of behavioral prediction to understand college students' hookup sex beliefs, intentions, and behaviors. *Journal of Health Communication* 33(9), 1078–87.

Daniels SR, Arnett DK, Eckel RH, Gidding SS, Hayman LL, Kumanyika S, Robinson TN, Scott BJ, St Jeor S & Williams CL (2005) Overweight in children and adolescents: Pathophysiology, consequences, prevention, and treatment. *Circulation* 111, 1999–2002.

David D, Cristea I & Hofmann SG (2018) Why cognitive behavioral therapy is the current gold standard of psychotherapy. *Frontiers in Psychiatry* 9, 4. https://doi.org/10.3389/fpsyt.2018.00004

Davis RAH, Plaisance EP & Allison DB (2018) Complementary hypotheses on contributors to the obesity epidemic. *Obesity (Silver Spring)* 26, 17–21.

Davis P (2017) *How the 'What-the-Hell' Effect Impacts Your Willpower*. https://www.psychologytoday.com/au/blog/pressure-proof/201701/how-the-what-the-hell-effect-impacts-your-willpower

De Baets L, Matheve T, Meeus M, Struyf F & Timmermans A (2019) The influence of cognitions, emotions and behavioral factors on treatment outcomes in musculoskeletal shoulder pain: A systematic review. *Clinical Rehabilitation* 33(6), 980–91.

De Rosa S, Arcidiacono B, Chiefari E, Brunetti A, Indolfi C & Foti D (2018) Type 2 diabetes mellitus and cardiovascular disease: Genetic and epigenetic links. *Frontiers in Endocrinology* 9, 2.

Dementia Australia (2020) Dementia prevalence data. https://www.dementia.org.au/information/statistics/prevalence-data

Deutz M, Geeraerts S, Belsky J, Deković M, van Baar A, Prinzie P & Patalay P (2020) General psychopathology and dysregulation profile in a longitudinal community sample: Stability, antecedents and outcomes. *Child Psychiatry & Human Development* 51(1), 114–26.

Dias KA, Ingul CB, Tjønna AE, Keating SE, Gomersall SR, Follestad T et al. (2018) Effect of high-intensity interval training on fitness, fat mass and cardiometabolic biomarkers in children with obesity: A randomised controlled trial. *Sports Medicine* 48(3), 733–46.

Dich N, Rozing MP, Kivimäki M & Doan SN (2020) Life events, emotions, and immune function: Evidence from Whitehall II Cohort Study. *Behavioral Medicine* 46(2), 153–60.

DiFusco LA, Schell KA & Saylor JL (2019) Risk-taking behaviors in adolescents with chronic cardiac conditions: A scoping review. *Journal of Pediatric Nursing* 48, 98–105.

Dimond E, Kittle C & Crockett J (1960) Comparison of internal mammary artery ligation and sham surgery for angina pectoris. *American Journal of Cardiology* 5, 483–6.

Ding X, Barban N, Tropf F & Mills M (2019) The relationship between cognitive decline and a genetic predictor of educational attainment. *Social Science & Medicine* 239, 112549.

Dinh TTH, Bonner A, Clark R, Ramsbotham J & Hines S (2016) The effectiveness of the teach-back method on adherence and self-management in health education for people with chronic disease: A systematic review. *JBI Evidence Synthesis* 14(1), 210–47.

Dishop C (2020) A simple, dynamic extension of temporal motivation theory. *Journal of Mathematical Sociology* 44(3), 147–62.

DiTomasso D (2019) Bearing the pain: A historic review exploring the impact of science and culture on pain management for childbirth in the United States. *Journal of Perinatal & Neonatal Nursing* 33(4), 322–30.

Dix L (1985) The effects of expectations on outcomes. Unpublished BMedSci thesis. Monash University.

DoH [Department of Health] (2019a) *Pregnancy Care Guidelines: Lifestyle Considerations—Alcohol.* https://www.health.gov.au/resources/pregnancy-care-guidelines/part-c-lifestyle-considerations/alcohol

DoH [Department of Health] (2019b) *Pregnancy Care Guidelines: Lifestyle Considerations—Tobacco Smoking.* https://www.health.gov.au/resources/pregnancy-care-guidelines/part-c-lifestyle-considerations/tobacco-smoking

DoH [Department of Health] (2019c) *National Asthma Strategy 2018.* https://www.health.gov.au/sites/default/files/documents/2019/09/national-asthma-strategy-2018_0.pdf

Doidge N (2008) *The Brain that Changes Itself: Stories of Personal Triumph from the Frontiers of Brain Science.* Scribe.

Doidge N (2016) *The Brain's Way of Healing: Remarkable Discoveries and Recoveries from the Frontiers of Neuroplasticity.* Penguin.

Dolan N, Simmonds-Buckley M, Kellett S, Siddell E & Delgadillo J (2021) Effectiveness of stress control large group psychoeducation for anxiety and depression: Systematic review and meta-analysis. *British Journal of Clinical Psychology* 60(3), 375–99.

Dorrian T, Di Benedetto M, Lane-Krebs K, Day M, Hutchinson A & Sherman K (2017) *Health Psychology in Australia.* Cambridge University Press.

Egger G (2006) Are meal replacements an effective clinical strategy for weight loss? *Medical Journal of Australia* 184(2), 52–3.

Ekman P (1980) *The Face of Man: Expressions of Universal Emotions in a New Guinea Village.* Garland STM Press.

El-Heneidy A, Abdel-Rahman M, Mihala G, Ross L & Comans T (2018) Milk other than breast milk and the development of asthma in children 3 years of age: A birth cohort study (2006–2011). *Nutrients* 10(11), 1798.

Engel G (1977) The need for a new medical model: A challenge for biomedicine. *Science* 196, 126–9.

Engeln R, Loach R, Imundo MN & Zola A (2020) Compared to Facebook, Instagram use causes more appearance comparison and lower body satisfaction in college women. *Body Image* 34, 38–45.

Epifanio MS, Ingoglia S, Alfano P, Lo Coco G & La Grutta S (2018) Type D personality and alexithymia: Common characteristics of two different constructs—implications for research and clinical practice. *Frontiers in Psychology* 9, 106. doi: 10.3389/fpsyg.2018.00106

Erikson E (1950) *Childhood and Society.* Norton.

Erikson EH (1968) *Identity: Youth and Crisis.* Norton.

Eskelinen M & Ollonen P (2011) Assessment of 'cancer-prone personality' characteristics in healthy study subjects and in patients with breast disease and breast cancer using the commitment questionnaire: A prospective case-control study in Finland. *Anticancer Research* 31(11), 4013–17.

Evers AWM, Colloca L, Blease C, Annoni M, Atlas LY, Benedetti F, Bingel U, Büchel C, Carvalho C, Colagiuri B, Crum AJ, Enck P, Gaab J, Geers AL, Howick J, Jensen KB, Kirsch I, Meissner K, Napadow V, Peerdeman KJ, Raz A, Rief W, Vase L, Wager TD, Wampold BE, Weimer K, Wiech K, Kaptchuk TJ, Klinger R & Kelley JM (2018) Implications of placebo and nocebo effects for clinical practice: Expert consensus. *Psychotherapy and Psychosomatics* 87, 204–10. doi: 10.1159/000490354

Evetts C (2017) Fight or flight versus tend and befriend behavioral response to stress. *American Journal of Occupational Therapy* 71(Supp.), 98.

Eysenck H (1976) Neuroticism. In S Krauss (Ed.) *Encyclopaedic Handbook of Medical Psychology.* Butterworths.

Farre A & Rapley T (2017) The new old (and old new) medical model: Four decades navigating the biomedical and psychosocial understandings of health and illness. *Healthcare* 5(4), 88.

Fava GA, McEwen BS, Guidi J, Gostoli S, Offidani E & Sonino N (2019) Clinical characterization of allostatic overload. *Psychoneuroendocrinology* 108, 94–101.

Felitti VJ, Anda RF, Nordenberg D, Williamson DF, Spitz AM, Edwards V & Marks JS (1998) Relationship of childhood abuse and household dysfunction to many of the leading causes of death in adults: The Adverse Childhood Experiences (ACE) Study. *American Journal of Preventive Medicine* 14(4), 245–58.

Ferguson RJ, Roy-Charland A, Rowe S, Perron M & Gallant J (2021) Examining featural processing of emotional facial expressions: Is trait anxiety a factor? *Canadian Journal of Behavioural Science* [advance online publication]. https://doi.org/10.1037/cbs0000250

Fernández-Aguilar C, Martín-Martín JJ, Minué Lorenzo S & Fernández Ajuria A (2021) Use of heuristics during the clinical decision process from family care physicians in real conditions. *Journal of Evaluation in Clinical Practice* 28(1), 135–41. https://doi.org/10.1111/jep.13608

Finkelstein-Fox L, Park C & Kalichman S (2020) Health benefits of positive reappraisal coping among people living with HIV/AIDS: A systematic review. *Health Psychology Review* 14(3), 394–426.

Fishbein M (2008) A reasoned action approach to health promotion. *Medical Decision Making* 28, 834–44.

Fishbein M & Ajzen I (1975) *Belief, Attitude, Intention and Behavior: An Introduction to Theory and Research.* Addison Wesley.

Fisher S (1986) *Stress and Strategy.* Lawrence Erlbaum.

Flanders Dunbar H (1947) *Mind and Body: Psychosomatic Medicine.* Random House.

Flegal KM, Graubard BI, Williamson DF & Gail MH (2005) Excess deaths associated with underweight, overweight, and obesity. *Journal of the American Medical Association* 293(15), 1861–7.

Fleischer T, Ulke C, Beutel M, Binder H, Brähler E, Johar H et al. (2021) The relation between childhood adversity and adult obesity in a population-based study in women and men. *Scientific Reports* 11(1), 1–10.

Flint S (2020) Stigmatizing media portrayal of obesity during the coronavirus (COVID-19) pandemic. *Frontiers in Psychology* 11, 2124. doi=10.3389/fpsyg.2020.02124

Flynn D (2020) Chronic musculoskeletal pain: Nonpharmacologic, non-invasive treatments. *American Family Physician* 102(8), 465–77.

Fordham B, Sugavanam T, Edwards K, Stallard P, Howard R, das Nair R, Copsey B, Lee H, Howick J, Hemming K & Lamb SE (2021) The evidence for cognitive behavioural therapy in any condition, population or context: A meta-review of systematic reviews and panoramic meta-analysis. *Psychological Medicine* 51(1), 21–9. https://doi.org/10.1017/S0033291720005292

Frank J (1973) *Persuasion and Healing* (rev. edn). Johns Hopkins University Press.

Frankenhaeuser M (1991) The psychophysiology of workload, stress and health: Comparison between the sexes. *Annals of Behavioral Medicine* 13, 197–201.

Friedman M & Rosenman R (1974) *Type A Behavior and Your Heart.* Knopf.

Friedrich MJ (2017) Global obesity epidemic worsening. *Journal of the American Medical Association* 318(7), 603.

Frier A & Devine S (2020) Poverty and inequality in Australia. *Australian Journal of Rural Health* 28(1), 94–5.

FTC [Federal Trade Commission] (2004) *Weighing the Evidence in Diet Ads*. www.ftc.gov/bcp/edu/pubs/consumer/health/hea03.shtm

Gainotti G (2019) The role of the right hemisphere in emotional and behavioral disorders of patients with frontotemporal lobar degeneration: An updated review. *Frontiers in Aging Neuroscience* 11, 55. doi: 10.3389/fnagi.2019.00055

Galaviz KI, Narayan KMV, Lobelo F, Weber MB (2015) Lifestyle and the prevention of type 2 diabetes: A status report. *American Journal of Lifestyle Medicine* 12(1),4–20.

Garakani A, Murrough JW, Freire RC, Thom RP, Larkin K, Buono FD & Iosifescu DV (2020) Pharmacotherapy of anxiety disorders: Current and emerging treatment options. *Frontiers in Psychiatry* 11, 595584. https://doi.org/10.3389/fpsyt.2020.595584

Garfin DR, Thompson RR & Holman EA (2018) Acute stress and subsequent health outcomes: A systematic review. *Journal of Psychosomatic Research* 112, 107–13.

Glick RM & Greco CM (2010) Biofeedback and primary care. *Primary Care* 37(1), 91–103.

Glozier N, Tofler G, Colquhoun D, Bunker S, Clarke D et al. (2013) Psychosocial risk factors for coronary heart disease. *Medical Journal of Australia* 199(3), 179–80.

Goh S (2017) Immorality of inaction on inequality. *BMJ* [online] 356, j556. doi: 10.1136/bmj.j556

Gore JS, Griffin DP & McNierney D (2016) Does internal or external locus of control have a stronger link to mental and physical health? *Psychological Studies* 61, 181–96. https://doi.org/10.1007/s12646-016-0361-y

Gu S, Wang F, Cao C, Wu E, Tang Y & Huang J (2019) An integrative way for studying neural basis of basic emotions with fMRI. *Frontiers in Neuroscience* 13, 628. doi: 10.3389/fnins.2019.00628

Guenther J (2021) Taken for a ride? The disconnect between high school completion, employment and income for remote Australian First Nations peoples. *Race, Ethnicity and Education* 24(1), 132–47.

Guidi J, Lucente M, Sonino N & Fava GA (2021) Allostatic load and its impact on health: A systematic review. *Psychotherapy and Psychosomatics* 90, 11–27. https://doi.org/10.1159/000510696

Hall KD (2018) Did the food environment cause the obesity epidemic? *Obesity* 26, 11–13.

Hall C (1979) *A Primer of Freudian Psychology* (25th anniv. edn). New American Library.

Hall J, Ambang T, Asante A, Mapira P, Craig A, Schuele E & Pervaz Iqbal M (2019) Poliomyelitis outbreak in Papua New Guinea: Health system and health security implications for PNG and Australia. *Medical Journal of Australia* 211(4), 161–2.e1.

Hamm JM, Heckhausen J, Shane J & Lachman ME (2020) Risk of cognitive declines with retirement: Who declines and why? *Psychology of Ageing* 35(3), 449–57. doi: 10.1037/pag0000453

Hart J (1971) The inverse care law. *Lancet*, 1, 405–12.

Harvey SB, Milligan-Saville JS, Paterson HM, Harkness EL, Marsh AM, Dobson M et al. (2016) The mental health of fire-fighters: An examination of the impact of repeated trauma exposure. *Australian and New Zealand Journal of Psychiatry* 50(7), 649–58.

Hashemipoor F, Jafari F & Zabihi R (2019) Maladaptive schemas and psychological well-being in premenopausal and postmenopausal women. *Przegląd Menopauzalny* 18(1), 33–8.

Health Direct (2019) *How to Get the Most Out of Your Doctor's Appointment*. https://www.healthdirect.gov.au/blog/how-to-get-the-most-out-of-your-doctors-appointment

Health Direct (2021) *7 Reasons People Don't Get COVID-19 Vaccinations*. https://www.healthdirect.gov.au/blog/7-reasons-people-dont-get-covid-19-vaccinations

Healthline (2021) *12 Healthy Foods High in Antioxidants*. https://www.healthline.com/nutrition/foods-high-in-antioxidants

Heath R (1964) *The Reasonable Adventurer*. University of Pittsburgh Press.

Heider F (1967) *The Psychology of Interpersonal Relations*. John Wiley & Sons.

Hetherington MM, Blundell-Birtill P, Caton SJ, Cecil JE, Evans CE, Rolls BJ & Tang T (2018) Understanding the science of portion control and the art of downsizing. *Proceedings of the Nutrition Society* 77(3), 347–55. https://doi.org/10.1017/S0029665118000435

Hing N, Browne M, Russell A, Rockloff M, Rawat V, Nicoll F & Smith G (2019) Avoiding gambling harm: An evidence-based set of safe gambling practices for consumers. *PloS One* 14(10), e0224083.

Hoffnung M, Hoffnung R, Seifert K, Hine A, Ward L, Pause C, Ward L, Sawbey K, Yates K & Smith R (2019) *Lifespan Development* (4th Australasian edn). John Wiley & Sons.

Holland J, Graves S, Klingspon K & Rozalski V (2016) Prolonged grief symptoms related to loss of physical functioning: Examining unique associations with medical service utilization. *Disability & Rehabilitation* 38(3), 205–10.

Holmes T & Rahe R (1967) The social readjustment rating scale. *Journal of Psychosomatic Research* 11, 213–18.

Howe LC, Goyer JP & Crum AJ (2017) Harnessing the placebo effect: Exploring the influence of physician characteristics on placebo response. *Health Psychology* 36(11), 1074–82. https://doi.org/10.1037/hea0000499

Howe P, Vargas-Sáenz A, Hulbert C & Boldero J (2019) Predictors of gambling and problem gambling in Victoria, Australia. *PloS One* 14(1), e0209277.

Howick J, Webster R, Kirby N et al. (2018) Rapid overview of systematic reviews of nocebo effects reported by patients taking placebos in clinical trials. *Trials* 19, 674. https://doi.org/10.1186/s13063-018-3042-4

Howie V, Lane-Krebs K & Wilson N (2021) Disability. In A Berman, G Frandsen, S Snyder, T Levett-Jones, A Burston, T Dwyer, M Hales, N Harvey, T Langtree, K Reid-Searl, F Rolf & D Stanley (Eds) (2021) *Kozier and Erb's Fundamentals of Nursing: Concepts, Processes and Practice* (5th Australian edn, pp. 1157–76). Pearson.

Huggins C, Donnan G, Cameron I & Williams J (2021) Emotional self-awareness in autism: A meta-analysis of group differences and developmental effects. *Autism* 25(2), 307–21.

Hull C (1943) *Principles of Behavior*. Appleton-Century-Crofts.

IASP [International Association for the Study of Pain] (2020) *IASP Announces Revised Definition of Pain*. https://www.iasp-pain.org/publications/iasp-news/iasp-announces-revised-definition-of-pain/

IISC [Interaction Institute for Social Change] (n.d.) *Illustrating Equality vs Equity*. https://interactioninstitute.org/illustrating-equality-vs-equity/

Isik K, Cengiz Z & Doğan Z (2020) The relationship between self-care agency and depression in older adults and influencing factors. *Journal of Psychosocial Nursing & Mental Health Services* 58(10), 39–47.

Jaaniste T, Yang J, Bang J, Yee R, Evans E, Aouad P, Champion G & Yee R (2021) Multidimensional self-report assessment of children's acute pain in an inpatient setting. *Clinical Journal of Pain* 37(6), 421–8.

Jacobs J, Peterson K, Allender S, Alston L & Nichols M (2018) Regional variation in cardiovascular mortality in Australia 2009–2012: The impact of remoteness and socioeconomic status. *Australian and New Zealand Journal of Public Health* 42(5), 467–73.

Jacobson E (1938) *Progressive Relaxation* (2nd edn). University of Chicago Press.

James D & Jowza M (2019) Treating opioid dependence: Pain medicine physiology of tolerance and addiction. *Clinical Obstetrics & Gynecology* 62(1), 87–97.

James W (1890) *Psychology*. Holt.

Jandackova V, Koenig J, Jarczok M, Fischer J & Thayer J (2017) Potential biological pathways linking type-D personality and poor health: A cross-sectional investigation. *PloS One* 12(4), e0176014.

Jandaghi G, Firoozi M & Zia-Tohidi A (2020) Psychological interventions for depression and anxiety: A systematic review and meta-analysis of Iranian chronic pain trials. *Health Promotion Perspectives* 10(3), 180–91.

Jarman HK, Marques MD, McLean SA, Slater A & Paxton SJ (2021) Social media, body satisfaction and well-being among adolescents: A mediation model of appearance-ideal internalization and comparison. *Body Image* 36, 139–48.

Jensen M, Mendoza M, Ehde D, Patterson D, Molton I, Dillworth T, Gertz K, Chan J, Hakimian S, Battalio S & Ciol M (2020) Effects of hypnosis, cognitive therapy, hypnotic cognitive therapy, and pain education in adults with chronic pain: A randomized clinical trial. *Pain* 161(10), 2284–98. doi: 10.1097/j.pain.0000000000001943

Jones K (1970) Role conflict: Perception and experience. PhD dissertation. University of Missouri.

Jones K (1991) Type A behavior as a generally available strategy: Varying activation by tasks and instructions. *Psychology and Health* 5, 289–96.

Jones K (2001) Encouraging the transition to teamwork learning communities. *Communities of Learning: Who, Where, How.* Proceedings of the 2001 ANZAME Annual Conference, Nelson, New Zealand.

Jones K, Copolov D & Outch K (1986) Type A, test performance and salivary cortisol. *Journal of Psychosomatic Research* 30, 699–707.

Jones N, Gilman S, Cheng T, Drury S, Hill C & Geronimus A (2019) Life course approaches to the causes of health disparities. *American Journal of Public Health* 109(S1), S48–55.

Kabat-Zinn J (2013) *Full Catastrophe Living: Using the Wisdom of Your Body and Mind to Face Stress, Pain and Illness*. Penguin RandomHouse.

Kany S, Vollrath JT & Relja B (2019) Cytokines in inflammatory disease. *International Journal of Molecular Sciences* 20(23), 6008. https://doi.org/10.3390/ijms20236008

Katon W, Lin EHB & Kroenke K (2007) The association of depression and anxiety with medical symptom burden in patients with chronic medical illness. *General Hospital Psychiatry* 29(2), 147–55.

Katsukawa F (2016) FITT principle of exercise in the management of lifestyle-related diseases. *Clinical Calcium* 26, 447–51.

Katzmarzyk PT, Chaput JP, Fogelholm M, Hu G, Maher C, Maia J et al. (2019) International Study of Childhood Obesity, Lifestyle and the Environment (ISCOLE): Contributions to understanding the global obesity epidemic. *Nutrients* 11(4), 848.

Keating CL, Moodie ML & Swinburn BA (2011) The health-related quality of life of overweight and obese adolescents: A study measuring body mass index and adolescent-reported perceptions. *International Journal of Pediatric Obesity* 6, 434–41.

Kennedy GC (1953) The role of depot fat in the hypothalamic control of food intake in the rat. *Proceedings of the Royal Society B: Biological Sciences* 140, 578–92.

Keys A, Fidanza F, Karvonen MJ, Kimura N & Taylor HL (1972) Indices of relative weight and obesity. *Journal of Chronic Disease* 25(6), 329–43.

Kimble D (1992) *Biological Psychology* (2nd edn). Harcourt Brace Jovanovich.

Kinlen D, Cody D & O'Shea D (2017) Complications of obesity. *QJM* 111(7), 437–43. https://doi.org/10.1093/qjmed/hcx152

Kinsman L, Radford J, Elmer S, Ogden K, Randles S, Jacob A, Delphin D, Burr N & Goss M (2021) Engaging 'hard-to-reach' men in health promotion using the OPHELIA principles: Participants' perspectives. *Health Promotion Journal of Australia* 32, 33–40.

Kleber RJ (2019) Trauma and public mental health: A focused review. *Frontiers in Psychiatry* 10, 451. https://doi.org/10.3389/fpsyt.2019.00451

Klein M (2021) Relapse into opiate and crack cocaine misuse: A scoping review. *Addiction Research & Theory* 29(2), 129–47. doi: 10.1080/16066359.2020.1724972

Kleinman A (1988) *The Illness Narratives*. Basic Books.

Klinger R, Stuhlreyer J, Schwartz M, Schmitz J & Colloca L (2018) Clinical use of placebo effects in patients with pain disorders. *International Review of Neurobiology* 139, 107–28. doi: 10.1016/bs.irn.2018.07.015.

Kloss O, Eskin N & Suh M (2018) Thiamine deficiency on fetal brain development with and without prenatal alcohol exposure. *Biochemistry and Cell Biology* 96(2), 169–77.

Kobasa S (1979) Stressful life events and health: An inquiry into hardiness. *Journal of Personality and Social Psychology* 37, 1–11.

Kok BE, Coffey KA, Cohn MA, Catalino LI, Vacharkulksemsuk T, Algoe SB, Brantley M & Fredrickson BL (2013) How positive emotions build physical health: Perceived positive social connections account for the upward spiral between positive emotions and vagal tone. *Psychological Science* 24(7), 1123–32. https://doi.org/10.1177/0956797612470827

Koziel N, Vigod S, Price J, Leung J & Hensel J (2022) Walking psychotherapy as a health promotion strategy to improve mental and physical health for patients and therapists: Clinical open-label feasibility trial. *Canadian Journal of Psychiatry* 67(2), 153–5. doi: 10.1177/07067437211039194

Kramer A (2020) An overview of the beneficial effects of exercise on health and performance. *Advances in Experimental Medicine and Biology* 1228, 3–22. doi: 10.1007/978-981-15-1792-1_1. PMID: 32342447

Krinner LM, Warren-Findlow J, Bowling J, Issel LM & Reeve CL (2021) The dimensionality of adverse childhood experiences: A scoping review of ACE dimensions measurement. *Child Abuse & Neglect* 121, 105270.

Krot K & Sousa J (2017) Factors impacting on patient compliance with medical advice: Empirical study. *Engineering Management in Production and Services* 9, 10.1515/emj-2017-0016.

Kübler-Ross E (1969) *On Death and Dying*. Macmillan.

Kuss DJ & Lopez-Fernandez O (2016) Internet addiction and problematic internet use: A systematic review of clinical research. *World Journal of Psychiatry* 6(1), 143–76.

Lalezari S, Barg A, Dardik R, Luboshitz J, Bashari D, Avishai E & Kenet G (2021) Women with hemophilia: Case series of reproductive choices and review of literature. *TH Open: Companion Journal to Thrombosis and Haemostasis* 5(2), e183–7.

Lancaster CL, Teeters JB, Gros DF & Back SE (2016) Post-traumatic stress disorder: Overview of evidence-based assessment and treatment. *Journal of Clinical Medicine* 5(11), 105. https://doi.org/10.3390/jcm5110105

Langham E, Thorne H, Browne M, Donaldson P, Rose J & Rockloff M (2016) Understanding gambling related harm: A proposed definition, conceptual framework, and taxonomy of harms. *BMC Public Health* 16(1), 80.

Lautenschlager N, Cox K & Ellis K (2019) Physical activity for cognitive health: What advice can we give to older adults with subjective cognitive decline and mild cognitive impairment? *Dialogues in Clinical Neuroscience* 21(1), 61–8.

Lazarus A (1971) *Behavior Therapy and Beyond*. McGraw-Hill.

Lazarus R & Alfert E (1964) The short-circuiting of threat by experimentally altering cognitive appraisal. *Journal of Abnormal and Social Psychology* 69, 195–205.

Lazarus R & Folkman S (1984) *Stress Appraisal and Coping*. Springer.

LeBlanc R & Jacelon C (2018) Self-care among older people living with chronic conditions. *International Journal of Older People Nursing* 13(3), e12191. doi: 10.1111/opn.12191

LeDoux JE & Brown R (2017) A higher-order theory of emotional consciousness. *Proceedings of the National Academy of Sciences of the United States of America* 114(10), e2016–25. https://doi.org/10.1073/pnas.1619316114

Lee T, Berg C, Baker A, Mello D, Litchman M & Wiebe D (2019) Health-risk behaviors and type 1 diabetes outcomes in the transition from late adolescence to early emerging adulthood. *Children's Health Care* 48(3), 285–300.

Lee R, Rashid A, Thomson W & Cordingley L (2020) Reluctant to assess pain: A qualitative study of health care professionals' beliefs about the role of pain in juvenile idiopathic arthritis. *Arthritis Care & Research* 72(1), 69–77.

Lei J, Ploner A, Elfström KM, Wang J, Roth A, Fang F, Sundström K, Dillner J & Sparén P (2020) HPV vaccination and the risk of invasive cervical cancer. *New England Journal of Medicine* 383(14), 1340–8. doi: 10.1056/NEJMoa1917338. PMID: 32997908

Leleu V, Douilliez C & Rusinek S (2014) Difficulty in disengaging attention from threatening facial expressions in anxiety: A new approach in terms of benefits. *Journal of Behavior Therapy and Experimental Psychiatry* 45(1), 203–7.

León-Valenzuela A, Palacios J & Del Pino Algarrada R (2020) IncobotulinumtoxinA for the treatment of spasticity in children with cerebral palsy: A retrospective case series focusing on dosing and tolerability. *BMC Neurology* 20(1), 126.

Leventhal H, Meyer D & Nerenz D (1980) The common sense representation of illness behaviour. In S Rachman (Ed.) *Contributions to Medical Psychology* (Vol. 2). Pergamon Press.

Levine J, Gordon N & Fields H (1978) The mechanism of placebo analgesia. *Lancet* 2(8091), 654–7.

Lewis GN & Bean DJ (2021) What influences outcomes from inpatient multidisciplinary pain management programs? A systematic review and meta-analysis. *Clinical Journal of Pain* 37(7), 504–23.

LFA [Lung Foundation of Australia] (n.d.) https://lungfoundation.com.au/lung-health/protecting-your-lungs/e-cigarettes-and-vaping/

Limbachia C, Morrow K, Khibovska A, Meyer C, Padmala S & Pessoa L (2021) Controllability over stressor decreases responses in key threat-related brain areas. *Communications Biology* 4, 42. https://doi.org/10.1038/s42003-020-01537-5

Linn A, Goot M, Brandes K, Weert J & Smit E (2019) Cancer patients' needs for support in expressing instrumental concerns and emotions. *European Journal of Cancer Care* 28(6). doi:10.1111/ecc.13138

LoCicero J (1991) *Grief Chart*. www.grief-chart.com

Loftus E & Loftus G (1980) On the permanence of stored information in the brain. *American Psychologist* 35, 409–20.

Lorenz L, Doherty A & Casey P (2019) The role of religion in buffering the impact of stressful life events on depressive symptoms in patients with depressive episodes or adjustment disorder. *International Journal of Environmental Research and Public Health* 16(7), 1238. https://doi.org/10.3390/ijerph16071238

Lorenzo-Luaces L & Dobson K (2019) Is behavioral activation (BA) more effective than cognitive therapy (CT) in severe depression? A reanalysis of a landmark trial. *International Journal of Cognitive Therapy* 12(2), 73–82.

Loxton D, Townsend N, Dolja-Gore X, Forder P & Coles J (2019) Adverse childhood experiences and healthcare costs in adult life. *Journal of Child Sexual Abuse* 28(5), 511–25.

Lynch KS & Lachman ME (2020) The effects of lifetime trauma exposure on cognitive functioning in midlife. *Journal of Traumatic Stress* 33, 773–82. https://doi.org/10.1002/jts.22522

Lynch S, Shuster G & Lobo M (2018) The family caregiver experience: Examining the positive and negative aspects of compassion satisfaction and compassion fatigue as caregiving outcomes. *Aging & Mental Health* 22(11), 1424–31.

MacCallum F & Bryant R (2011) Imagining the future in complicated grief. *Depression and Anxiety* 28(8), 658–65.

Mackley AM, Winter U, Guillen DA & Locke PR (2016) Health literacy among parents of newborn infants. *Advances in Neonatal Care* 16(4), 283–8.

Madison AA, Way BM, Beauchaine TP & Kiecolt-Glaser JK (2021) Risk assessment and heuristics: How cognitive shortcuts can fuel the spread of COVID-19. *Brain, Behavior, and Immunity* 94, 6–7. https://doi.org/10.1016/j.bbi.2021.02.023

Manderscheid R, Ryff CD, Freeman EJ, McKnight-Eily LR, Dhingra S & Strine TW (2010) Evolving definitions of mental illness and wellness. *Prevention of Chronic Diseases* 7(1), A19.

Markham F & Biddle N (2018) *Income, Poverty and Inequality: 2016 Census*. Paper no. 2. Centre for Aboriginal Economic Policy Research, Australian National University.

Marlatt G & Gordon J (1985) *Relapse Prevention: Maintenance Strategies in the Treatment of Addictive Behaviours*. Guilford Press.

Maslow AH (1943) A theory of human motivation. *Psychological Review* 50(4), 370–96. https://doi.org/10.1037/h0054346 (/doi/10.1037/h0054346)

Maslow A (1970) *Motivation and Personality* (2nd edn). Harper & Row.

McClelland D (1961) *The Achieving Society.* Van Nostrand.

McEwen BS (1998) Protective and damaging effects of stress mediators. *New England Journal of Medicine* 338, 171–9.

McEwen BS (2005) Stressed or stressed out: What is the difference? *Journal of Psychiatry & Neuroscience* 30(5), 315–18.

McKay F, Haines B & Dunn M (2019) Measuring and understanding food insecurity in Australia: A systematic review. *International Journal of Environmental Research and Public Health* 16(3), 476.

McKimmie BM, Butler T, Chan E, Rogers A & Jimmieson NL (2020) Reducing stress: Social support and group identification. *Group Processes & Intergroup Relations* 23(2), 241–61. doi:10.1177/1368430218818733

Medew J (2011) SensaSlim banned for advertising breach. *The Age,* 25 November. www.theage.com.au/national/sensaslim-banned-for-advertising-breach-20111124-1nwxk.html

MedlinePlus (2020) *Down Syndrome.* https://medlineplus.gov/genetics/condition/down-syndrome/#inheritance

Melzack R & Wall P (2003) *Handbook of Pain Management.* Churchill Livingstone.

Miguet M, Fearnbach NS, Metz L, Khammassi M, Julian V, Cardenoux C et al. (2020) Effect of HIIT versus MICT on body composition and energy intake in dietary restrained and unrestrained adolescents with obesity. *Applied Physiology, Nutrition, and Metabolism* 45(4), 437–45.

Miller GA (1956) The magical number seven plus or minus two: Some limits on our capacity for processing information. *Psychological Review* 63(2), 81–97.

Miller G (1990) The assessment of clinical skills/competence/performance. *Academic Medicine* 65, S63–7.

Miller WR & Rollnick S (2012) *Motivational Interviewing: Helping People Change* (3rd edn). Guilford Press.

Milligan E, West R, Saunders V, Bialocerkowski A, Creedy DK & Rowe-Minnis F (2021) Achieving cultural safety for Australia's First Peoples: A review of AHPRA registered health practitioners' codes of conduct and codes of ethics. *Australian Health Review* 45(4), 398–406. doi:10.1071/AH20215

Mills K, Creedy DK, Sunderland N & Allen J (2021) Examining the transformative potential of emotion in education: A new measure of health students' emotional learning in First Peoples' cultural safety. *Nurse Education Today* 100, 104854. doi.org/10.1016/j.nedt.2021.104854

Mills K & Creedy DK (2019) The 'pedagogy of discomfort': A qualitative exploration of student learning in a First Peoples health course. *Australian Journal of Indigenous Education* [online] 1–8. doi.org/10.1017/jie.2019.16

Mitchell NS, Catenacci VA, Wyatt HR & Hill JO (2011) Obesity: Overview of an epidemic. *Psychiatric Clinics of North America* 34(4), 717–32. https://doi.org/10.1016/j.psc.2011.08.005

Mols F & Denollet J (2010) Type D personality in the general population: A systematic review of health status, mechanisms of disease, and work-related problems. *Health and Quality of Life Outcomes* 8, 9. www.hqlo.com/content/8/1/9

Moss D (2020) Biofeedback-assisted relaxation training: A clinically effective treatment protocol. *Biofeedback* 48(2), 32–40.

Mouraux A & Iannetti G (2018) The search for pain biomarkers in the human brain. *Brain: A Journal of Neurology* 141(12), 3290–307.

MSAustralia (2021) *Symptoms.* https://www.msaustralia.org.au/about-ms/symptoms

Müller MJ, Geisler C, Heymsfield SB & Bosy-Westphal A (2018) Recent advances in understanding body weight homeostasis in humans. *F1000Research* 7, 1025. https://doi.org/10.12688/f1000research.14151.1

Murray H (1938) *Explorations in Personality.* Oxford University Press.

Murrup-Stewart C, Whyman T, Jobson L & Adams K (2021) 'Connection to culture is like a massive lifeline': Yarning with Aboriginal young people about culture and social and emotional wellbeing. *Qualitative Health Research* 31(10), 1833–46.

Myers D (2012) *Social Psychology* (11th edn). McGraw-Hill Education.

Nash S & Arora A (2021) Interventions to improve health literacy among Aboriginal and Torres Strait Islander peoples: A systematic review. *BMC Public Health* 21, 248. https://doi.org/10.1186/s12889-021-10278-x

NCD Risk Factor Collaboration (2019) Rising rural body-mass index is the main driver of the global obesity epidemic in adults. *Nature* 569(7755), 260.

NDRI [National Drug Research Institute] (2019) https://ndri.curtin.edu.au/NDRI/media/documents/publications/T273.pdf

Neff LA, Gleason MEJ, Crockett EE & Ciftci O (2021) Blame the pandemic: Buffering the association between stress and relationship quality during the COVID-19 pandemic. *Social Psychological and Personality Science* [online] June. doi:10.1177/19485506211022813

Neter E, Brainin E & Baron-Epel O (2015) The dimensionality of health literacy and eHealth literacy. *European Health Psychologist* 17(6), 275–80.

Nisbett R & Ross L (1980) *Human Inference: Strategies and Shortcomings of Social Judgment.* Prentice-Hall.

Noar S & Zimmerman R (2005) Health behavior theory and cumulative knowledge regarding health behaviors: Are we moving in the right direction? *Health Education Research* 20(3), 275–90.

Norberg J, Alexanderson K, Framke E, Rugulies R & Farrants K (2020) Job demands and control and sickness absence, disability pension and unemployment among 2,194,692 individuals in Sweden. *Scandinavian Journal of Public Health* 48(2), 125–33.

Norelli SK, Long A & Krepps JM (2021) *Relaxation Techniques.* Statpearls Publishing.

Norris FH, Friedman MJ, Watson PJ, Byrne CM, Diaz E & Kaniasty K (2002) 60,000 disaster victims speak: Part I. An empirical review of the empirical literature, 1981–2001. *Psychiatry* 65(3), 207–39. doi: 10.1521/psyc.65.3.207.20173

Nuss T, Morley B, Scully M et al. (2021) Energy drink consumption among Australian adolescents associated with a cluster of unhealthy dietary behaviours and short sleep duration. *Nutrition Journal* 20, 64.

O'Brien PE, Hindle A, Brennan L, Skinner S, Burton P, Smith A, Crosthwaite G & Brown W (2019) Long-term outcomes after bariatric surgery: A systematic review and meta-analysis of weight loss at 10 or more years for all bariatric procedures and a single-centre review of 20-year outcomes after adjustable gastric banding. *Obesity Surgery* 29(1), 3–14. https://doi.org/10.1007/s11695-018-3525-0

Ogbeiwi O (2017) Why written objectives need to be really SMART. *British Journal of Healthcare Management* 23, 324–36.

Ogden J (2003) Some problems with social cognitive models: A pragmatic and conceptual analysis. *Health Psychology* 22(4), 424–8.

Ogden J (2007) *Health Psychology: A Textbook* (4th edn). Open University Press.

Ogunsiji O, Wilkes L & Chok H (2018) 'You take the private part of her body … you are taking a part of her life': Voices of circumcised African migrant women on female genital circumcision (FGC) in Australia. *Health Care for Women International* 39(8), 906–18.

O'Kane G (2020) COVID-19 puts the spotlight on food insecurity in rural and remote Australia. *Australian Journal of Rural Health* 28(3), 319–20.

Okano K, Kaczmarzyk JR, Dave N, Gabrieli J & Grosman J (2019) Sleep quality, duration, and consistency are associated with better academic performance in college students. *NPJ Science of Learning* 4, 16.

Olusanya OA, Ammar N, Davis RL, Bednarczyk RA & Shaban-Nejad A (2021) A digital personal health library for enabling precision health promotion to prevent human papilloma virus-associated cancers. *Frontiers in Digital Health* 3. https://doi.org/10.3389/fdgth.2021.683161

Ornish D & Ornish A (2019) *Undo It! How Simple Lifestyle Changes Can Reverse Most Chronic Diseases*. Penguin Random House.

Osborne R, Buchbinder R, Elsworth G & Batterham R (2013) The grounded psychometric development and initial validation of the Health Literacy Questionnaire (HLQ). *BMC Public Health* 13, 658.

Østergaard C, Pedersen N, Thomasen A, Mechlenburg I & Nordbye-Nielsen K (2021) Pain is frequent in children with cerebral palsy and negatively affects physical activity and participation. *Acta Paediatrica* 110(1), 301–6.

Pan S, Smith M, Carpiano R, Fu H, Ong J, Huang W, Tang W & Tucker J (2020) Supernatural explanatory models of health and illness and HIV antiretroviral therapy use among young men who have sex with men in China. *International Journal of Behavioral Medicine* 27(5), 602–8.

Park N, Peterson C, Szvarca D, Vander Molen RJ, Kim ES & Collon K (2016) Positive psychology and physical health: Research and applications. *American Journal of Lifestyle Medicine* 10(3), 200–6. doi:10.1177/1559827614550277

Parsons T (1951) *The Social System*. Free Press.

Pascoe MC, Bailey AP, Craike M, Carter T, Patten RK, Stepto NK & Parker AG (2021) Single session and short-term exercise for mental health promotion in tertiary students: A scoping review. *Sports Medicine Open* 7(1), 1–24.

Pascoe M, Hetrick S & Parker A (2020) The impact of stress on students in secondary school and higher education. *International Journal of Adolescence and Youth* 25(1), 104–12. doi: 10.1080/02673843.2019.1596823

Pavlov IP (1927) *Conditioned Reflexes: An Investigation of the Physiological Activity of the Cerebral Cortex* (trans. and ed. GV Anrep). Oxford University Press.

Peck B & Terry D (2021) The kids are alright: Outcome of a safety programme for addressing childhood injury in Australia. *European Journal of Investigation in Health, Psychology and Education* 11(2), 546–56.

Peck C (1982) *Controlling Chronic Pain: A Self Help Guide*. Fontana.

Penfield W (1969) Consciousness, memory and man's conditioned reflexes. In K Pribram (Ed.) *On the Biology of Learning*. Harcourt Brace Jovanovich.

Petric G, Atanasova1 S & Kamin T (2017) Ill literates or illiterates? Investigating the eHealth literacy of users of online health communities. *Journal of Medical Internet Research* 19(10), e331. doi: 10.2196/jmir.7372

Pfefferbaum B & North CS (2020) Mental health and the COVID-19 pandemic. *New England Journal of Medicine* 383, 510–12. doi: 10.1056/NEJMp2008017

Philibert R, Dawes K, Philibert W, Andersen AM & Hoffman EA (2022) Alcohol use intensity decreases in response to successful smoking cessation therapy. *Genes* 13(1), 2. doi:10.3390/genes13010002

Piaget J (1985) *The Equilibration of Cognitive Structures: The Central Problem of Intellectual Development*. University of Chicago Press.

Pilowsky I (1978) A general classification of abnormal illness behaviours. *British Journal of Medical Psychology* 51, 131–7.

Poirier B, Hedges J, Smithers L, Moskos M & Jamieson L (2021) 'What are we doing to our babies' teeth?' Barriers to establishing oral health practices for Indigenous children in South Australia. *BMC Oral Health* 21(1), 434.

Pozza C & Isidori AM (2018) What's behind the obesity epidemic. In A Laghi & M Rengo (Eds) *Imaging in Bariatric Surgery* (pp. 1–8). Springer.

Prochaska J & DiClemente C (1984) *The Transtheoretical Approach: Crossing Traditional Boundaries of Therapy*. Dow Jones/Irwin.

QFCC [Queensland Family and Child Commission] (2019) *Real Skills for Real Life Survey*. https://www.qfcc.qld.gov.au/real-skills-real-life

Qin K, Paynter J, Wang L, Mollah T & Qu L (2021) Early childhood circumcision in Australia: Trends over 20 years and interrupted time series analysis. *ANZ Journal of Surgery* 91(7–8), 1491–6.

Queensland Health (2018) *Guidelines: Translating Evidence into Best Clinical Practice*. https://www.health.qld.gov.au/__data/assets/pdf_file/0033/139947/g-epl.pdf

Querstret D, Morison L, Dickinson S, Cropley M & John M (2020) Mindfulness-based stress reduction and mindfulness-based cognitive therapy for psychological health and well-being in nonclinical samples: A systematic review and meta-analysis. *International Journal of Stress Management* 27(4), 394–411.

Rafferty AP, Winterbauer NL, Luo H, Bell RA & Little NRG (2021) Diabetes self-care and clinical care among adults with low health literacy. *Journal of Public Health Management & Practice* 27(2), 144–53.

Ravussin E & Ryan DH (2018) Three new perspectives on the perfect storm: What's behind the obesity epidemic? *Obesity* 26(1), 9–10.

Razgonova M, Zakharenko A, Golokhvast K, Thanasoula M, Sarandi E, Nikolouzakis K, Fragkiadaki P, Tsatsakis D, Spandidos D & Tsatsakis A (2020) Telomerase and telomeres in aging theory and chronographic aging theory (review). *Molecular Medicine Reports* 22(3), 1679–94.

Reynolds DV (1969) Surgery in the rat during electrical analgesia induced by focal brain simulation. *Science* 164, 444–5.

Ridoutt B, Baird D, Anastasiou K & Hendrie G (2019) Diet quality and water scarcity: Evidence from a large Australian population health survey. *Nutrients* 11(8), 1846.

Rimm D & Masters R (1979) *Behavior Therapy Techniques and Empirical Findings*. Academic Press.

Rodriguez J, Karlamangla A, Gruenewald T, Miller-Martinez D, Merkin S & Seeman T (2019) Social stratification and allostatic load: Shapes of health differences in the MIDUS study in the United States. *Journal of Biosocial Science* 51(5), 627–44.

Rogers R (1985) Attitude change and information integration in fear appeals. *Psychological Reports* 56, 179–82.

Rosenstock I (1974) Historical origins of the health belief model. *Health Education Monographs* 2, 328–35.

Rotter JB (1966) Generalized expectancies for internal versus external control of reinforcement. *Psychological Monographs*, 80 [whole issue].

Rugnetta M (2020) Phantom limb syndrome. *Encyclopædia Britannica* [online].

Russell G (2016) Holism and holistic. *BMJ* 353, i1884. doi: https://doi.org/10.1136/bmj.i1884

Ryan R & Deci E (2000) Self-determination theory and the facilitation of intrinsic motivation, social development, and well-being. *American Psychologist* 55(1), 68–78.

Ryder A, Azcarate P & Cohen BE (2018) PTSD and physical health. *Current Psychiatry Reports* 20, 116. doi 10.1007/s11920-018-0977-9

Rymarczyk K, Turbacz A, Strus W & Cieciuch J (2020) Type C personality: Conceptual refinement and preliminary operationalization. *Frontiers in Psychology* 11, 552740. doi: 10.3389/fpsyg.2020.552740

Sahni PS, Singh K, Sharma N & Garg R (2021) Yoga: An effective strategy for self-management of stress-related problems and wellbeing during COVID-19 lockdown—a cross-sectional study. *Plos One* 16(2), e0245214.

Sahoo S, Padhy SK, Padhee B, Singla N & Sarkar S (2018). Role of personality in cardiovascular diseases: An issue that needs to be focused too! *Indian Heart Journal* 70(Suppl. 3), S471–7.

Salari N, Hosseinian-Far A, Jalali R, Vaisi-Raygani A, Rasoulpoor S, Mohammadi M, Rasoulpoor S & Khaledi-Paveh B (2020) Prevalence of stress, anxiety and depression among the general population during the COVID-19 pandemic: A systematic review and meta-analysis. *Global Health* 16, 57. https://doi.org/10.1186/s12992-020-00589-w

Salazar H (2018) *The Philosophy of Spirituality: Analytic, Continental, and Multicultural Approaches to a New Field of Philosophy.* Brill Rodopi.

Samdal GB, Eide GE, Barth T, Williams G & Meland E (2017) Effective behaviour change techniques for physical activity and healthy eating in overweight and obese adults: Systematic review and meta-regression analyses. *International Journal of Behavioral Nutrition and Physical Activity* 14, 42. https://doi.org/10.1186/s12966-017-0494-y

Sandweiss D (2019) How different topical ingredients hit their targets: Analgesics and the gate-control theory of pain. *Chiropractic Economics* 65(12), 50–4.

Santos A, Nunes B, Kislaya I, Gil A & Ribeiro O (2021) Exploring the correlates to depression in elder abuse victims: Abusive experience or individual characteristics? *Journal of Interpersonal Violence* 36, 115–34.

Santos-Salas S, Fuentes Contreras J, Armijo-Olivo S, Saltaji H, Watanabe S, Chambers T, Walter L & Cummings G (2016) Non-pharmacological cancer pain interventions in populations with social disparities: A systematic review and meta-analysis. *Supportive Care in Cancer* 24(2), 985–1000.

Sattler KM, Deane FP, Tapsell L & Kelly PJ (2018) Gender differences in the relationship of weight-based stigmatisation with motivation to exercise and physical activity in overweight

individuals. *Health Psychology Open* 5(1), 2055102918759691. https://doi.org/10.1177/2055102918759691Sastytler

Scaglioni S, De Cosmi V, Ciappolino V, Parazzini F, Brambilla P & Agostoni C (2018) Factors influencing children's eating behaviours. *Nutrients* 10(6), 706. https://doi.org/10.3390/nu10060706

Scarborough P, Burg MR, Foster C, Swinburn B, Sacks G, Rayner M, Webster P & Allender S (2011) Increased energy intake entirely accounts for increase in body weight in women but not in men in the UK between 1986 and 2000. *British Journal of Nutrition* 105, 1399–404.

SCHA [Sollis Clarity Health Analytics] (2021) *Integrated Care Systems and the Demon of Health Inequality.* https://www.sollis.co.uk/

Schachter S & Singer J (1962) Cognitive, social and physiological determinants of emotional state. *Psychological Review* 69, 379–99.

Schachter S (1964) The interaction of cognitive and physiological determinants of emotional state. In L Berkowitz (Ed.) *Advances in Experimental Social Psychology* (Vol. 1). Academic Press.

Schachter S (1971) Some extraordinary facts about obese humans and rats. *American Psychologist* 26, 129–44.

Scheier M & Carver C (2018) Dispositional optimism and physical health: A long look back, a quick look forward. *American Psychologist* 73(9), 1082–94. doi:10.1037/amp0000384

Scherr CL, Jensen JD & Christy K (2017) Dispositional pandemic worry and the health belief model: Promoting vaccination during pandemic events. *Journal of Public Health* 39(4), e242–50. doi: 10.1093/pubmed/fdw101. PMID: 27679662

Schnurr P & Green B (Eds) (2004) *Trauma and Health: Physical Health Consequences of Exposure to Extreme Stress.* American Psychiatric Association.

Schöpf AC, Martin GS & Keating MA (2017) Humor as a communication strategy in provider–patient communication in a chronic care setting. *Qualitative Health Research* 27(3), 374–90.

Schreiber J (2016) *Motivation 101.* Springer.

Seaman CE, Green E & Smith B (2021) Reaching at-risk rural men: An evaluation of a health promotion activity targeting men at a large agricultural event. *Health Promotion Journal of Australia* 32, 65–71.

Segerstrom SC (2010) Resources, stress, and immunity: An ecological perspective on human psychoneuroimmunology. *Annals of Behavioral Medicine* 40(1), 114–25.

Segerstrom S (2012) *The Oxford Handbook of Psychoneuroimmunology.* Oxford University Press.

Seligman M & Maier S (1967) Failure to escape traumatic shock. *Journal of Experimental Psychology* 74, 1–9.

Seow H, Guthrie D, Stevens T, Barbera L, Burge F, McGrail K, Chan K, Peacock S & Sutradhar R (2021) Trajectory of end-of-life pain and other physical symptoms among cancer patients receiving home care. *Current Oncology* 28(3), 1641–51.

Shahram SZ, Smith ML, Ben-David S, Feddersen M, Kemp TE & Plamondon K (2021) Promoting 'zest for life': A systematic literature review of resiliency factors to prevent youth suicide. *Journal of Research on Adolescence* 31(1), 4–24.

Shapiro A & Morris L (1978) Placebo effects in medical and psychological therapies. In A Bergin & S Garfield (Eds) *Handbook of Psychotherapy and Behavior Change* (2nd edn). Wiley.

Sharifi N, Sharifi F, Jamali J & Khajeh Z (2019) The impact of education on modification of lifestyle personality dimensions associated with osteoporosis in female students. *Journal of Midwifery & Reproductive Health* 7(4), 1888–95.

Shelton S (1994) The doctor–patient relationship. In A Stoudemire (Ed.) *Human Behavior: An Introduction for Medical Students* (2nd edn). JB Lippincott.

Sheridan SL, Halpern DJ, Viera AJ, Berkman ND, Donahue KE & Crotty K (2011) Interventions for individuals with low health literacy: A systematic review. *Journal of Health Communication* 16, 30–54.

Shin W, Lwin M, Yee A & Kee K (2020) The role of socialization agents in adolescents' responses to app-based mobile advertising. *International Journal of Advertising* 39(3), 365–86.

Shulman R, Arora R, Geist R, Ali A, Ma J, Mansfield E, Martel S, Sandercock J & Versloot J (2021) Integrated community collaborative care for seniors with depression/anxiety and any physical illness. *Canadian Geriatrics Journal* 24(3), 251–7.

Simon C, Lentz T, Bishop M, Riley J, Fillingim R & George SZ (2016) Comparative associations of working memory and pain catastrophizing with chronic low back pain intensity. *Physical Therapy* 96, 1049–56.

Sin N, Wen J, Klaiber P, Buxton O & Almeida D (2020) Sleep duration and affective reactivity to stressors and positive events in daily life. *Health Psychology* 39(12), 1078–88.

Skinner BF (1938) *The Behavior of Organisms: An Experimental Analysis*. Appleton.

Smart Richman L, Kubzansky L, Maselko J, Kawachi I, Choo P & Bauer M (2005) Positive emotion and health: Going beyond the negative. *Health Psychology* 24(4), 422–9.

Smith M, Thompson A, Hall L, Allen S & Wetherell M (2018) The physical and psychological health benefits of positive emotional writing: Investigating the moderating role of type D (distressed) personality. *British Journal of Health Psychology* 23(4), 857–71.

Solomon RL (1980) The opponent–process theory of acquired motivation: The costs of pleasure and the benefits of pain. *American Psychologist* 35, 691–712.

Sonneborn O & Williams A (2020) How does the 2020 revised definition of pain impact nursing practice? *Journal of Perioperative Nursing* 33(4), e25–8.

Soto-Rubio A, Giménez-Espert MDC & Prado-Gascó V (2020) Effect of emotional intelligence and psychosocial risks on burnout, job satisfaction, and nurses' health during the COVID-19 pandemic. *International Journal of Environmental Research and Public Health* 17(21), 7998.

Speakman JR, Levitsky DA, Allison DB, Bray MS, de Castro JM, Clegg DJ, Clapham JC, Dulloo AG, Gruer L, Haw S, Hebebrand J, Hetherington MM, Higgs S, Jebb SA, Loos RJF, Luckman S, Luke A, Mohammed-Ali V, O'Rahilly S, Pereira M, Perusse L, Robinson TN, Rolls B, Symonds ME & Westerterp-Plantenga MS (2011) Set points, settling points and some alternative models: Theoretical options to understand how genes and environments combine to regulate body adiposity. *Disease Models and Mechanisms* 4(6), 733–45.

Spence C (2017) Comfort food: A review. *International Journal of Gastronomy and Food Science* 9, 105–9. https://doi.org/10.1016/j.ijgfs.2017.07.001

Spielberger CD (1975) Anxiety: State-trait-process. In CD Spielberger & IG Sarason (Eds) *Stress and Anxiety* (Vol. 1). Hemisphere/Wiley.

Spiro H (1986) *Doctors, Patients, and Placebos*. Yale University Press.

Standfield L, Comans T & Scuffham P (2018) Simulation of health care and related costs in people with dementia in Australia. *Australian Health Review* 43(5), 531–9.

Steca P, D'Addario M, Magrin M, Miglioretti M, Monzani D, Pancani L, Marcello S, Marta S, Vecchio L, Fattirolli F, Giannattasio C, Cesana F, Riccobono S & Greco A (2016) A type A and type D combined personality typology in essential hypertension and acute coronary syndrome patients: Associations with demographic, psychological, clinical, and lifestyle indicators. *PLoS One* 11(9), e01618. https://doi.org/10.1371/journal.pone.0161840

Storms M & Nisbett R (1970) Insomnia and the attribution process. *Journal of Personality and Social Psychology* 16, 319–28.

Stubbs B, Vancampfort D, Rosenbaum S, Firth J, Cosco T, Veronese N, Salum GA & Schuch FB (2016) An examination of the anxiolytic effects of exercise for people with anxiety and stress-related disorders: A meta-analysis. *Psychiatry Research* 246, 102–8. doi: 10.1016/j.psychres.2016.12.020

Stubbs B, Vancampfort D, Veronese N, Kahl K, Mitchell A, Lin P, Tseng P, Mugisha J, Solmi M, Carvalho A & Koyanagi A (2017) Depression and physical health multimorbidity: Primary data and country-wide meta-analysis of population data from 190 593 people across 43 low- and middle-income countries. *Psychological Medicine* 47(12), 2107–17.

Su L, Fu J, Sun S, Zhao G, Cheng W, Dou C & Quan M (2019) Effects of HIIT and MICT on cardiovascular risk factors in adults with overweight and/or obesity: A meta-analysis. *PLoS One* 14(1), e0210644.

Sudore RL, Landefeld CS, Williams BA, Barnes DE, Lindquist K & Schillinger D (2006) Use of a modified informed consent process among vulnerable patients: A descriptive study. *Journal of General Internal Medicine* 21(8), 867–73.

Suh M (2018) Salivary cortisol profile under different stressful situations in female college students: Moderating role of anxiety and sleep. *Journal of Neuroscience Nursing* 50(5), 279–85.

Sulat JS, Prabandari YS, Sanusi R, Hapsari ED & Santoso B (2018) The validity of health belief model variables in predicting behavioral change: A scoping review. *Health Education* 118(6), 499–512. https://doi.org/10.1108/HE-05-2018-0027

Sumner JA, Hagan K, Grodstein F, Roberts AL, Harel B & Koenen KC (2017) Post-traumatic stress disorder symptoms and cognitive function in a large cohort of middle-aged women. *Depression and Anxiety* 34(4), 356–66. https://doi.org/10.1002/da.22600

SWA [Safe Work Australia] (2015) *Cost of Work-related Injury and Disease*. https://www.safeworkaustralia.gov.au/system/files/documents/1702/cost-of-work-related-injury-and-disease-2012-13.docx.pdf

Swinburn B, Egger G & Raza F (1999) Dissecting obesogenic environments: The development and application of a framework for identifying and prioritising environmental interventions for obesity. *Preventive Medicine* 29, 563–70.

Tan J, Sharpe L & Russell H (2021) The impact of ovarian cancer on individuals and their caregivers: A qualitative analysis. *Psycho-oncology* 30(2), 212–20.

Taylor EB (1871) *Primitive Culture*. Murray.

Taylor S (2021) *Health Psychology* (11th edn). McGraw-Hill.

Terry PC, Parsons-Smith RL & Terry VR (2020) Mood responses associated with COVID-19 restrictions. *Frontiers in Psychology* 11, 589598. doi: 10.3389/fpsyg.2020.589598

TGA [Therapeutic Goods Administration] (2019) *Addressing Prescription Opioid Use and Misuse in Australia*. Pub. no. D196309644. Australian Government.

Thompson D, Antcliff D & Woby S (2020) Cognitive factors are associated with disability and pain, but not fatigue among physiotherapy attendees with persistent pain and fatigue. *Physiotherapy* 106(1), 94–100.

Thompson NJ, Fiorillo D, Rothbaum BO, Ressler KJ & Michopoulos V (2018) Coping strategies as mediators in relation to resilience and post-traumatic stress disorder. *Journal of Affective Disorders* 225, 153–9. doi: 10.1016/j.jad.2017.08.049

Tolgou T, Rohrmann S, Stockhausen C, Krampen D, Warnecke I & Reiss N (2018) Physiological and psychological effects of imagery techniques on health anxiety. *Psychophysiology* 55(2). doi: 10.1111/psyp.12984

Tolman E (1932) *Purposive Behavior in Animals and Men*. Appleton-Century-Crofts.

Toohill J, Fenwick J, Sidebotham M, Gamble J & Creedy DK (2019) Trauma and fear in Australian midwives. *Women & Birth* 32(1), 64–71.

Toombs E, Kowatch KR, Dalicandro L, McConkey S, Hopkins C & Mushquash CJ (2021) A systematic review of electronic mental health interventions for Indigenous youth: Results and recommendations. *Journal of Telemedicine and Telecare* 27(9), 539–52.

Toussaint L, Nguyen QA, Roettger C, Dixon K, Offenbächer M, Kohls N, Hirsch J & Sirois F (2021) Effectiveness of progressive muscle relaxation, deep breathing, and guided imagery in promoting psychological and physiological states of relaxation. *Evidence Based Complementary Alternative Medicine* July, 5924040. doi: 10.1155/2021/5924040

Townshend T & Lake AA (2017) Obesogenic environments: Current evidence of the built and food environments. *Perspectives in Public Health* 137(1), 38–44.

Turner K, Weinberger M, Renfro C, Powell BJ, Ferreri S, Trodgon JG et al. (2021) Stages of change: Moving community pharmacies from a drug dispensing to population health management model. *Medical Care Research and Review* 78(1), 57–67.

Tyrer P, Wang D, Tyrer H, Crawford M, Loebenberg G, Cooper S, Barret B & Sanatinia R (2021) Influence of apparently negative personality characteristics on the long-term outcome of health anxiety: Secondary analysis of a randomized controlled trial. *Personality and Mental Health* 15(1), 72–86.

UNESCO (2016) *UNESCO Strategy on Education for Health and Well-being*. https://unesdoc.unesco.org/ark:/48223/pf0000246453

Unger CA, Busse D & Yim IS (2017) The effect of guided relaxation on cortisol and affect: Stress reactivity as a moderator. *Journal of Health Psychology* 22(1), 29–38. https://doi.org/10.1177/1359105315595511

US BDC [Burden of Disease Collaborators] (2018) The state of US health, 1990–2016: Burden of diseases, injuries, and risk factors among US states. *Journal of the American Medical Association* 319(14), 1444–72. doi: 10.1001/jama.2018.0158

USC [University of South Carolina] (2021) *Resiliency Project*. https://sc.edu/about/offices_and_divisions/housing/documents/resiliencyproject/7keyattitudesofmindfulness.pdf

van Achterberg T, Huisman-de Waal GGJ, Ketelaar NABM, Oostendorp RA, Jacobs JE & Wollersheim HCH (2011) How to promote healthy behaviours in patients? An overview of evidence for behaviour change techniques. *Health Promotion International* 26(2), 148–62.

Van Dyke BP, Newman AK, Moraís CA, Burns JW, Eyer JC & Thorn BE (2019) Heterogeneity of treatment effects in a randomized trial of literacy-adapted group cognitive behavioral therapy, pain psychoeducation, and usual medical care for multiply disadvantaged patients with chronic pain. *Journal of Pain* 20(10), 1236–48. https://doi.org/10.1016/j.jpain.2019.04.006

Van Zutven K, Mond J, Latner J & Rodgers B (2015) Obesity and psychosocial impairment: Mediating roles of health status, weight/shape concerns and binge eating in a community sample of women and men. *International Journal of Obesity* 39(2), 346–52.

Vicary D & Westerman T (2004) 'That's just the way he is': Some implications of Aboriginal mental health beliefs. *Australian e-Journal for the Advancement of Mental Health* 3(3), 1–10.

Vina J (2019) The free radical theory of frailty: Mechanisms and opportunities for interventions to promote successful aging. *Free Radical Biology & Medicine* 134, 690–4.

Vitaliano PP, Maiuro RD, Russo J, Katon W, De Wolfe D & Hall G (1990) Coping profiles associated with psychiatric, physical health, work and family problems. *Health Psychology* 9, 348–76.

Voit M & Meyer-Ortmanns H (2019) How aging may be an unavoidable fate of dynamical systems. *New Journal of Physics* 21(4), 43045.

Vroom VH (1964) *Work and Motivation*. Jossey-Bass.

Walters G & Grusec J (1977) *Punishment*. Freeman.

Wantonoro (2020) Cognitive-behavioural therapy improved quality of sleep and reducing pain among elderly with osteoarthritis: Literature review. *International Journal of Caring Sciences* 13(3), 2309–16.

Wehner SK, Tjørnhøj-Thomsen T, Bonnesen CT, Madsen KR, Jensen MP & Krølner RF (2021) Peer mentors' role in school-based health promotion: Qualitative findings from the Young & Active study. *Health Promotion International* daab089. https://doi.org/10.1093/heapro/daab089

Weinberg M, Seton C & Cameron N (2018) The measurement of subjective wellbeing: Item-order effects in the personal wellbeing index—adult. *Journal of Happiness Studies* 19(1), 315–32.

Weinstein N (1984) Why it won't happen to me: Perceptions of risk factors and susceptibility. *Health Psychology* 3, 431–57.

Weinstein N (2007) Misleading tests of health behavior theories. *Annals of Behavioral Medicine* 33(1), 1–10.

Werth S & Brownlow C (2018) *Work and Identity*. Springer.

Wettasinghe P, Allan W, Garvey G, Timbery A, Hoskins S, Veinovic M, Daylight G, Mack G, Minogue C, Donovan T, Broe G, Radford K & Delbaere K (2020) Older Aboriginal Australians' health concerns and preferences for healthy ageing programs. *International Journal of Environmental Research and Public Health* 17(20), 7390.

White K, Issac M, Kamoun C, Leygues J & Cohn S (2018) The THRIVE model: A framework and review of internal and external predictors of coping with chronic illness. *Health Psychology Open* 5(2), 2055102918793552.

WHO [World Health Organization] (1986) *Ottawa Charter for Health Promotion*. https://www.who.int/publications/i/item/ottawa-charter-for-health-promotion

WHO [World Health Organization] (2016) *Health Literacy: 9th Global Conference on Health Promotion*. www.who.int/teams/health-promotion/enhanced-wellbeing/ninth-global-conference/health-literacy

WHO [World Health Organization] (2018) *Global Status Report on Alcohol and Health*. World Health Organization.

WHO [World Health Organization] (2021a) *Constitution*. https://www.who.int/about/governance/constitution

WHO [World Health Organization] (2021b) *Breastfeeding*. https://www.who.int/health-topics/breastfeeding#tab=tab_1

WHO [World Health Organization] (2022) *1st International Conference on Health Promotion, Ottawa, 1986*. https://www.who.int/teams/health-promotion/enhanced-wellbeing/first-global-conference

Wieseler B, McGauran N & Kaiser T (2019) New drugs: Where did we go wrong and what can we do better? *BMJ* 366, l4340. doi:10.1136/bmj.l4340

Wilkie DJ & Keefe FJ (1991) Coping strategies of patients with lung cancer-related pain. *Clinical Journal of Pain* 7(4), 292–9.

Wolfe MS, Davis TC, Curtis LM, Webb JA, Bailey SC, Shrank WH et al. (2011) Effect of standardised patient-centred label instructions to improve comprehension of prescription drug use. *Medical Care* 49(1), 96–100.

Wolfe MS, Williams MV, Parker RM, Parikh NS, Nowlan AW & Baker DW (2007) Patients' shame and attitudes toward discussing the result of literacy screening. *Journal of Health Communication: International Perspectives* 12(8), 721–32.

Wolpe J (1973) *The Practice of Behavior Therapy* (2nd edn). Pergamon.

Worley SL (2018) The extraordinary importance of sleep: The detrimental effects of inadequate sleep on health and public safety drive an explosion of sleep research. *Pharmacy and Therapeutics* 43(12), 758–63.

Wortley E & Hagell A (2021) Young victims of youth violence: Using youth workers in the emergency department to facilitate 'teachable moments' and to improve access to services. *Archives of Disease in Childhood: Education and Practice* 106(1), 53–9.

Wouk K, Morgan I, Johnson J, Tucker C, Carlson R, Berry D & Stuebe A (2021) A systematic review of patient-, provider-, and health system-level predictors of postpartum health care use by people of color and low-income and/or uninsured populations in the United States. *Journal of Women's Health* 30(8), 1127–59.

Wyse JJ, Ganzini L, Dobscha SK, Krebs EE & Morasco BJ (2019) Setting expectations, following orders, safety, and standardization: Clinicians' strategies to guide difficult conversations about opioid prescribing. *Journal of General Internal Medicine* 34(7), 1200–6.

Yam M, Loh Y, Tan C, Khadijah S, Manan A & Basir R (2018) General pathways of pain sensation and the major neurotransmitters involved in pain regulation. *International Journal of Molecular Science* 19, 2164. doi:10.3390/ijms19082164

Yang C, Chen A & Chen Y (2021) College students' stress and health in the COVID-19 pandemic: The role of academic workload, separation from school, and fears of contagion. *PLoS One* 16(2), e0246676. https://doi.org/10.1371/journal.pone.0246676

Yerkes RM & Dodson JD (1908) The relation of strength of stimulus to rapidity of habit-formation. *Journal of Comparative Neurology and Psychology* 18, 459–82.

Zander-Schellenberg T, Collins IM, Miché M, Guttmann C, Lieb R & Wahl K (2020) Does laughing have a stress-buffering effect in daily life? An intensive longitudinal study. *PLoS One* 15(7), e0235851. https://doi.org/10.1371/journal.pone.0235851

Zarcadoolas C, Pleasant AF & Greer DS (2006) *Advancing Health Literacy*. John Wiley & Sons.

Zeliger HI (2016) Predicting disease onset in clinically healthy people. *Interdisciplinary Toxicology* 9(2), 39–54. doi: 10.1515/intox-2016-0006

Zhang J, Ma C, Yang A, Zhang R, Gong J & Mo F (2018) Is preterm birth associated with asthma among children from birth to 17 years old? A study based on 2011–2012 US National Survey of Children's Health. *Italian Journal of Pediatrics* 44(1), 151.

Ziada A, Smith M & Côté H (2020) Updating the free radical theory of aging. *Frontiers in Cell and Developmental Biology* 8, 575645.

INDEX

abnormal illness behaviour 57
acceptance 230, 291
  cognitive response 78
  stages of dying 47
access to health 287
accommodation 25
acute illness 166
addiction
  addictive behaviours 94
  families, running in 60
  gambling 156–8
  non-prescription drugs 232
  opponent-process theory 144
  prescription drugs 231
  sick role 56–7
adolescence 29–34
  chronic conditions in 74
  development in 29–34
  Erikson's stages of development 24
  First Peoples 27–8
  health in 33
  personal fable 32
  Piaget's stages of development 25
  socialisation 248
adulthood 36–45
  cognitive development and decline 41
  health in 41
  legal status 36
  middle 37
  older 37
  transition to 36
  young adults 37
advance health care directive 46
affective support 82
age, measurements of 20–1
ageing 37, 42–5
  Australian population, of 13, 44
  chronic conditions and 74
  stress and 43
  theories of 42–4
agents 124
alcohol use
  lifestyle diseases 91
  regulation of emotion/stress
    management 187, 231, 232, 234
  relationship abuse 96
  risky behaviour 91, 93
alcoholism
  sick role and 56–7
  treatment for 101–2
algorithms 116
allostasis 216
allostatic load 216
Alzheimer's disease 44, 109
  grief 45, 48

reactions to 59
  see also dementia
antioxidants 42–3
anti-social influences 247
anxiety 179, 191–2, 213–14
  adolescent development 33
  behavioural strategies 65
  child development 23, 62
  chronic conditions and 76, 84
  chronic pain sufferers, in 200
  emotions and 186–7
  illness and 58
  immune function and 133
  MS and 76
  negative health outcomes and 65
  stress and 213
  systematic desensitisation 297
  Type D (distressed) personality 189
appraisal
  appraisal theory of emotion 184
  definition 13
  primary appraisal 210, 217
  secondary appraisal 210–11
  stress process and 210–12, 214, 215
  trauma 217
arousal
  cognition and 183–4
  definition 63, 223
  emotion and 182–3
  performance, and 208–9
  reduction strategies 65
  stress management 225, 227, 231
arthritis 73, 74
  behavioural activation 203
  expectations and 128
  gender and 74
  impact on daily life 75, 84–5, 289
assimilation 25
asthma 73
  breastfeeding and 61
  controllability 79
  fitness 166
  impact on daily life 64
  prematurity and 62
  quality of life and 79
  self-regulation 80, 83
  stress and 239
  tertiary prevention 281
attitudes 14, 59, 120
aversive conditioning 101–2
avoidance learning 101–2

balance theory 128
bariatric surgery 163–4

behaviour
  antecedents 147
  biological factors 140–2
  cognitive factors 142
  determinant of health 251
  emotions and 182, 187
  gender and 253–4
  genetic factors 60, 140
  health behaviours 149, 161–71, 288
  health literacy and 264, 270–1
  low-awareness behaviours 149, 150–1
  observation of 148
  pain and 197
  past 147
  psychological responses and 200–1
  psychophysiology and 63–4, 188–90
  risky behaviours 149
  socialisation and 247–9
  stress and 209, 215
  trauma and 217–18
  see also behavioural change
behavioural activation 203–5
behavioural change 138–59
  expectations 145–6
  health professionals and 284–5
  increasing and decreasing 149–51
  lapses, managing 156
  motivation for 138–40
  positive reinforcement 152–5
  punishment 154
  reinforcements, changing 151
  stimuli, changing 147–9
  strategies for 144–7
  stress management and 225–30, 232–7
behavioural predispositions 60
behavioural strategies 64–5
biofeedback 202, 229
biopsychosocial model 14, 18
biopsychosocial-spiritual model 15
birth
  health risks 253
  pain control techniques 9–10, 202
  prematurity 62
  perinatal events 61–2
  trauma and 217
birth defects 13, 28, 61
birth rates 27, 39–40
body image 67, 171–2
body mass index (BMI) 161–2
breastfeeding 61–2, 281–2
breathing 227

cancer 73
  ageing and 44
  childhood 28

cervical cancer   94, 284
  deaths from   91
  diagnosis, responses to   68–9, 78, 84
  epidemic   14
  errors in copying   43
  genetic predisposition   60, 247
  hormone replacement therapy   262
  obesity and   91
  pain management   197, 200, 202, 203–5
  positive emotions and   190
  psychophysiology   63, 189–90
  reactions to   59
  screening for   280
  type C (cancer prone) behaviour pattern   63, 189–90
capabilities
  coping strategies and   65
  definition   60
  genetic predisposition   60
  illness behaviour   53, 59
cardiovascular disease
  chronic condition   73
  deaths from   14, 273
  socio-economic status and   251
cardiovascular psychophysiology   188–9
catastrophising   211, 236
cerebral palsy   19–20, 21–2, 26, 28–9, 32–3, 38
  MS and   75
  multidisciplinary approach   82
cerebrovascular disease   91
cervical cancer   94
chemotherapy
  reactions to   59, 204
children
  adversity   62
  child abuse   102
  chronic conditions   74, 76–7
  development milestones   20–1
  developmental stages   22–9
  early life events   62
  First Nations people   27
  genetic conditions   28
  health   27–8
  measurement of age   20–1
  obesity in   163
  prepubertal growth spurt   22
cholesterol
  genetic predisposition   60
  levels   8
  stress   188
chronic conditions   73–87
  adolescence, in   74
  childhood, in   74, 76–7
  coping strategies   75
  daily life, impact on   75–7
  disability, causing   73
  gender and   74
  grief and   76
  interventions   81, 84
  models of care   79–85

  positive emotions   76
  prevalence of   74
chronic fatigue syndrome   12, 73
chronic strain   213
circumcision   11
classical conditioning   99–100
Closing the Gap   28, 252
cognition   14–15, 114–36
  attitudes   120–2
  chronic conditions and   78
  development   24–5, 30–1, 41
  emotion and   183–5
  expectations   128
  rational decision-making   115–16
cognitive behavioural therapy (CBT)   65, 232
  sleep problems   96
cognitive decline   41
  see also Alzheimer's disease, dementia
cognitive development
  adolescence, in   30–1
  adulthood, in   41
  childhood, in   24–5
  Piaget's stages of   25
cognitive distortions   235–6
cognitive load   266–8
cognitive reframing   84
cognitive responses   78
cognitive restructuring   236
collaborative model   80
comfort food   170
communication disabilities   252
compassion fatigue   77
compliance   127
confabulation   109
conservation withdrawal   65
control   124
  abuse and   96
  coping and   224–5
  decision-making and   122
  emotions and   181–2
  perceptions of   79, 123
controllability   79
coping strategies   223–39
  capabilities and   65
  chronic conditions   75
  individual, variations in   78
cortisol   60, 188
COVID-19
  attitudes of others to   59
  chronic fatigue syndrome   12
  genome sequencing   8
  health and behaviour   88–9, 138
  obesity and   162
  risk-reduction behaviours   95
  socialisation and   248–9
  stress and coping   213, 237
  unimmunised people and treatment   57
cultural literacy   260
culture
  cultural safety in health care   249–50

  definition   197, 243
  pain tolerance and   197–8
  perceptions of health and illness   68
  responsibility-oriented   57
  sick role and   56–7
cytokines   190

dangerous activities   94–5
death   45–8
  accidents, due to   276–7
  cardiovascular events, due to   189
  death rates and gender   253
  dementia, due to   44, 109
  five stages of dying   46–7
  preventable causes of   94–5
  smoking, due to   276
dementia   41, 73, 97, 109–10
  ageing population and   44, 109
  cause of death   44
  causes of   109–10
  frustration, anger and anxiety   97
  memory and   105, 109
  personality changes and   110
  prevalence of   44, 109
  types of   109
depression
  adolescence and   33
  chronic pain sufferers, in   74, 200–1
  emotions and   186
  gender and   74
  heart disease and   188–9
  illness and   58
  learned helplessness and   104
  MS and   76
  negative health outcomes and   65
  postnatal   62
  post-traumatic stress disorder and   218
  stages of grief   46
  type D (distressed) personality   189
diabetes   73, 265–6
  anxiety about   79
  breastfeeding and   61
  childhood   27–8
  deaths from   14
  genetic predisposition   60
  humour as a coping mechanism   76
  lifestyle changes   145
  obesity and   91, 163
  reactions to   59
  self-regulation   80
diet   168–171
  food restriction   170
  self-care behaviour   80
disability   19, 252–3
  children with   20, 24
  chronic conditions causing   73–5
  coping with   78–9
  definition   19, 73
  grief   45, 48
  health promotion and   82–3
  mothers living with   62

persistence of reactions 52
physical, due to chronic condition 76
tertiary prevention 281
disease 8–12
absence of 12
ageing and 44
determinants of 19–20
genetic predisposition to 60
health literacy and 269
measurements of 13
models of health 14–15, 82
obesity and 163
prevention of 280–1, 284
reactions to 59
disengagement theory of ageing 43
domestic and family violence 96
Down Syndrome 19, 28
drugs 231–2

eating 168–71
control and 170
disordered 171
intervention 172
stimulus control 168, 170
efficacy beliefs 79
electronic health (e-Health) literacy 259
emotional intelligence 31
emotions 180–7
appraisal theory of 184
arousal and 182–3
attribution theory of 184
brain and 182
cognition and 183–4
dysregulation of 187
expression of 185
health and 186
negative 65
physiology of 181
positive 76, 190
end of life (EoL) 45–7
endogenous opioid peptides 199
endorphins 133
energy balance 163
environments
adolescence home 30, 31
childhood home 23, 26, 29, 247
determinant of health 18–20
eating and 170–1
illness behaviour 53
in utero 60–1
inequitable distribution 288
learning 99–101
perception and 68–9
epidemiology 13
epilepsy 59, 79
equity 287
Erikson's stages of development 24, 37
errors in copying theory 43
ethnicity 244–5
ethnocentrism 243
euthanasia 46

exercise 165, 166
FIIT principle 227
long-term benefits 152
risk-reduction behaviour 95
self-care behaviour 80
stress management and 227
expectancy-value theory 55, 115–16
expectations 127, 128
extinction, conditioned response of 144

family 39–40
fight or flight response 209
First Peoples 244, 252
Country 246
cultural safety 249–50, 255
health disparities 27–8, 252, 260
life expectancy 39, 252
rituals and traditions 36
fitness 166
FITT principle 227
foetal alcohol spectrum disorder
(FASD) 61
foetus 60–1
folic acid 19
food insecurity 251
food pyramid 168
forgetting 108–9
free radical theory 42–3

gambling 94, 154
gate-control theory 198–9
gender 253–4
chronic conditions and 74
overweight and obesity 162–3
generalised anxiety disorder (GAD) 214
genetic conditions 28
genetic predispositions 19, 60
Gestalt School 67
gestation 60–1
good behaviour bond 155
goodness of fit 214, 224
grief 47–9
complicated or chronic 76
stages of 47–9, 76

habits 96
low-awareness 149–51
habituation 143–4
haemophilia 60
hardiness 66
hassles 213
health 5, 12
adolescence, in 33
beliefs 120–2
childhood, in 27–9
culture and 68
determinants of 18–20
education and 263
emotion and 186
heuristics 118

measurement of 13–14
memory and 109
models of 14–16
social determinants of 251–4
health behaviours 95
strategies for changing 125, 138,
144–59
health belief model 121
health care 249–50
cultural safety in 249–50, 255
geography and living conditions 251
inequalities in 255–6
institutional racism 249
models of 14–16
health literacy 259, 263–71
Health Literacy Questionnaire 261
interventions to enhance 266–70
socio-cultural factors 263
health professionals 54–5, 284–5
health promotion 283–8
chronic conditions 82–3
health professionals and 284–5
primary, secondary and tertiary 284
heart disease
cardiovascular
psychophysiology 188–9
deaths from 91
depression and 189
genetic predisposition 60
lifestyle changes 145
see also cardiovascular disease
helplessness 78
heuristics 116
HIV/AIDS 9, 78
holism 180
homeostasis 141, 216
human papillomavirus (HPV) 94
hypertension 10–11
genetic predisposition 60
psychosomatic 179
hypnosis 202
hypothalamus 141, 182

illegal drugs 232
risky behaviour 91, 93–4
illness 5, 6–7
acute 166
culture and 68
determinants of 18–20
disease, comparison with 10–12
explanatory models 245
factors affecting reactions to 59
measurement of 13–14
models of 14–16
nature of 59
psychological challenges 58
reactions to 51–3
secondary gains from 103–4
illness behaviour 53–6, 57
illness perceptions 66–70
illness prevention 276, 279

levels of   282–3
primary   279–80
secondary   280–1
tertiary   281
incentives   141
incidence   13, 74
indigenous populations   244
    health conditions in   27
    see also First Peoples
inequality   250
    health care, in   255–6
inequity   250
injury, preventing   276–8
instincts   140
instrumental support   82
intellectual disabilities   253
intelligence   41
    breastfeeding and   61
    emotional   31
internet addiction   94

kidney disease   73

laughter   190
learned helplessness   104
learning   68, 99–105, 266–8
    aggression, of   102
    basis of   97
    five steps of   266
    learning to be sick   103–4
    models of   99–103
life expectancy   39
    First Peoples   252
lifestyle diseases   91, 92–5
lifestyle factors   41, 57, 91–6
lifestyle programs   145
living wills   46
locus of control   53, 224–5

mania   7
marriage rates   39–40
Maslow's hierarchy of needs   138–9
mastery learning   268–9
medical model   14–15, 80
medication   144, 231–2
meditation   229–30
memory   97, 105–11
    cognitive load and   266–8
    dementia patients, in   109–10
    health and   109
    long-term   107
    measuring   108
    organisation of   107
    sensory memory   105–6
    short-term   106–7
    working memory   267
mental health conditions   73, 74
    anxiety disorders   214
    cognitive behaviour techniques   232–7
    genetic predisposition   60

regulation of emotion and   186–7
    social selection   252
    social support   236–7
    symptoms of   187
mental imagery   235
mind–body dualism   179
mindfulness   229–30
morbidity   13
mortality   13
motivation   138–40
    eating and   169–71
motivational interviewing (MI)   142–3
mourning *see* grieving
multimorbidity   73
multiple sclerosis (MS)   75–6
    individual coping   78–9
myelination   22

National Disability Insurance Scheme
    (NDIS)   253
nervous system   97–8
neuroplasticity   67, 98
    memory and   107
nocebo effects   132
nociceptors   198

obesity   91, 161, 162–7
    breastfeeding and   61
    children, in   163
    COVID-19 pandemic and   162
    ecological model   164
    gender and   162–3
    high cortisol levels   60
    treatment of disorders   57
obesogenic environments   170
obsessive compulsive disorder
    (OCD)   214
obsolescence theories of ageing   43–4
operant conditioning   100–1
opiates   199–200
opioids   200
opponent-process theory   144
optimal level theory   143
optimism   65–6, 79
Ornish program   145
osteoarthritis   74, 84–5
    expectations   128
    obesity and   91
    pain management   203
osteoporosis   39, 73, 74
    prevention of   82–3
Ottawa Charter for Health
    Promotion   283
overweight   161
    gender and   162–3
    see also obesity

pain   195–205
    acute   198–200
    avoidance   141

chronic   103–4, 200–1
    complaints of   103–4
    culture and   197
    pain control techniques   197–8, 201–2
    pain management programs   203
    relievers   103–4
    reporting   196–8
    understanding   195
panic disorder (PD)   214
patient, process of becoming   54–5
Pavlov's dogs   99
perceived benefit   78
perceptions   66–70
    basic perceptual processes   67–8
    expectation and   68
    illness, of   66
    other people, of   68–9
    perceptual constancy   68
perinatal events   61–2
persistent (chronic) pain syndrome
    200–1
personality   63–4
pessimism   65
phantom limb syndrome   67
phobias   100, 233–4
physical activity   165, 166
physical disabilities   19–20, 73, 74–5,
    252–3
placebo effects   129–34
    perception explanations   132
    physiological explanations   133
    therapeutic uses of   133–4
post-traumatic stress disorder
    (PTSD)   214, 218
postnatal depression   62
pregnancy   60–1, 94
    risks associated with   253
premature birth   62
prevalence   13, 74
primary drives   140
professional help   54–5
prosocial influences   247
psychological traits   60
psychoneuroimmunology   190
psychophysiology   188–92
psychosocial interventions   83–4
psychosomatic illness   179
puberty   29–30
punishment   101–2, 154

quality of life (QoL)   5
    improving   14
    chronic conditions   28
    older people, for   46

race   244–5, 252
reaction range   19
reflexes   22
reinforcement   101, 151–6
    positive   101, 152–6

schedule of   152
summary of methods   155–6
relaxation   225–30
    benefits of   145
    pain control management   202
    pharmacological approaches to   231–2
    training   84, 202
religion   15, 243
risk-reduction behaviours   95–6
risky behaviours   57, 91–5
road rage   96
rooting reflex   22

schemas   266
scientific literacy   259
self-agency model   80–1
self-care   39, 79
    models of   79–81
self-efficacy   153–4
    beliefs, enhancing   84
self-esteem   51, 146
self-regulation   79–80
self-reinforcement   153–4
sensation, study of   67–8
sensory disabilities   253
set point theory   170
settling point theory   170–1
sex   94, 141
sexually transmitted infections
    (STIs)   94
shaping   101
sick role   56–7
sickness   5–10
    see also illness
sleep   95
SMART model   145
smoking   91, 92, 276

sick role and   56–7
social capital   255
social cognitive theory   124–5
social phobia   214
social support   59, 236–7
socialisation   247–9
    adolescence   31
    childhood   23–4
    primary agents of   247–8
    secondary agents of   248
    tertiary agents of   248–9
socio-cultural indicators   36
socio-economic status (SES)   251
spirituality   15, 224
stereotyping   69, 131
stigma   197
stimulus   100
stimulus control   148–9
    eating   168, 170
stress   207–17
    adverse clinical outcomes   190
    ageing and   43
    anxiety and   213–14
    'eustress'   209
    management   84, 225–39
    process, as   210–12
    response, as   208–9
    response to   214–15
    stimulus, as   207
    styles of dealing with   60
stressors   208, 211
substance abuse
    adolescence, in   33
    illness as trigger for   58
    see also alcohol, drugs, smoking
symptoms   6–7
    normalisation of   54

responses to   51
synaptic cleft   98
systematic desensitisation   233–4

teach to goal   271
teachable moments   285
teach-back   269
telomeres   43
tend and befriend   215
thalidomide   61
trauma   217–18
type A (coronary prone) behaviour
    pattern   188–9
type C (cancer prone) behaviour
    pattern   189–90
type D (distressed) personality   189

unsafe sex   94

validation   132
vulnerabilities   60–4
    genetic predispositions   60
    impact of health behaviour   59

wear and tear theory of ageing   42
well-being   12–16
    self-care   39
    subjective   12
wellness   5
wonder drug effect   131
work   40

Yerkes–Dodson Law   208–9
young adulthood   29–34, 37